WU 101.5

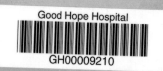

Hypodontia

A Team Approach to Management

John A. Hobkirk
BDS (Hons), PhD, DrMed.hc, FDSRCS (Ed), FDSRCS (Eng), CSci, MIPEM, ILTM, FHEA
Emeritus Professor of Prosthetic Dentistry, UCL Eastman Dental Institute, University College London
Honorary Consultant in Restorative Dentistry, Eastman Dental Hospital, UCLH NHS Foundation Trust, London

Daljit S. Gill
BDS (Hons), MSc, BSc (Hons), FDSRCS (Eng), MOrthRCS (Eng), FDS (Orth) RCS (Eng)
Consultant in Orthodontics, Eastman Dental Hospital, UCLH NHS Foundation Trust
Honorary Consultant in Orthodontics, Great Ormond Street Hospital, London
Honorary Senior Lecturer in Orthodontics, UCL Eastman Dental Institute, University College London

Steven P. Jones
BDS (Hons), MSc, LDSRCS (Eng), FDSRCS (Ed), FDSRCS (Eng), FDSRCPS (Glasg), DOrthRCS (Eng), MOrthRCS (Eng), ILTM, FHEA
Consultant in Orthodontics, Eastman Dental Hospital, UCLH NHS Foundation Trust
Honorary Senior Lecturer in Orthodontics, UCL Eastman Dental Institute, University College London

Kenneth W. Hemmings
BDS (Hons), MSc, DRDRCS (Ed), MRDRCS (Ed), FDSRCS (Eng), ILTM, FHEA
Consultant in Restorative Dentistry, Eastman Dental Hospital, UCLH NHS Foundation Trust
Honorary Lecturer in Conservative Dentistry, UCL Eastman Dental Institute, University College London

G. Steven Bassi
BDS, LDSRCS (Eng), FDSRCPS (Glasg), FDSRCS (Ed), FDS (Rest Dent) RCPS (Glasg), MDentSci
Consultant in Restorative Dentistry, Eastman Dental Hospital, UCLH NHS Foundation Trust

Amanda L. O'Donnell
BDS, MFDSRCS (Eng), MClinDent, MPaedDent, FDS (Paed Dent) RCS (Eng)
Consultant in Paediatric Dentistry, Eastman Dental Hospital, UCLH NHS Foundation Trust, London
Honorary Lecturer in Paediatric Dentistry, UCL Eastman Dental Institute, University College London

Jane R. Goodman
BDS, FDSRCS (Ed), FDSRCS (Eng), FRCPCH, FCDSHK, ILTM, FHEA
Former Consultant in Paediatric Dentistry, Eastman Dental Hospital, UCLH NHS Foundation Trust, and Honorary Senior Lecturer in Paediatric Dentistry, UCL Eastman Dental Institute, University College London

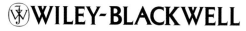
WILEY-BLACKWELL
A John Wiley & Sons, Ltd., Publication

This edition first published 2011
© 2011 J.A. Hobkirk, D.S. Gill, S.P. Jones, K.W. Hemmings, G.S. Bassi, A.L. O'Donnell and J.R. Goodman

Blackwell Publishing was acquired by John Wiley & Sons in February 2007. Blackwell's publishing programme has been merged with Wiley's global Scientific, Technical, and Medical business to form Wiley-Blackwell.

Registered office
John Wiley & Sons Ltd, The Atrium, Southern Gate, Chichester, West Sussex, PO19 8SQ, United Kingdom

Editorial offices
9600 Garsington Road, Oxford, OX4 2DQ, United Kingdom
The Atrium, Southern Gate, Chichester, West Sussex, PO19 8SQ, UK
2121 State Avenue, Ames, Iowa 50014-8300, USA

For details of our global editorial offices, for customer services and for information about how to apply for permission to reuse the copyright material in this book please see our website at www.wiley.com/wiley-blackwell.

Library of Congress Cataloging-in-Publication Data

Hypodontia: a team approach to management/J.A. Hobkirk ... [et al.].
     p. ; cm.
  Includes bibliographical references and index.
  ISBN 978-1-4051-8859-3 (hardcover: alk. paper)   1. Hypodontia.   I. Hobkirk, John A.
  [DNLM: 1. Anodontia. WU 101.5]
  RK305.H96 2011
  617.6–dc22
                                                      2010040510

A catalogue record for this book is available from the British Library.

Set in 9.5/11.5 pt Palatino by Toppan Best-set Premedia Limited
Printed and bound in Singapore by Fabulous Printers

1   2011

Contents

Acknowledgements   v
Introduction   vii

Part 1 Background   1

1 Definitions, Prevalence and Aetiology   3

2 Features   14

3 Providing Care   28

Part 2 Key Issues   43

4 Space   45

5 Occlusion   60

6 Supporting Tissues   82

Part 3 Age-Related Approaches to Treatment   103

7 Primary/Early Mixed Dentition   105

8 Late Mixed and Early Permanent Dentition   124

9 The Established Dentition with Hypodontia   150

Glossary of Terms   188
Index   193

Acknowledgements

Over the 33 years since the establishment of the Multidisciplinary Hypodontia Clinic at the Eastman Dental Hospital, we have had the privilege of working with many talented colleagues to whom we owe a great debt of gratitude. The late Ian Reynolds was one of the three founding members of the Clinic and contributed greatly to its development, as did Paul King, who was a member of the team for many years. We would particularly like to acknowledge the support of the Head Dental Nurses from our respective departments, Lesley Cogan, Alex Moss and Helen Richardson, all of whom have been key members of the Clinic. We are also grateful to Manish Patel, Akit Patel, Nicholas Lewis, Zahra Hussain, Akil Gulamali, Joanne Collins and Amal Abu Maizar who have provided some of the treatment that is illustrated in this book. Much dental care is dependent on the support of technical colleagues, and in this respect we have been superbly assisted by the work of the staff in the Prosthodontic and Orthodontic laboratories at the Eastman Dental Hospital. The Clinic has also enjoyed a close working relationship with the Ectodermal Dysplasia Society, the UK's national patient support group. Many of its members have been our patients and we have learnt much from them.

We are grateful to Anatomage Inc., San Jose, California, for allowing us to use the skull image on the front cover of the book.

JAH
DSG
SPJ
KWH
GSB
ALO'D
JRG
London 2010

Introduction

This book has its origins in the establishment in 1977 of a multidisciplinary hypodontia clinic at the Eastman Dental Hospital in London. In subsequent years both the number of clinicians in the team and their range of activities has expanded such that by 2007 over 3000 patients had been treated. They and their patients' collective journeys form the basis of this book.

This text has been written for senior undergraduate students, graduate students and specialist trainees from the range of specialisms that can form part of a multidisciplinary hypodontia team, and it assumes a basic level of knowledge of subjects outside a given speciality. Its aim is to develop greater knowledge and understanding of the causes and features of hypodontia, the key issues in its management, and potential approaches to helping those with the condition at the various stages of dental development. Throughout the book emphasis is placed on the potential contributions of the different members of the hypodontia team, and the manner in which each of these can contribute to an integrated care pathway for the patient throughout their life.

The text has been divided into three broad areas, namely background topics, key issues, and age-related approaches to treatment. The content of each of these sections has been influenced by the views of the entire team, as would occur in a hypodontia clinic. Consequently there are cross-references between the various chapters, with some topics appearing in different contexts for the sake of clarity and completeness. This avoids needless movement between sections when reading a particular chapter.

The first section, on background topics, considers issues that are fundamental to treatment. It addresses the aetiology and prevalence of hypodontia and the troublesome issue of terminology. The characteristics of the condition are also explored and the section concludes by considering the various ways in which treatment for patients with hypodontia might best be organised using both a specialist hypodontia team and local care providers.

Key issues are addressed in the second section, exploring the fundamentals of space, occlusion and supporting tissues. Assessment and management of space are major factors in the treatment of patients with hypodontia since the size and distribution of space largely determine the feasibility of many treatment procedures and their final outcomes. Modifications to spaces within the arches and between opposing teeth may require orthodontic, prosthodontic and surgical approaches, guided by a clear collective understanding of the ultimate treatment objectives. Patients with hypodontia frequently require treatment that necessitates changes to their occlusion and which may employ a range of principles, philosophies and techniques as work progresses. Hypodontia is characterised not only by missing teeth but also by deficits in the tissues that are often used to support fixed and removable prostheses; their significance and potential management are also considered in this section.

The third section brings the first two together in the context of treating patients with hypodontia, drawing on the contributions that various specialisms may collectively make to achieve the optimum outcome. While treatment is in practice a continuum, the section has been divided into chapters that consider patients in three consecutive stages of dental development: firstly the primary/early mixed dentition, secondly the late mixed dentition/early permanent dentition, and thirdly the established dentition with hypodontia.

The lists of key points found in every chapter are intended to help readers who are revising and provide a link between chapters, each of which also has its own list of references. These references contribute to an evidence-based approach, supporting various statements in the text and pointing the reader towards further reading. Individual references are not unique to any one chapter since some issues are referred to in more than one context.

Working within a multidisciplinary team can be an extremely rewarding experience both for clinicians and for their patients; it is the authors' hope that readers will find this book of help in initiating, developing and running such clinics.

Part 1

Background

1

Definitions, Prevalence and Aetiology

Introduction

Disturbances during the early stages of tooth formation may result in the developmental or congenital absence of one or more teeth. This condition has been described in the literature using a range of terms that can be a source of confusion since they are frequently neither synonymous nor mutually exclusive, and no single name is universally accepted.

The most widely employed general term is *hypodontia*, used by many to describe the whole spectrum of the disorder from the absence of a single tooth to the rare absence of all teeth (termed *anodontia*). Absent third permanent molars are generally not considered when assessing the presence and severity of hypodontia. To assist in diagnostic classification, the degree of severity of hypodontia has been arbitrarily described as:

- Mild: 1–2 missing teeth
- Moderate: 3–5 missing teeth
- Severe: 6 or more missing teeth

(From Goodman *et al.*, 1994; Dhanrajani, 2002; Nunn *et al.*, 2003; Jones, 2009).

In contrast, some authors have suggested that the term *hypodontia* should be employed solely to describe the absence of a few teeth, preferring the term *oligodontia* to describe the absence of a larger number of teeth (Nunn *et al.*, 2003). This has been further refined with the suggestion that the absence of one to six teeth should be termed *hypodontia*, while the absence of more than six teeth should be termed *oligodontia* (Arte and Pirinen, 2004; Polder *et al.*, 2004). Others have proposed that the term *oligodontia* should be further limited to describe the absence of six or more teeth with associated systemic manifestations, as seen in several syndromes (Goodman *et al.*, 1994; Nunn *et al.*, 2003). To reflect the differences in terminology, a further subdivision of hypodontia and oligodontia has been proposed into *isolated hypodontia/oligodontia* (non-syndromic) and *syndromic hypodontia/oligodontia* (associated with syndromes) (Schalk van der Weide *et al.*, 1992; Arte and Pirinen, 2004).

Current terminology also demonstrates geographical variations. The term *oligodontia* is often preferred in Europe, whereas the descriptive terms *agenesis* or *multiple dental agenesis* are often used in the USA. One historic and self-contradictory descriptor, which was once widely used but is now

Table 1.1   Terms used to describe the developmental or congenital absence of teeth.

Term	Definition	Common usage	Used in this book
Hypodontia	A developmental or congenital condition characterised by fewer than normal teeth	As defined Often sub-divided into mild (fewer than six teeth missing) and severe (six or more missing) forms*	A developmental or congenital condition characterised by fewer than normal teeth
Severe hypodontia	A developmental or congenital condition characterised by absence of six or more teeth	As defined Often used synonymously with oligodontia	A developmental or congenital condition characterised by absence of six or more teeth*
Oligodontia	A developmental or congenital condition characterised by fewer than normal teeth	As defined Often used synonymously with severe hypodontia	A developmental or congenital condition characterised by fewer than normal teeth in the presence of systemic manifestations
Anodontia	A developmental or congenital condition characterised by absence of all teeth	Sometimes sub-divided into anodontia and partial anodontia (now obsolete, but equates to hypodontia or oligodontia)	A developmental or congenital condition characterised by absence of all teeth

*By convention, third molars are excluded from the definition.

considered largely obsolete (and deprecated), is *partial anodontia* (Jones, 2009).

In this book we use the terms *hypodontia, oligodontia* and *anodontia* (Table 1.1). They are simple to employ and provide convenient labels for the relevant conditions, being of particular value in epidemiological studies. They are, however, defined solely by the number of missing teeth and take no account of the patterns of dental agenesis. In addition they do not include frequently encountered clinical features of hypodontia such as variations in the form and size of the teeth, delayed eruption, connective tissue changes, malpositioning of teeth, and occlusal disharmony, which means they are of limited value when assessing treatment needs.

Hypodontia is one factor in the clinical indices used by orthodontists when prioritising treatment, so reflecting the clinical importance of the condition for the patient concerned. The Index of Orthodontic Treatment Need (Dental Health Component) uses a five-point scale in which Category 5 indicates the greatest need for treatment (Shaw *et al.*, 1991; Waring and Jones, 2003; Ferguson, 2006). The absence of more than a single tooth in any one quadrant is assigned to Category 5, while cases in which there are fewer missing teeth are assigned to Category 4. These categories are based on a need for multidisciplinary care for

more severe hypodontia, with the possibility of closure of spaces in milder cases. Other indices have also considered hypodontia as a factor with a high impact on dental status (Otuyemi and Jones, 1995; Shelton *et al.*, 2008).

Many societies now place considerably greater emphasis on oral health than they have done in the past. As a result, individuals with hypodontia are increasingly requesting treatment for their condition. It can be complex and expensive, particularly where advanced restorative care results in the need for lifetime dental maintenance (Forgie *et al.*, 2005; Thind *et al.*, 2005; Hobkirk *et al.*, 2006). It also often involves a number of specialist services, and consequently data on the prevalence of hypodontia within a given population are important for planning and allocating healthcare resources both at regional and national levels. Knowledge of the prevalence of hypodontia is also important when counselling patients and their carers (Lucas, 2000; Gill *et al.*, 2008).

Prevalence

Primary dentition

In the primary dentition, hypodontia is relatively uncommon. The prevalence of 0.1–0.9% is equally distributed between males and females (Grahnen and Granath, 1961; Järvinen and Lehtinen, 1981; Carvalho et al., 1998; Dhanrajani, 2002; Nunn et al., 2003). It is most common in the anterior maxilla, with the lateral incisors being most frequently affected (Daugaard-Jensen et al., 1997). Hypodontia in the primary dentition is often associated with hypodontia in the permanent dentition (Whittington and Durward, 1996; Daugaard-Jensen et al., 1997; Arte and Pirinen, 2004), and can be used in the early counselling of affected individuals and their carers. In mild cases, hypodontia of the primary dentition often goes unnoticed or may be wrongly dismissed as of some interest but seemingly unimportant. Diagnosis in a younger patient is frequently made by general dental practitioners, who should have knowledge of the condition and be prepared to refer the patient early for specialist investigation and family counselling (Hobson et al., 2003; Gill et al., 2008).

Permanent dentition

Studies into the prevalence of hypodontia in the permanent dentition have frequently suffered from relatively small sample sizes (Polder et al., 2004) which is probably one of the reasons why reported prevalence often varies, even within similar populations, with ranges as wide as 0.3–36.5%. Although data on missing teeth are only available for a small number of racial groups (and inevitably some have been studied more thoroughly than others), it has been shown that the prevalence of hypodontia in females is higher in Europe and Australia than in North America (Flores-Mir, 2005). The same difference was also noted for males (Polder et al., 2004). The most extensive studies have been of Caucasian people, with a reported prevalence of hypodontia in the range 4.0–6.0% and among whom females are more frequently affected than males in the ratio of 3:2 (Egermark-Eriksson and Lind, 1971; Dhanrajani, 2002; Nunn et al., 2003; Larmour et al., 2005). In contrast, the prevalence of severe hypodontia, defined as the developmental absence of six or more teeth, has been reported at 0.14–0.3% in Caucasian people (Hobkirk and Brook, 1980; Polder et al., 2004).

In order to increase the sample size and thus improve the reliability of population data, Polder et al. (2004) conducted a meta-analysis which has added significantly to our knowledge. It included data from 33 studies, with a total sample size of approximately 127,000 individuals, and concluded that the prevalence of hypodontia in the permanent dentition varied between continents, racial groups and genders.

The reported prevalence in the population for different racial groups included white Europeans (4.6–6.3%), white North Americans (3.2–4.6%), black African–Americans (3.2–4.6%), white Australians (5.5–7.6%), Arabs (2.2–2.7%) and Chinese people (6.1–7.7%) (Polder et al., 2004). Other studies have examined the prevalence among white Scandinavians (4.5–6.3%) and Japanese people (7.5–9.3%) (Niswander and Sujaku, 1963; Endo et al., 2006a, 2006b). The data analysed confirmed that hypodontia was more prevalent in females than males (1.37:1), which closely approximates to the previously cited ratio of 3:2 found in smaller studies. Table 1.2 summarises the prevalence data in relation to ethnicity.

Table 1.2 Prevalence of dental agenesis by gender in different ethnic groups and male to female ratios in each ethnic group.

Ethnic group	Mean % males (CI)	Mean % females (CI)	Male to female ratio
European (white)	4.6% (4.5, 4.8)	6.3% (6.1, 6.5)	1:1.4
North American (white)	3.2% (2.9, 3.5)	4.6% (4.2, 4.9)	1:1.4
North American (African-American)	3.2% (2.2, 4.1)	4.6% (3.5, 5.8)	1:1.4
Australian (white)	5.5% (4.4, 6.6)	7.6% (6.0, 9.2)	1:1.4
Saudi Arabian (white)	2.7% (2.0, 3.4)	2.2% (1.2, 3.1)	1:0.8
Chinese (Mongoloid)	6.1% (4.0, 8.1)	7.7% (5.4, 10.0)	1:1.3

CI, confidence intervals. Data from Polder et al. (2004).

The reported sites and frequency of missing teeth both vary between studies. To evaluate the prevalence of absence of an individual tooth within a normal population, Polder *et al.* (2004) carried out a meta-analysis. This considered 10 studies with an aggregate sample of over 48,000 people. The frequency of absent teeth in *descending* order was:

- Mandibular second premolar (3.0%)
- Maxillary lateral incisor (1.7%)
- Maxillary second premolar (1.5%)
- Mandibular central incisor (0.3%)
- Mandibular lateral incisor and maxillary first premolar (0.2%)
- Mandibular first premolar (0.15%)
- Mandibular second molar and maxillary canine (0.1%)
- Maxillary second molar (0.05%)
- Maxillary first molar (0.03%)
- Mandibular canine (0.02%)
- Mandibular first molar (0.01%)
- Maxillary central incisor (0.005%)

This supports one of the widely accepted sequences of missing teeth as:

- Mandibular second premolar >
- Maxillary lateral incisor >
- Maxillary second premolar >
- Mandibular incisors

To consider the frequency of missing teeth within a sample of hypodontia patients, a meta-analysis examined data from 24 studies reporting on individuals with hypodontia with a total of approximately 11,500 absent teeth (Polder *et al.*, 2004). The absence of individual teeth within the hypodontia group had the same sequence as that described above, namely: mandibular second premolar (41.0%) > maxillary lateral incisor (22.9%) > maxillary second premolar (21.2%) > mandibular central incisor (3.5%) > maxillary first premolar (2.8%) > mandibular lateral incisor (2.5%). The remaining teeth were within the range 0.2–1.4%, supporting a previously expressed view that the absence of maxillary central incisors, canines and first molars is rare and principally occurs in patients with severe hypodontia, where there is the concomitant absence of the most frequently missing teeth (Hobkirk and Brook, 1980; Rózsa *et al.*, 2009).

Table 1.3 summarises data relating to the frequency of absent teeth within a group of hypodontia patients.

The majority of patients with developmentally missing teeth (83%) had only one or two teeth missing. Patients with three to five teeth missing represented 14.4% of the group, while severe hypodontia with six or more absent teeth was present in 2.6% of the sample. This was equated to a population prevalence of 0.14%.

The bilateral absence of a particular tooth in one jaw has been reported to be 54% for maxillary lateral incisors. These are the only teeth with a prevalence that is greater than 50% (with values of 49.25% for maxillary second premolars, 45.6% for mandibular second premolars and 41.2% for mandibular central incisors), hence it can be concluded that it is more common for maxillary lateral incisors to be absent bilaterally and other teeth to be absent unilaterally. Table 1.4 summarises data relating to the frequency of bilaterally absent teeth.

Table 1.3   Distribution of individual missing teeth for each jaw in patients with hypodontia.

Tooth	Maxilla	Mandible
I1	0.2%	3.5%
I2	22.9%	2.5%
C	1.3%	0.3%
P1	2.8%	1.4%
P2	21.2%	41.0%
M1	0.7%	0.3%
M2	0.6%	1.2%

Data from Polder *et al.* (2004).

Table 1.4   Frequency of the bilateral absence of teeth.

Tooth	Frequency %	(95% CI)
MAXILLA		
I2	54.0%	(50.9, 57.0)
P2	49.25%	(46.3, 52.2)
MANDIBLE		
I1	41.2%	(30.5, 51.9)
P2	45.6%	(43.5, 47.7)

Data from Polder *et al.* (2004).

Aetiology

Environmental and genetic factors

Several theories concerning the aetiology of hypodontia have been proposed, including suggestions that both genetic and environmental factors may play a role. Hypodontia may appear as an isolated non-syndromic feature or as part of a complex syndrome with developmental defects of other ectodermal organs (Lucas, 2000). Early workers investigating the aetiology of isolated non-syndromic hypodontia proposed an anthropological viewpoint, one that reflected an ongoing process of evolution. Butler's Field Theory for the evolutionary development of mammalian teeth (Butler, 1939), when applied to the human dentition by Dahlberg (1945), suggested that the most mesial tooth in each morphological series was the most genetically stable and consequently was rarely missing. Such teeth were designated as 'key teeth' and included the central incisors, canines, first premolars and first molars. In contrast, teeth at the end of each field showed less genetic stability. This led to the concept of *stable* and *unstable* elements of the dentition (Bailit, 1975).

This principle was further supported by Bolk's Theory of Terminal Reduction (de Beer, 1951; Rózsa *et al.*, 2009). This proposed that the evolutionary process was leading to the reduction of the distal element of tooth groups, resulting in the more frequent absence of second premolars, lateral incisors and third molars (Muller *et al.*, 1970; Jorgenson, 1980; Brook, 1984; Schalk van der Weide *et al.*, 1994; Fekonja, 2005; Gábris *et al.*, 2006; Rózsa *et al.*, 2009).

It was also suggested that intra-uterine conditions were involved, and Bailit (1975) encouraged good maternal antenatal nutrition and medical care, but considered that postnatal nutrition, disease, general health and climatic conditions had little influence on hypodontia. The intra-uterine effects of drugs such as thalidomide have been associated with the development of hypodontia (Axrup *et al.*, 1966) as have radiotherapy and chemotherapy in early infancy (Maguire *et al.*, 1987; Dahllöf *et al.*, 1994; Kaste and Hopkins, 1994; Näsman *et al.*, 1997; Nunn *et al.*, 2003; Oğuz *et al.*, 2004).

Other environmental factors that may cause arrested tooth development include a local effect of trauma, such as alveolar fracture or jaw fracture, jaw surgery or iatrogenic damage to the developing tooth germ from traumatic extraction of the overlying primary tooth (Grahnen, 1956; Nunn *et al.*, 2003).

Hypodontia has also been associated with cleft lip and palate, usually localised to the maxillary lateral incisor in the line of the alveolar cleft (Dhanrajani, 2002). This was initially considered to be a physical obstruction of the developing dental lamina from which the tooth germ develops, however more recently a defect in the *Msx1* gene has been identified, which is associated with both isolated cleft lip and cleft palate, and hypodontia (Satokata and Maas, 1994; van den Boogaard *et al.*, 2000; Alappat *et al.*, 2003).

Although occasionally hypodontia is associated with environmental factors, in the majority of cases it has a genetic basis, which has been the subject of intensive research. Hypodontia is frequently identified as a familial trait, with several generations affected within families, although the genetic mechanisms are still poorly understood. In family studies, a greater frequency of hypodontia has been demonstrated among the relatives of probands than in the general population (Brook, 1984).

As well as the familial nature of hypodontia, it often presents as an isolated diagnosis with no detectable family history, which suggests it can occur as a result of a spontaneous genetic mutation (Kupietzky and Houpt, 1995; Dhanrajani, 2002).

Inheritance patterns

Examination of monozygotic twins and triplets indicates there is a familial pattern in hypodontia (Gravely and Johnson, 1971). This is thought to occur by an autosomal dominant process with incomplete penetrance of up to 86% (Arte and Pirinen, 2004). A polygenic model was proposed that involved interaction between epistatic genes and environmental factors (Suarez and Spence, 1974; Bailit, 1975). A link was also proposed to explain the commonly observed association between hypodontia and microdontia. This multifactorial model (Suarez and Spence, 1974; Brook, 1984) was based on an underlying continuum of tooth size with thresholds, whereby there is a progressive reduction in the size of the tooth which reaches a certain threshold below which the developing tooth germ degenerates, so producing hypodontia.

Tooth development

Tooth development is a complex process, which commences in the developing embryo as an interaction between the oral epithelium and ectomesenchyme derived from the neural crest. A thickening of the epithelium develops into a dental placode and invagination then occurs to produce a tooth bud (Dassule *et al.*, 2000). A collection of cells within the tooth bud, known as the primary enamel knot, manages this process through genetically controlled signalling pathways (Vaahtokari *et al.*, 1996). The mesenchyme begins to surround the epithelium to initially produce a cap stage, and later a bell stage. Mesenchymal cells adjacent to the basement membrane differentiate into odontoblasts, which begin to secrete an organic dentine matrix into which hydroxyapatite crystals are deposited. The epithelial cells adjacent to the dentine differentiate into ameloblasts, which secrete the enamel matrix and control the mineralisation and subsequent maturation of the enamel (Dassule *et al.*, 2000).

The formation and morphology of the cusps in premolars and molars is controlled by secondary enamel knots, which develop at the sites where the cusps are to form. These produce folding of the developing tooth germ to the pre-determined crown morphology (Zhang *et al.*, 2008). Root formation continues with the formation of dentine under the control of Hertwig's root sheath, which later degenerates and leads to the development of cementoblasts. The cementoblasts, in turn, deposit cementum on the root surface (Nakatomi *et al.*, 2006; Khan *et al.*, 2007). Cells in the adjacent dental follicle differentiate into fibroblasts and osteoblasts, and these cells contribute to the formation of the periodontal ligament (Fleischmannova *et al.*, 2008).

Genes involved in odontogenesis

As can be seen, the development of the dentition is a complex process involving a series of epithelial–mesenchymal interactions, and involving growth factors, transcription factors, signalling pathways and other morphogens (Thesleff, 2000). With such

complexity, it is not surprising that disturbances can occur in the process, potentially resulting in tooth agenesis (Kapadia *et al.*, 2007). At the molecular level during odontogenesis, epithelial–mesenchymal signalling is under the control of members of the *Wnt* (wingless), *Hh* (hedgehog), *Fgf* (fibroblast growth factor) and *Bmp* (bone morphogenic protein) gene families (Cobourne, 1999; Dassule *et al.*, 2000). Defects in any of these pathways can result in disorders of tooth number (hypodontia or supernumerary teeth), tooth morphology (tooth size and shape) and tooth mineralisation (amelogenesis imperfecta or dentinogenesis imperfecta) (Fleischmannova *et al.*, 2008).

Of particular interest in hypodontia are the genes called *Msx1* (muscle segment homeobox 1) and *Pax9* (paired box 9), which are homeobox transcription factors involved in early odontogenesis under the control of *Bmp* and *Fgf* signalling (Satokata and Maas, 1994; Vastardis *et al.*, 1996; Dahl, 1998; Lidral and Reising, 2002; Alappat *et al.*, 2003; Mostowska *et al.*, 2003; Nunn *et al.*, 2003; Cobourne, 2007; Kapadia *et al.*, 2007; Fleischmannova *et al.*, 2008; Matalova *et al.*, 2008).

A review by Fleischmannova *et al.* (2008) has highlighted the progress that has been made over the last decade in understanding the genetic basis of hypodontia using the transgenic mouse model incorporating selective gene deletions. These have concentrated on the role of homeobox genes, which were originally identified in the fruit fly, *Drosophila*. Homeobox genes code for specific transcription factors, which regulate downstream target genes. Studies have suggested that mutations in the homeobox genes *Msx1* and *Pax9*, which interact during odontogenesis, are associated with tooth agenesis in mice and may be associated with hypodontia in humans. *Msx1* is expressed in regions of condensing ectomesenchyme within the tooth germ. Mice lacking a functional *Msx1* gene demonstrate arrested tooth development at the bud stage. *Pax9* is expressed in the mesenchymal element of the developing tooth germ and is essential during later stages of tooth development. Mice with targeted mutations of *Pax9* show arrested tooth development at the bud stage. More recently, defects in a third gene, *Axin2*, have been identified as having a possible association with severe hypodontia (Lammi *et al.*, 2004; Cobourne, 2007).

Syndromic associations

Several syndromes exhibit hypodontia as one of their features, and many of these have demonstrated gene defects (*Online Mendelian Inheritance in Man* (OMIM) database). Mutations in the homeobox transcription factor *Pitx2* (paired-like homeodomain transcription factor 2) are associated with Rieger syndrome, an autosomal dominant disorder with ocular, umbilical and dental defects. Mutations in *p63* are associated with syndromes involving hypodontia that include digital disorders like syndactyly and ectrodactyly, facial clefts, cleft lip and palate, and ectodermal dysplasia. Mutations in *Msx1* have also been associated with isolated cleft lip and palate, and Witkop (tooth and nail) syndrome (Jumlongras *et al.*, 2001).

The genetic inheritance of the family of ectodermal dysplasias has been investigated. There are over 190 different types of this condition, and while several genes have been implicated, the exact numbers of genes have yet to be determined. Hypohidrotic ectodermal dysplasia (HED) is a disorder in which the sweat glands are reduced in number, which has received the greatest attention. Defects in the *Xq12–Xq13* site on the X chromosome, which encodes for the protein ectodysplasin-A (*Eda*), have been shown to be associated with an X-linked inheritance pattern (XHED). The same chromosome site defects have been identified in non-syndromic isolated X-linked hypodontia. Mutations in the modulator gene *Nemo*, a downstream target of *Eda* signalling, have also been associated with X-linked HED. *Eda* has a role in epithelial–mesenchymal signalling, and is expressed in the development of the ectodermal structures that develop from epithelial placodes, including skin, sweat glands, hair, nails and teeth. In severe cases, the dental effects can result in anodontia. Hypohidrotic ectodermal dysplasia is also associated with both autosomal dominant and autosomal recessive patterns of inheritance through mutations in the ectodysplasin-A receptor (*Eda-R*), and an autosomal recessive pattern of inheritance through mutations in the EdaR-associated death domain (*Edaradd*).

Studies in mice have shown that defects in the *Eda* pathway result in disorders of tooth number, tooth size and tooth morphology, with a reduction in the number of molar cusps. This suggests a mechanism for the relationship of hypodontia and microdontia, and in particular the conical shape of the teeth in individuals with ectodermal dysplasia. Table 1.5 presents further information relating to syndromes associated with hypodontia, including the current understanding of inheritance patterns, the gene loci associated with the syndrome and affected gene pathways.

The genetic processes and signalling pathways involved in hypodontia are complex and frequently rely on data extrapolated from transgenic mice to humans (Kronmiller *et al.*, 1995; Vaahtokari *et al.*, 1996; Hardcastle *et al.*, 1999; Dassule *et al.*, 2000; Zhang *et al.*, 2000; Cobourne *et al.*, 2001, 2004; Miletich *et al.*, 2005; Nakatomi *et al.*, 2006; Khan *et al.*, 2007; Zhang *et al.*, 2008). Understanding the genetics of hypodontia is important for diagnostic and counselling purposes (Gill *et al.*, 2008) and offers the opportunity of genetic screening for affected families. It also presents the challenges of employing tissue engineering and stem cell technology as therapeutic alternatives. Initial studies have suggested that arrested tooth development in *Pax9*- or *Msx1*-deficient mice can be rescued by the transgenic expression of *Bmp4*, an influential signalling factor in a number of developmental processes (Zhang *et al.*, 2000; Fleischmannova *et al.*, 2008).

Identifying the genes and pathways associated with hypodontia and associated syndromes, opens an exciting possibility for the future, one that may hold the potential for direct postnatal gene therapy on developing tooth germs and the prospect of treating hypodontia at a molecular level (Fleischmannova *et al.*, 2008). This concept has so far been investigated in animal models, whereby teeth have been successfully bioengineered in mice, rats and pigs using stem cell biology and biodegradable scaffolds for potential use in organ replacement therapy (Young *et al.*, 2005a, 2005b; Yelick and Vacanti, 2006; Nakahara and Ide, 2007; Duailibi *et al.*, 2008; Honda *et al.*, 2008; Ikeda and Tsuji, 2008; Ikeda *et al.*, 2009; Zhang *et al.*, 2009).

These developments support the feasibility of bioengineering the formation of replacement teeth in the jaws of humans in the future. Such practical application of bioengineering could provide a novel approach to the management of patients with hypodontia through tissue regenerative therapy.

Table 1.5 Syndromic associations of hypodontia (including genetic data).

Syndrome	Affected areas/structures	Mode of inheritance	Gene map loci	Genes affected
Hypohidrotic ectodermal dysplasia 1 (HED)	Skin, sweat glands, hair, nails, teeth (hypodontia)	X-linked recessive	. Xq12–q13.1	Ectodysplasin A (Eda)
Hypohidrotic ectodermal dysplasia 3 (EDA3)	Skin, sweat glands, hair, nails, teeth (hypodontia)	Autosomal dominant	2q11–q13 1q42–q43	Ectodysplasin anhidrotic receptor gene (Edar); EDAR-associated death domain (Edaradd)
Hypohidrotic ectodermal dysplasia with immune deficiency (HED-ID)	Skin, sweat glands, hair, nails, teeth (hypodontia), dysgammaglobulinaemia	X-linked recessive	Xq28	IKK-gamma gene (IKBKG or Nemo)
Incontinentia pigmenti (Bloch–Sulzberger syndrome)	Skin (hyperpigmented patches), hair, eyes, central nervous system, teeth (hypodontia)	Male-lethal X-linked dominant	Xq28	IKK-gamma gene (IKBKG or Nemo)
Ectrodactyly, ectodermal dysplasia and cleft lip/palate syndrome 1 (EEC1)	Digits (split hand/foot), hair, skin, nails, mouth (cleft lip/palate), teeth (hypodontia)	Autosomal dominant	7q11.2–q21.3	TP63
Cleft lip/palate-ectodermal dysplasia syndrome (CLPED1)	Mouth (cleft lip/palate), nails, hair, digits (syndactyly), teeth (hypodontia)	Autosomal recessive	11q23–q24	PVRL 1
Witkop syndrome (tooth and nail syndrome)	Nails, teeth (hypodontia)	Autosomal dominant	4p16.1	Msx1
van der Woude syndrome (lip-pit syndrome)	Mouth (pits in lower lip, cleft lip/palate/ uvula), teeth (hypodontia)	Autosomal dominant	1q32–q41	Interferon regulatory factor 6 (IRF6)
Oral-facial-digital syndrome (OFD)	Mouth (cleft palate, cleft tongue), digits (polydactyly), kidneys, central nervous system, teeth (hypodontia)	Male-lethal X-linked dominant	Xp22.3–p22.2	OFD1 protein gene (CXorf5)
Rieger syndrome	Eyes, umbilical cord, growth hormone (deficiency), teeth (hypodontia)	Autosomal dominant	4q25–q26	Paired-like homeodomain transcription factor-2 gene (Pitx2)
Down syndrome (trisomy 21)	Face, eyes, heart, blood (leukaemia), central nervous system, endocrine system, hearing, teeth (hypodontia)	Isolated cases	21q22.3 1q43 Xp11.23	–
Book syndrome	Hair (premature greying), hyperhidrosis, teeth (hypodontia)	Autosomal dominant	–	–
Holoprosencephaly	Cyclopia, face (facial clefts), mouth (cleft lip/palate, midline maxillary central incisor	Autosomal recessive	21q22.3	–

Data from Online Mendelian Inheritance in Man (OMIM) at www.ncbi.nlm.nih.gov/Omim/.

References

Alappat S, Zhang ZY, Chen YP. *Msx* homeobox gene family and craniofacial development. *Cell Res* 2003;13: 429–442.

Arte S, Pirinen S. Hypodontia. *Orphanet Encyclopedia* 2004. Available at www.orpha.net/data/patho/GB/uk-hypodontia.pdf [/](last accessed July 2010.

Axrup K, D'Avignon M, Hellgren K, *et al.* Children with thalidomide embryopathy: odontological observations and aspects. *Acta Odontol Scand* 1966;24:3–21.

Bailit HL. Dental variation among populations. An anthropologic view. *Dent Clin North Am* 1975;19:125–139.

Brook AH. A unifying aetiological explanation for anomalies of human tooth number and size. *Arch Oral Biol* 1984;29:373–378.

Butler PM. Studies of the mammalian dentition. Differentiation of the post-canine dentition. *Proc Zoolog Soc Lond* 1939;109B:1–36.

Carvalho JC, Vinker F, Declerck D. Malocclusion, dental injuries and dental anomalies in the primary dentition of Belgian children. *Int J Paediatr Dent* 1998;8: 137–141.

Cobourne MT. The genetic control of early odontogenesis. *Br J Orthod* 1999;26:21–28.

Cobourne MT. Familial human hypodontia – Is it all in the genes? *Br Dent J* 2007;203:203–208.

Cobourne MT, Hardcastle Z, Sharpe PT. *Sonic hedgehog* regulates epithelial proliferation and cell survival in the developing tooth germ. *J Dent Res* 2001;80:1974–1979.

Cobourne MT, Miletich I, Sharpe PT. Restriction of *sonic hedgehog* signalling during early tooth development. *Development* 2004;131:2875–2885.

Dahl N. Genetics of ectodermal dysplasia syndromes. In: B Bergendal, G Koch, J Kurol, G Wänndahl (eds) *Consensus Conference on Ectodermal Dysplasia with Special Reference to Dental Treatment*. Gothia, Stockholm, 1998, pp. 22–31.

Dahlberg AA. The changing dentition of man. *J Am Dent Assoc* 1945;32:676–690.

Dahllöf G, Rozell B, Forsberg CM, Borgström B. Histologic changes in dental morphology induced by high dose chemotherapy and total body irradiation. *Oral Surg Oral Med Oral Pathol* 1994;77:56–60.

Dassule HR, Lewis P, Bei M, Maas R, McMahon AP. *Sonic hedgehog* regulates growth and morphogenesis of the tooth. *Development* 2000;127:4775–4785.

Daugaard-Jensen J, Nodal M, Skovgaard LT, Kjaer I. Comparison of the pattern of agenesis in the primary and permanent dentitions in a population characterized by agenesis in the primary dentition. *Int J Paediatr Dent* 1997;7:143–148.

de Beer GR. *Embryos and Ancestors*. Clarendon Press, Oxford 1951; pp 58–59.

Dhanrajani PJ. Hypodontia: Etiology, clinical features, and management. *Quintessence Int* 2002;33:294–302.

Duailibi SE, Duailibi MT, Zhang W, *et al.* Bioengineered dental tissues grown in the rat jaw. *J Dent Res* 2008;87: 745–750.

Egermark-Eriksson I, Lind V. Congenital numerical variation in the permanent dentition. Sex distribution of hypodontia and hyperodontia. *Odontol Revy* 1971;22: 309–315.

Endo T, Ozoe R, Kubota M, Akiyama M, Shimooka S. A survey of hypodontia in Japanese orthodontic patients. *Am J Orthod Dentofacial Orthop* 2006a;129:29–35.

Endo T, Ozoe R, Yoshino S, Shimooka S. Hypodontia patterns and variations in craniofacial morphology in Japanese orthodontic patients. *Angle Orthod* 2006b;76: 996–1003.

Fekonja A. Hypodontia in orthodontically treated children. *Eur J Orthod* 2005;27:457–460.

Ferguson JW. IOTN (DHC): Is it supported by evidence? *Dent Update* 2006;33:478–486.

Fleischmannova J, Matalova E, Tucker AS, Sharpe PT. Mouse models of tooth abnormalities. *Eur J Oral Sci* 2008;116:1–10.

Flores-Mir C. More women in Europe and Australia have dental agenesis than their counterparts in North America. *Evid Based Dent* 2005;6:22–23.

Forgie AH, Thind BS, Larmour CJ, Mossey PA, Stirrups DR. Management of hypodontia: restorative considerations. Part III. *Quintessence Int* 2005;36: 437–445.

Gábris K, Fábián G, Kaán M, Rózsa N, Tarján I. Prevalence of hypodontia and hyperdontia in paedodontic and orthodontic patients in Budapest. *Community Dent Health* 2006;23:80–82.

Gill DS, Jones S, Hobkirk J, *et al.* Counselling patients with hypodontia. *Dent Update* 2008;35:344–352.

Goodman JR, Jones SP, Hobkirk JA, King PA. Hypodontia:1. Clinical features and the management of mild to moderate hypodontia. *Dent Update* 1994;21:381–384.

Grahnen H. Hypodontia in the permanent dentition. A clinical and genetical investigation. *Odontol Revy* 1956; 7(Suppl.3):1–100.

Grahnen H, Granath LE. Numerical variations in primary dentition and their correlation with the permanent dentition. *Odontol Revy* 1961;12:348–357.

Gravely JF, Johnson, DB. Variation in the expression of hypodontia in monozygotic twins. *Dent Pract Dent Rec* 1971;21:212–220.

Hardcastle Z, Hui CC, Sharpe PT. The *Shh* signalling pathway in early tooth development. *Cell Mol Biol* 1999;45:567–578.

Hobkirk JA, Brook AH. The management of patients with severe hypodontia. *J Oral Rehabil* 1980;7: 289–298.

Hobkirk JA, Nohl F, Bergendal B, Storhaug K, Richter MK. The management of ectodermal dysplasia and severe hypodontia. International conference statements. *J Oral Rehabil* 2006;33:634–637.

Hobson RS, Carter NE, Gillgrass TJ, *et al.* The interdisciplinary management of hypodontia: The relationship between an interdisciplinary team and the general dental practitioner. *Br Dent J* 2003;194:479–482.

Honda MJ, Fong H, Iwatsuki S, Sumita Y, Sarikaya M. Tooth-forming potential in embryonic and postnatal tooth bud cells. *Med Mol Morphol* 2008;41:183–192.

Ikeda E, Tsuji T. Growing bioengineered teeth from single cells: potential for dental regenerative medicine. *Expert Opin Biol Ther* 2008;8:735–744.

Ikeda E, Morita R, Nakao K, *et al.* Fully functional bioengineered tooth replacement as an organ replacement therapy. *Proc Natl Acad Sci USA* 2009;106:13475–13480.

Järvinen S, Lehtinen L. Supernumerary and congenitally missing primary teeth in Finnish children. An epidemiologic study. *Acta Odontol Scand* 1981;39:83–86.

Jones SP. The multidisciplinary management of hypodontia. *Dental Nursing* 2009;5:678–682.

Jorgenson RJ. Clinician's view of hypodontia. *J Am Dent Assoc* 1980;101:283–286.

Jumlongras D, Bei M, Stimson JM, *et al.* A nonsense mutation in *MSX1* causes Witkop syndrome. *Am J Hum Genet* 2001;69:67–74.

Kapadia H, Mues G, D'Souza R. Genes affecting tooth morphogenesis. *Orthod Craniofac Res* 2007;10:237–244.

Kaste SC, Hopkins KP. Micrognathia after radiation therapy for childhood facial tumors. Report of two cases with long-term follow-up. *Oral Surg Oral Med Oral Pathol* 1994;77:95–99.

Khan M, Seppala M, Zoupa M, Cobourne MT. *Hedgehog* pathway gene expression during early development

of the molar tooth root in the mouse. *Gene Expr Patterns* 2007;7:239–243.

Kronmiller JE, Nguyen T, Berndt W, Wickson A. Spatial and temporal distribution of *sonic hedgehog* mRNA in the embryonic mouse mandible by reverse transcription/polymerase chain reaction and in situ hybridization analysis. *Arch Oral Biol* 1995;40: 831–838.

Kupietzky A, Houpt M. Hypohidrotic ectodermal dysplasia: characteristics and treatment. *Quintessence Int* 1995;26:285–291.

Lammi L, Arte S, Somer M, *et al.* Mutations in *AXIN2* cause familial tooth agenesis and predispose to colorectal cancer. *Am J Hum Genet* 2004;74:1043–1050.

Larmour CJ, Mossey PA, Thind BS, Forgie AH, Stirrups DR. Hypodontia - a retrospective review of prevalence and etiology. Part I. *Quintessence Int* 2005;36:263–270.

Lidral AC, Reising BC. The role of *MSX1* in human tooth agenesis. *J Dent Res* 2002;81:274–278.

Lucas J. The syndromic tooth–the aetiology, prevalence, presentation and evaluation of hypodontia in children with syndromes. *Ann R Australas Coll Dent Surg* 2000; 15:211–217.

Maguire A, Craft AW, Evans RG, *et al.* The long-term effects of treatment on the dental condition of children surviving malignant disease. *Cancer* 1987;60: 2570–2575.

Matalova E, Fleischmannova J, Sharpe PT, Tucker AS. Tooth agenesis: from molecular genetics to molecular dentistry. *J Dent Res* 2008;87:617–623.

Miletich I, Cobourne MT, Abdeen M, Sharpe PT. Expression of the *Hedgehog* antagonists *Rab23* and *Slimb/betaTrCP* during mouse tooth development. *Arch Oral Biol* 2005;50:147–151.

Mostowska A, Kobielak A, Trzeciak WH. Molecular basis of non-syndromic tooth agenesis: mutations of *MSX1* and *PAX9* reflect their role in patterning human dentition. *Eur J Oral Sci* 2003;111:365–370.

Muller TP, Hill IN, Petersen AC, Blayney JR. A survey of congenitally missing permanent teeth. *J Am Dent Assoc* 1970;81:101–107.

Nakahara T, Ide Y. Tooth regeneration: implications for the use of bioengineered organs in first-wave organ replacement. *Hum Cell* 2007;20:63–70.

Nakatomi M, Morita I, Eto K, Ota MS. *Sonic hedgehog* signaling is important in tooth root development. *J Dent Res* 2006;85:427–431.

Näsman M, Forsberg CM, Dahllöf G. Long-term dental development in children after treatment for malignant disease. *Eur J Orthod* 1997;19:151–159.

Niswander JD, Sujaku C. Congenital anomalies of teeth in Japanese children. *Am J Phys Anthropol* 1963;21: 569–574.

Nunn JH, Carter NE, Gillgrass TJ, *et al.* The interdisciplinary management of hypodontia: background and role of paediatric dentistry. *Br Dent J* 2003;194: 245–251.

Oğuz A, Cetiner S, Karadeniz C, *et al*. Long-term effects of chemotherapy on orodental structures in children with non-Hodgkin's lymphoma. *Eur J Oral Sci* 2004; 112:8–11.

Online Mendelian Inheritance in Man (OMIM). Available at: www.ncbi.nlm.nih.gov/Omim/ (last accessed July 2010).

Otuyemi OD, Jones SP. Methods of assessing and grading malocclusion: A review. *Aust Orthod J* 1995;14: 21–27.

Polder BJ, Van't Hof MA, Van der Linden FPGM, Kuijpers-Jagtman AM. A meta-analysis of the prevalence of dental agenesis of permanent teeth. *Community Dent Oral Epidemiol* 2004;32:217–226.

Rózsa N, Nagy K, Vajó Z, *et al*. Prevalence and distribution of permanent canine agenesis in dental paediatric and orthodontic patients in Hungary. *Eur J Orthod* 2009;31:374–379.

Satokata I, Maas R. *MSX1* deficient mice exhibit cleft palate and abnormalities of craniofacial and tooth development. *Nat Genet* 1994;6:348–356.

Schalk van der Weide Y, Beemer FA, Faber JAJ, Bosman F. Symptomatology of patients with oligodontia. *J Oral Rehabil* 1994;21:247–261.

Schalk van der Weide Y, Steen WH, Bosman F. Distribution of missing teeth and tooth morphology in patients with oligodontia. *J Dent Child* 1992;59:133–140.

Shaw WC, Richmond S, O'Brien KD, Brook P, Stephens CD. Quality control in orthodontics: Indices of treatment need and treatment standards. *Br Dent J* 1991; 170:107–112.

Shelton AT, Hobson RS, Slater D. A preliminary evaluation of pre-treatment hypodontia patients using the Dental Aesthetic Index: how does it compare with other commonly used indices? *Eur J Orthod* 2008;30: 244–248.

Suarez BK, Spence MA. The genetics of hypodontia. *J Dent Res* 1974;53:781–785.

Thesleff I. Genetic basis of tooth development and dental defects. *Acta Odontol Scand* 2000;58:191–194.

Thind BS, Stirrups DR, Forgie AH, Larmour CJ, Mossey PA. Management of hypodontia: orthodontic considerations. (II). *Quintessence Int* 2005;36:345–353.

Vaahtokari A, Aberg T, Jernvall J, Keränen S, Thesleff I. The enamel knot as a signaling center in the developing mouse tooth. *Mech Dev* 1996;54:39–43.

van den Boogaard MJ, Dorland M, Beemer FA, van Amstel HK. *MSX1* mutation is associated with orofacial clefting and tooth agenesis in humans. *Nat Genet* 2000;24:342–343.

Vastardis H, Karimbux N, Guthua SW, Seidman JG, Seidman CE. A human *MSX1* homeodomain missense mutation causes selective tooth agenesis. *Nat Genet* 1996;13:417–421.

Waring D, Jones JW. Does the GDP need to know about IOTN? *Dent Update* 2003;30:123–130.

Whittington BR, Durward CS. Survey of anomalies in primary teeth and their correlation with the permanent dentition. *N Z Dent J* 1996;92:4–8.

Yelick PC, Vacanti JP. Bioengineered teeth from tooth bud cells. *Dent Clin North Am* 2006;50:191–203.

Young CS, Abukawa H, Asrican R, *et al*. Tissue-engineered hybrid tooth and bone. *Tissue Eng* 2005a; 11:1599–1610.

Young CS, Kim SW, Qin C, *et al*. Developmental analysis and computer modelling of bioengineered teeth. *Arch Oral Biol* 2005b;50:259–265.

Zhang L, Hua F, Yuan GH, Zhang YD, Chen Z. *Sonic hedgehog* signaling is critical for cytodifferentiation and cusp formation in developing mouse molars. *J Mol Histol* 2008;39:87–94.

Zhang W, Abukawa H, Troulis MJ, *et al*. Tissue engineered hybrid tooth-bone constructs. *Methods* 2009;47: 122–128.

Zhang Y, Zhang Z, Zhao X, *et al*. A new function of *BMP4*: dual role for *BMP4* in regulation of *Sonic hedgehog* expression in the mouse tooth germ. *Development* 2000;127:1431–1443.

2 Features

Introduction

Individuals with hypodontia typically have a number of complaints related to their condition, depending on its predominant features and the patient's (and, where relevant, their carers') reactions to them. The following description of the oral features of hypodontia includes many of those that may be encountered, but note that it is very unusual for all to be present in one person, and that any one feature may be present to a greater or lesser extent.

It has been reported that severe hypodontia is associated with a reduction in the oral health-related quality of life index (Wong et al., 2006), however a feature that is of great significance to one individual may appear to be only of passing interest to another (Hobkirk et al., 1994; Gill et al., 2008; Laing et al., 2008). The dental team frequently sees patients with hypodontia over the course of many years (Nunn et al., 2003). During the earlier part of their lives, it may be expected that a young patient's perception of (and reaction to) a particular symptom will change over time, and this must be allowed for when developing, reviewing and updating their potential treatment plan.

Poor aesthetics is the most common complaint of patients with hypodontia (Hobkirk et al., 1994). There is some preliminary evidence linking the aesthetic impact of hypodontia to the number of missing teeth (Laing et al., 2008). From the patient's viewpoint the aesthetic consequences of hypodontia depend on the number of missing teeth, the sizes and shape of the remaining teeth and the dimensions of the jaws, as well as the location of the spacing. A patient may consider a small gap in the molar region to be of little significance compared with a similar space in the maxillary incisor region. The patient's view of the effects of the condition on his or her appearance will also be greatly influenced by age and personality. Social pressures reflecting cultural values, the need to conform, and the value placed on the possession of a dentition appropriate to the patient's age group can also be significant. Individual reactions to hypodontia can also vary widely, from extreme concern to apparent indifference, which may mask an underlying anxiety about the condition (Hobkirk et al., 1994; Gill et al., 2008).

Missing teeth can give rise to difficulties with mastication and speech, although these are much

Hypodontia: A Team Approach to Management, First Edition
© J.A. Hobkirk, D.S. Gill, S.P. Jones, K.W. Hemmings, G.S. Bassi, A.L. O'Donnell and J.R. Goodman
Published 2011 by Blackwell Publishing Ltd

less commonly identified as problems by patients attending specialist clinics for the management of hypodontia (Hobkirk *et al.*, 1994). There is anecdotal evidence that where many teeth are missing in a young child, his or her speech development may be affected, and diet is sometimes restricted due to a reduced masticatory ability. If hypodontia is associated with an ectodermal dysplasia, there may be reduced salivary flow, which can influence dietary intake. However, it is unusual for patients to complain of this unless it is particularly severe, because they do not experience normal oral lubrication.

Treatment issues

Carers of patients with hypodontia, and some older patients, are often concerned about the ramifications of the condition, in terms of its implications for their siblings and future children, as well as any possible syndromic associations. Hypodontia is, for example, a frequent feature of the ectodermal dysplasias and dental problems are a common concern in this group of patients. A number of syndromes have hypodontia as one of their characteristics (see Table 1.5) and the clinician needs to be aware of these relationships (Lucas, 2000; Kotsiomiti *et al.*, 2007; Gill *et al.*, 2008; Matalova *et al.*, 2008). Where a patient has developmentally missing teeth, an investigation should be carried out to assess any potential syndromic association. An appropriate referral for further assessment should be arranged where indicated.

Oral features

Missing teeth

This characteristic is inherent to the condition, yet robust population-level data have only started to become available quite recently due to the difficulties of accurately sampling sufficient numbers of subjects (rather than relying on subsets such as patients referred for orthodontic treatment). In addition, the criteria for data collection have not always been consistent, and consequently findings have tended to be rather variable (Brook, 1975; Larmour *et al.*, 2005). More recently the results of

several meta-analyses have been published and these have considerably extended our knowledge of the topic (Polder *et al.*, 2004). Patterns of missing teeth in hypodontia are very variable with regards to number and form and the jaw that is affected, even within siblings, although certain characteristics do tend to predominate (Hobkirk and Brook, 1980; Chung *et al.*, 2000; Dhanrajani, 2002; Tavajohi-Kermani *et al.*, 2002).

Number

Some 5% of populations reported to date have at least one missing tooth (excluding third molars) with a range of between 2.2% and 7.7% (Polder *et al.*, 2004) (Table 1.2). The majority of patients with hypodontia have one or two teeth missing and the percentage with larger numbers of missing teeth is much smaller (Hobkirk *et al.*, 1994; Polder *et al.*, 2004) (Figure 2.1). These data relate principally to the permanent dentition and there is little information available for prevalence in the primary dentition, although it does appear to be much less common with a reported prevalence of approximately 0.5%. There are very limited published data for the prevalence of anodontia (Figure 2.2), which is very uncommon. While hypodontia appears to be more frequently reported than was historically the case, meta-analysis of the data on prevalence has not demonstrated an increase in its incidence in Caucasian people.

Dentition

Hypodontia is much less common in the primary dentition, although where it occurs it does seem to

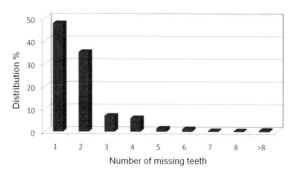

Figure 2.1   Percentage of hypodontia patients (n = 1365) with different numbers of missing teeth (courtesy of Eastman Hypodontia Clinic).

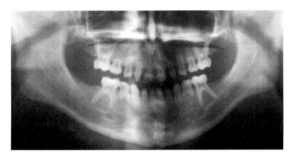

Figure 2.2 Anodontia of the permanent dentition.

be succeeded by missing teeth in the permanent dentition (Daugaard-Jensen *et al.*, 1997). Despite this association, the patterns of absent teeth in the two dentitions are very different in these circumstances, with incisors being most commonly missing in the primary dentition and premolars in the permanent. In addition, the number of developmentally absent teeth appears to be markedly greater in the permanent dentition than in the primary dentition. Furthermore, in these circumstances there is often hypodontia of the permanent teeth which are much less frequently missing in people whose primary dentition is unaffected.

Gender

Hypodontia of the permanent dentition is more common in females than in males, and while the male to female ratios reported vary they are typically of the order of 1 to 1.4 (Goodman *et al.*, 1994; Polder *et al.*, 2004; Nunn *et al.*, 2003; Larmour *et al.*, 2005). In the primary dentition, both genders are equally affected (Goodman *et al.*, 1994; Polder *et al.*, 2004).

Racial group

The data on missing teeth are only available for a small number of racial groups, some of which have been studied more thoroughly than others. However, it has been shown that the prevalence of hypodontia in women is higher in Europe and Australia than in women in North America (Polder *et al.*, 2004; Flores-Mir, 2005). Bailit (1975) commented on the anthropological aspects of these variations, suggesting that they reflect evolutionary change.

Patterns within jaws

While the overall prevalence of hypodontia in the maxilla is comparable to that in the mandible, there are marked differences between the jaws with regards to the types of missing teeth (Tavajohi-Kermani *et al.*, 2002). In addition, with the exception of maxillary lateral incisors, the bilateral absence of a given tooth in either jaw occurs on average in less than 50% of cases (Polder *et al.*, 2004).

Tooth form

The teeth most likely to be absent in hypodontia are the last members of a morphological group to form. Thus the lateral incisor, second premolar and third molar teeth are most commonly absent, while the maxillary central incisor, canine, and first molar teeth are least likely to be absent (Hobkirk and Brook, 1980; Goodman *et al.*, 1994). This pattern, which reflects Butler's Field Theory (Butler, 1939), is not invariable and indeed it can differ on opposite sides of the dental arch in the same individual.

Microdontia

This is a condition characterised by smaller than normal teeth and is a widely reported feature of hypodontia (Brook, 1984; Goodman *et al.*, 1994; Hobkirk *et al.*, 1994) (Figure 2.3). There are limited data on prevalence and severity, and the available material is largely based on case reports or short case series. It may be seen in both the primary and in the permanent dentitions, and can affect one or more teeth. In addition to microdontia the affected teeth often have crowns with abnormal contours. These include parallel sides, or forms that taper towards the occlusal surface or incisal edge, with the absence of undercuts on posterior teeth. Affected lateral incisors tend to have ovate or incisally tapered crown forms. The roots of the teeth are similarly reduced in size and other abnormalities of form may be seen (Garn and Lewis, 1970; Schalk-van der Weide *et al.*, 1993, 1994; Ooshima *et al.*, 1996; Schalk-van der Weide and Bosman 1996; Buckley and Doran, 2001; Pinho *et al.*, 2005).

Microdontia is genetically determined and can be seen in its most severe form in the ectodermal

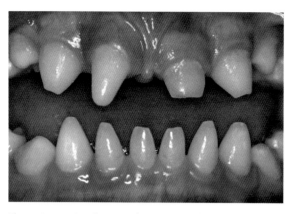

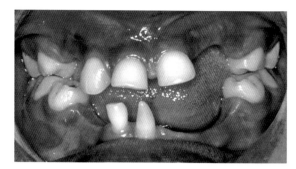

Figure 2.4   Microdontia with missing teeth resulting in significant spacing in arches, markedly tapered LR1, and lack of alveolar bone (where permanent teeth have failed to develop).

Figure 2.3   Microdontia and tapering teeth associated with hypodontia.

dysplasias and the many other syndromes linked with hypodontia, although one does not invariably accompany the other. It has also been reported in patients who have had chemotherapy (Dahllöf et al., 1994; Oğuz et al., 2004) and those with hypodontia caused by local factors such as irradiation of the jaws in early life (Kaste and Hopkins, 1994). Brook (1984) proposed that microdontia and hypodontia were genetically linked as reflections of a continuum of tooth size, with a 'threshold' size of tooth germ below which a tooth failed to develop.

Microdontia affects the relationships between the lengths of the dental bases and those of the dental arches, introducing a tooth–arch discrepancy that may result in spacing of the teeth. It may be generalised whereby all or several teeth are affected, or more localised whereby only one or two (typically the maxillary lateral incisors) are microdont. The condition can be challenging to manage as it may require orthodontic redistribution of spaces and prosthodontic procedures to alter the apparent size of the tooth by adding restorative materials. Extreme circumstances may require the use of overlay removable prostheses. Microdont teeth present a reduced surface area of enamel that can be insufficient for adhesive prosthodontic techniques, and the loss of undercuts may present further treatment challenges. The use of restorative material can also produce an unsatisfactory appearance if the addition is extensive due to disparity between the diameter of the root as it emerges through the gingivae and the modi-

fied crown. In addition, the patient may find it difficult to clean the re-shaped tooth at the gingival margin. Where a primary tooth is modified in this manner, root resorption may also occur more rapidly than normal. This is because of the increased mechanical loads on the root due to the unfavourable crown to root ratio. In a young patient, the procedure may be considered as an interim measure in such circumstances, until skeletal maturity occurs and tooth replacement with an implant-stabilised restoration may be considered.

Conical teeth

Conical teeth have a tapered form that narrows towards the incisal edge or occlusal surface. Sometimes the teeth have a needle-like appearance (Figure 2.4). Affected teeth may also be microdont and, as with microdontia, the condition may affect some or all of the teeth. The condition is usually genetically determined, but it can have other systemic or local causes as previously described for microdontia.

Tapered teeth produce an appearance that many patients consider unsatisfactory because of their shape and the apparent increase in spacing between them. The tooth form often benefits from modification using restorative procedures such as the addition of composite resin or placement of an adhesive restoration. The former has the merits of simplicity and is largely reversible, making it well suited to younger patients or those seeking less extensive treatment. Temporary acrylic overdentures can also be useful for changing the tooth form, especially where it is desirable to alter the occlusal vertical dimension (OVD) or where several teeth are missing, such that alteration of tooth form in itself will not adequately change the appearance.

Very pointed teeth may require re-shaping to reduce the risk of accidental trauma to the soft tissues of the mouth. In addition to the techniques described above, this may be done by smoothing the tip of the tooth. Caution should be exercised when making such adjustments as the affected teeth often contain a narrow strand of pulpal tissue extending into the crown, increasing the risk of inadvertent pulp exposure. Re-contouring by adding a composite resin is therefore preferable. Where it is desired to prepare the tooth for a conventional 'permanent' restoration then it may be difficult to obtain adequate retention form while preserving sufficient tooth substance for structural integrity, especially in anterior teeth.

Ectopic eruption

Ectopic eruption of permanent teeth is common in hypodontia (Figures 2.5 and 2.6) and is probably caused both by the lack of adjacent teeth to guide the eruptive process and of spaces into which they may erupt. The eruption of maxillary canine teeth into the positions of the lateral incisors when these teeth are absent has been well documented, while transposition of teeth is also seen (Becker *et al.*, 1981; Brin *et al.*, 1986; Zilberman *et al.*, 1990; Pirinen *et al.*, 1996; Brenchley and Oliver, 1997; Peck *et al.*, 1998, 2002; Shapira and Kuftinec, 2001).

Ectopic eruption can give rise both to spaces that are inappropriate for aesthetically satisfactory restoration, and to an unattractive appearance where a tooth is transposed (Peck *et al.* 1998, 2002). Where teeth erupt some distance from the desired position, they may need to be orthodontically moved a considerable distance, often with uncertain anchorage. Transpositions may be difficult (or even impossible) to correct and therefore place limitations on treatment outcomes. Where such teeth are unerupted, they may need surgical exposure.

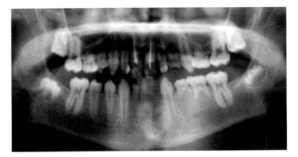

Figure 2.5 Radiograph showing ectopic eruption of UL3 in a patient with hypodontia. UR1 and UL1 have been endodontically treated as a result of trauma.

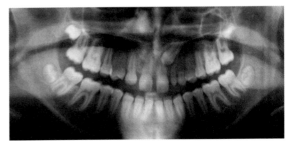

Figure 2.6 Radiograph showing anterior path of eruption of UL3.

Retained primary teeth

If primary teeth lack a permanent successor then the normal resorption of their roots is delayed. They may be retained for considerable periods, sometimes even into the fourth and fifth decades (Haselden *et al.*, 2001) (Figure 2.7). It should be noted that delayed eruption of the permanent teeth is a feature of hypodontia, and the primary predecessor may be retained for longer than normal (Goodman *et al.*, 1994) – this is not in itself diagnostic of hypodontia of the permanent successor.

The rate of resorption of the root in a primary tooth that lacks a permanent successor is highly variable. In the case of primary canine and molar teeth, resorption is more likely to be delayed in the mandible than in the maxilla. In both jaws the probability of resorption of the roots of primary teeth without a permanent successor is likely to occur in the sequence shown in Figure 2.8.

Of the primary canines (C_P) and primary molars (M_P) without permanent successors retained to any given age, some general predictions can be made

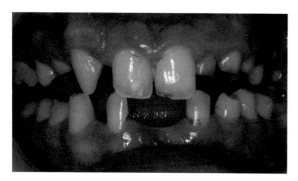

Figure 2.7   Primary teeth may be retained for many years but often become infra-occluded and suffer from tooth wear.

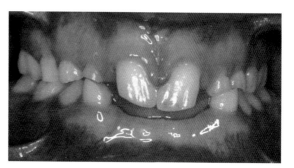

Figure 2.9   Wear of primary teeth and overeruption of unopposed UR1 and UL1, resulting in a greatly reduced prosthetic envelope in the anterior mandible.

Jaw	Tooth	Root resorption
Mandible	C$_P$	
Maxilla	C$_P$	
Mandible	M$_P$2	
Maxilla	M$_P$2	
Mandible	M$_P$1	
Maxilla	M$_P$1	

Figure 2.8   Relative probability of root resorption of different primary teeth when lacking a permanent successor (base of triangle represents highest probability).

about the levels of root resorption that might be expected. It is important nevertheless to recognise that individual variations can be large.

Up to the age of 35 years, 60–80% of primary canines might be expected to have minimal root resorption, with the remaining balance of 20–40% having less than half of their roots resorbed. After the age of 35, root resorption is likely to become more significant. In contrast, primary first molars

appear to undergo root resorption earlier and more extensively. Only 20% of these teeth might be expected to have minimal root resorption by the age of 12 years, with the balance having more than half their roots resorbed. Some 40–60% of primary second molars might be expected to have minimal root resorption up to the age of 24 years, with the balance predominantly having root resorption in the range of 25–50%. After the age of 25 years, root resorption becomes much more marked (Haselden et al., 2001).

Retained primary teeth can give satisfactory service for many years, despite significant root resorption. The decision to retain or remove them must be taken on a case-by-case basis within the framework of a long-term treatment strategy (Ekim and Hatibovic-Kofman, 2001).

The retention of primary teeth beyond their normal span can result in marked tooth surface loss, causing an unsatisfactory appearance (Figure 2.9), as well as problems with mastication and an increased risk of supra-eruption of an opposing permanent tooth. Retained primary teeth frequently become ankylosed, and consequently infra-occluded (Rune and Sarnäs, 1984; Kurol, 2006) as a result of localised failure of alveolar development and the relative eruption of adjacent permanent teeth (Figure 2.10).

Severely infra-occluded primary teeth may eventually become covered with oral mucosa and can be troublesome to remove in these circumstances. Tipping of adjacent permanent teeth can result in apparent impaction of the ankylosed tooth beneath their contact points, increasing the risk of caries where access for oral hygiene is difficult. The

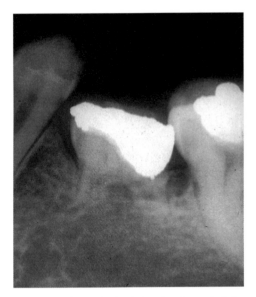

Figure 2.10   Radiograph of ankylosed, infra-occluded second primary molar.

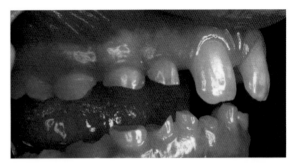

Figure 2.11   Severe wear of primary teeth and hypodontia affecting most of the permanent teeth, with marked aesthetic and functional effects.

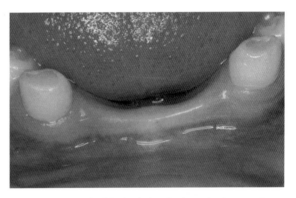

Figure 2.12   Marked lack of alveolar bone in the anterior region of the mandible, with missing permanent teeth.

removal of ankylosed, infra-occluded primary teeth can be difficult due to their position, thin resorbed roots and brittle dentine, in addition to the need to preserve as much alveolar bone as possible, which is often crucial to the orthodontic or restorative treatment of such patients.

Tooth surface loss (TSL)

Tooth surface loss in excess of what might be normally expected is frequently seen in patients with hypodontia. It is especially likely to affect retained primary teeth, although if there are few occluding pairs of permanent posterior teeth, these can also be affected due abrasion and attrition caused by excessive loading. Tooth surface loss can lead to an increase in the freeway space (FWS), which detracts from the patient's appearance, and may be challenging to manage (Figure 2.11). Methods of managing TSL are discussed in Chapter 9.

Reduced alveolar development

Patients with hypodontia may have alveolar processes that are less well developed than normal, both in those parts of the arch with teeth and those

parts where they are absent. In the latter situation the appearance of the alveolar ridge is similar to that of an elderly edentulous person who has suffered from extensive alveolar resorption. The reduced growth of the alveolar process may be localised to one part of the jaw or it may be generalised. Where it is localised there may be resulting effects on the appearance and occlusion due to the disparity within the arch, and where it is generalised both of these effects plus an increased freeway space may result.

A further feature of alveolar growth in the edentulous regions of the jaw is that of marked narrowing of the ridge below its crest (Figure 2.12).

Sometimes this is referred to colloquially as 'waisting'. It can arise in three principal ways:

1.   Where there is anodontia, then alveolar development will not occur and the jaw has a similar

intra-oral appearance to that of a formerly dentate patient who has been edentulous for some time.

2. Where the primary teeth have no permanent successors, then alveolar development will be restricted. There is no need to accommodate the larger tooth, so the stimulus for alveolar growth is lost and the primary teeth often become ankylosed when retained beyond the time that they would normally be shed. In these circumstances alveolar growth largely ceases and the tooth becomes infra-occluded. The problem may be further compounded by iatrogenic loss of alveolar volume as a result of the surgical procedure of removing the ankylosed primary tooth.

3. In some individuals with hypodontia, alveolar development is less than normal, even in the presence of permanent teeth.

Reduced alveolar development can have aesthetic and functional effects due to the hard-tissue deficit. While small deficiencies can be managed with fixed restorations, larger ones require either the use of removable prostheses or surgical procedures to augment the bone prior to restorative treatment. These are often preceded by orthodontic procedures to optimise the positions of the teeth. In more severe situations correction may be best achieved by orthognathic surgery.

Reduced alveolar development can also create problems when contemplating implant treatment because the small surgical envelope may be suboptimal or inadequate for placement of an ideally sized implant body, while its outline may dictate a less than favourable orientation of the device. Sub-crestal narrowing of the alveolar ridge can also create difficulties in implant treatment. While the crest of the alveolar ridge may be sufficiently wide to accommodate a device, it may fenestrate the bone on its labial or lingual aspects further apically.

A reduction in the bulk of the alveolar bone may also place limitations on orthodontic tooth movement. There must be an adequate volume of bone into which to move a tooth. Where attempts are made to move a permanent tooth into an area of 'waisted' alveolus, the root is likely to come into contact with the buccal and lingual cortical plates (which will be in close approximation). This may result in cessation of root movement under orthodontic forces and consequent tipping of the crown into the space. If excessive forces are applied in an attempt to move the root into the space, root resorption may occur. Where the 'waisting' is mild, moving the root into this area may produce deposition of alveolar bone and an improvement in bony contour (Kokich, 2004).

Reduced alveolar development can also result in an increased freeway space, which is discussed below.

Increased freeway space

An increased freeway space is unusual in patients with hypodontia and accurate data are lacking. However, it has been reported that 10% of patients referred to a specialist clinic for the management of hypodontia had a clinically determined freeway space of 5–7 mm and a further 4% a freeway space in excess of this (Hobkirk et al., 1994). The condition results in either or both occlusal planes being closer to the basal bone than normal. Consequently, in addition to an 'over-closed' facial appearance in the intercuspal position (ICP), the anterior teeth may not be visible in normal function. An increased freeway space may also occur due to extensive loss of tooth surface. This is especially likely to occur where retained primary teeth are in occlusion.

The principal effects of a significantly increased freeway space are on appearance, although speech and mastication may also be affected. Correction in younger patients may often be achieved by treatment with overdentures, which can produce a significant change in both appearance and function in a relatively straightforward and reversible manner. In older patients, more complex procedures using fixed restorations with possible implant stabilisation may be more suitable, where necessary in conjunction with bone grafting and orthognathic procedures to correct major jaw discrepancies and facilitate long-term restorative care.

Delayed eruption of permanent teeth

This is another recognised feature of hypodontia, although few data are available about the phenomenon (Schalk-van der Weide et al., 1993;

Taylor, 1998; Dhanrajani, 2002). The delayed eruption of permanent teeth may have implications for the timing of treatment where interventions are dependent on the eruption of particular teeth. Treatment may include orthodontic or restorative procedures. It is also important to confirm radiographically the definitive absence of a permanent tooth that has failed to erupt at the anticipated time before planning treatment based on its presumed absence.

Altered craniofacial morphology

There is evidence to suggest that people with hypodontia have significantly different craniofacial morphology from those with a normal number of teeth. Reported differences include reduced maxillary and mandibular lengths, as demonstrated by reductions in the cephalometric angles SNA and SNB, with a reduced mandibular–cranial base length ratio (Wisth et al., 1974; Øgaard and Krogstad, 1995; Ben-Bassat and Brin, 2009; Chan et al., 2009). There may be a tendency to a Class III skeletal relationship with reduced angle ANB, resulting from maxillary retrusion with relative mandibular prognathism and the chin positioned more anteriorly (Roald et al., 1982; Woodworth et al., 1985; Nodal et al., 1994; Chung et al., 2000; Bondarets et al., 2002; Endo et al., 2004, 2006).

The overall anterior face height has also been described as being reduced due to a forward mandibular growth rotation, with a reduced Frankfort–mandibular plane angle (FMPA) and cranial base–mandibular plane angle (SNMP), and shortening of both upper and lower anterior face heights (Sarnäs and Rune, 1983; Woodworth et al., 1985; Nodal et al., 1994; Øgaard and Krogstad, 1995; Bondarets and McDonald, 2000: Chung et al., 2000). The reduced vertical facial height in conjunction with an increased freeway space may make patients appear over-closed. This has been related to changes in dental and functional compensation due to a lack of posterior dental support (Dermaut et al., 1986; Øgaard and Krogstad, 1995).

In general, these craniofacial changes appear to be most obvious in patients with severe hypodontia, although there have been different findings with respect to the relationships between the numbers and patterns of missing teeth and any

possible associations with craniofacial morphology (Øgaard and Krogstad, 1995; Chung et al., 2000; Tavajohi-Kermani et al., 2002; Endo et al., 2006; Ben-Bassat and Brin, 2009; Chan et al., 2009). An altered craniofacial morphology impacts on facial (and in particular oral) appearance, with the consequent potential need for correction, often requiring complex orthodontic and restorative procedures. Severe deviations from normal may require orthognathic surgery.

Patients' complaints

The features of hypodontia in an individual patient will be recorded during an initial consultation, but it is his or her understanding of the condition, its implications and potential treatment and the personal relationship with the healthcare team that will influence any complaints and expectations. These factors will ultimately drive the treatment process, often over many years. Most patients with hypodontia are first seen specifically for the management of the condition when their lack of teeth first starts to become evident; however occasionally patients with hypodontia do not seek professional advice until much later. This has implications for treatment planning, and it also reflects the patient's personal views on the significance of their dental status, as well as their dental history. The complaints are therefore of considerable importance and time needs to be spent in elucidating them. The most common problems are listed in Figure 2.13 (Hobkirk et al., 1994).

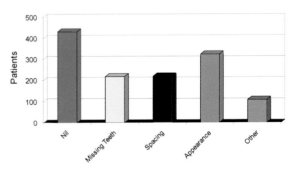

Figure 2.13   Complaints made by 1365 hypodontia patients at first attendance at a multidisciplinary clinic. Complaints were not mutually exclusive (courtesy of Eastman Hypodontia Clinic).

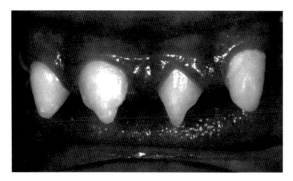

Figure 2.14 Severe tapering of permanent anterior maxillary teeth in a patient with hypodontia.

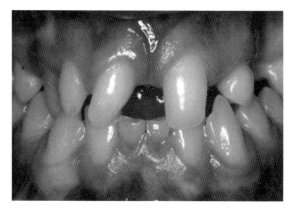

Figure 2.15 Missing teeth and narrow tapering permanent central incisors, resulting in significant spacing in the anterior maxilla.

Appearance

Appearance is the prime concern for many patients. It can be the effect of a number of factors so these need to be carefully explored with the patient, who may not always be precise when indicating a complaint. The problem may be principally related to:

- The appearance of the teeth themselves
- Spacing
- Excessive freeway space

Appearance of the teeth

This can arise as a result of factors related to hypodontia, such as microdontia, retained primary teeth possibly with tooth surface loss and a tapering tooth form (Figure 2.14). The complaint may also reflect some other condition that is unrelated to hypodontia but has affected dental development (such as amelogenesis or dentinogenesis imperfecta).

Spacing

Spacing between the teeth as a result of microdontia, retained primary teeth or missing teeth can significantly affect appearance (Figures 2.15 and 2.16). As stated above it is also important to recognise that the patient may have another condition, unrelated to hypodontia (such as an unfavourable skeletal pattern), that is causing spaces between the teeth.

Excessive freeway space

This, as previously described, can result in the typical appearance of a 'collapsed' lower third of the face – typically associated with the edentulous

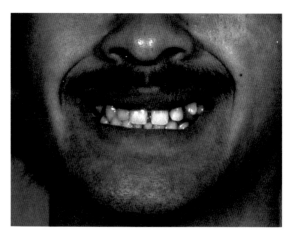

Figure 2.16 Hypodontia in the maxilla and spacing of the anterior maxillary teeth, detracting from the appearance when smiling.

state in elderly people – and can give rise to embarrassment and ridicule. Where either of the occlusal planes is abnormally close to the relevant jaw then the teeth will not be evident when smiling, supporting the assumption of edentulism. This is less of a problem in the lower jaw, as the mandibular incisors are normally less evident than their maxillary counterparts, especially in younger people.

Clinical significance

Concerns about appearance are the most common complaint of patients with hypodontia, and will frequently require multidisciplinary management over many years. A range of procedures will be carried out to meet changing needs and reflect the feasibility of various treatment options at different ages. A patient with severe hypodontia may be provided with overdentures when young, orthodontic therapy in the mixed dentition phase, followed by treatment with adhesive restorations, and implant-stabilised prostheses when skeletal maturity has been reached.

Speech problems

Complaints about speech problems are relatively uncommon in patients with hypodontia, although the missing teeth and supporting tissues can make pronunciation of some words difficult.

In younger patients the missing teeth and tissue deficit may interfere with normal speech development. In these circumstances there is evidence that treatment with removable prostheses confers some benefits, especially in patients with few teeth who often improve with complete overdentures (Miller, 1995; Kotsiomiti et al., 2000; Tarjan et al., 2005; He et al., 2007). There are, however issues relating to consent. Not all young children with severe hypodontia want this type of treatment, which potentially brings the patient into conflict with his or her carer or dentist. Problems may arise if there is a difference of opinion between patients and carers regarding the desirability, necessity and appropriateness of early interventions of this type.

Difficulties with mastication

Having a reduced number of pairs of occluding posterior teeth makes an individual more likely to have a restricted diet. Little work has been reported on the impact of hypodontia on food choices, however, and it has been reported that complaints about mastication are infrequent among patients referred to a specialist clinic for the management of hypodontia (Hobkirk et al., 1994). Nevertheless the evidence from studies of partially dentate patients with several teeth missing (as opposed to those with hypodontia) suggests that patients with a number of missing teeth in the posterior region of the jaws may be at risk of a restricted diet (Walls et al., 2000). Such studies of diet and being partially dentate tend to involve people who are older than

---

Key Points: Oral features

Missing teeth
Missing teeth define hypodontia, but other features may be present, including:
- Microdontia
- Conical teeth
- Ectopic eruption
- Retained primary teeth
- Tooth surface loss
- Reduced alveolar development
- Abnormally large freeway space
- Delayed eruption of permanent teeth
- Altered craniofacial morphology

Prevalence
- About 5% of the population have one or more permanent tooth missing
- Most people with hypodontia have one or two teeth missing

Dentition
- Prevalence of hypodontia in the primary dentition is about 10% of that in the permanent
- Hypodontia in the permanent dentition is more common in females than males
- The male to female ratio in the permanent dentition varies, but is typically 1:1.4
- Hypodontia of the primary dentition affects both genders equally

Racial group
- Prevalence of hypodontia in Europe and Australia is higher than that in North America

Patterns within jaws
- The overall prevalence is comparable in both jaws
- The pattern of missing teeth differs between jaws
- Bilateral absence of a given tooth in one jaw is less than 50% except for maxillary lateral incisors

Tooth form
P2 in the mandible, I2 and P2 in the maxilla are most commonly missing in the order:
- Mandibular P2 >
- Maxillary I2 >
- Maxillary P2

Patients' complaints
The most common complaints are:
- Appearance (frequent)
- Speech problems (less frequent)
- Mastication difficulties (less frequent)

the patients predominantly referred to a specialist clinic for the management of hypodontia. This means the findings may not be directly transferable to a hypodontia group. There is also the possibility that patients with hypodontia accommodate to the lack of teeth better than people who lose teeth in later life.

Pain

Hypodontia rarely gives rise to complaints of pain, although this can arise because of food packing between spaced teeth, sensitivity from primary teeth with extreme tooth surface loss, and inadvertent self-injury from sharp teeth. Occasionally, patients may present complaining of pain in an attempt to mask concerns relating to aesthetics, for fear that an aesthetic complaint could be viewed by the clinical team as vanity and may be less likely to result in an offer of treatment. A careful and sympathetic approach to history-taking usually exposes the true complaint and confirms the presence or absence of pain.

References

Bailit HL. Dental variation among populations. An anthropologic view. *Dent Clin North Am* 1975;19:125–139.

Becker A, Smith P, Behar R. The incidence of anomalous maxillary lateral incisors in relation to palatally-displaced cuspids. *Angle Orthod* 1981;51:24–29.

Ben-Bassat Y, Brin I. Skeletal and dental patterns in patients with severe congenital absence of teeth. *Am J Orthod Dentofacial Orthop* 2009;135:349–356.

Bondarets N, Jones RM, McDonald F. Analysis of facial growth in subjects with syndromic ectodermal dysplasia: a longitudinal analysis. *Orthod Craniofac Res* 2002;5:71–84.

Bondarets N, McDonald F. Analysis of the vertical facial form in patients with severe hypodontia. *Am J Phys Anthropol* 2000;111:177–184.

Brenchley Z, Oliver RG. Morphology of anterior teeth associated with displaced canines. *Br J Orthod* 1997;24:41–45.

Brin I, Becker A, Shalhav M. Position of the maxillary permanent canine in relation to anomalous or missing lateral incisors: a population study. *Eur J Orthod* 1986;8:12–16.

Brook AH. Variables and criteria in prevalence studies of dental anomalies of number, form and size. *Community Dent Oral Epidemiol* 1975;3:288–293.

Brook AH. A unifying aetiological explanation for anomalies of human tooth number and size. *Arch Oral Biol* 1984;29:373–378.

Buckley JK, Doran GA. True oligodontia with microdontia in monozygous twins: implications for reappraisal of Butler's Field Theory. *Bull Group Int Rech Sci Stomatol Odontol* 2001;43:1–10.

Butler PM. Studies of the mammalian dentition. – Differentiation of the post-canine dentition. *Proc Zool Soc Lond Ser B* 1939;109:1–36.

Chan DW, Samman N, McMillan AS. Craniofacial profile in Southern Chinese with hypodontia. *Eur J Orthod* 2009;31:300–305.

Chung LK, Hobson RS, Nunn JH, Gordon PH, Carter NE. An analysis of the skeletal relationships in a group of young people with hypodontia. *J Orthod* 2000;27:315–318.

Dahllöf G, Rozell B, Forsberg CM, Borgström B. Histologic changes in dental morphology induced by high dose chemotherapy and total body irradiation. *Oral Surg Oral Med Oral Pathol* 1994;77:56–60.

Daugaard-Jensen J, Nodal M, Skovgaard LT, Kjaer I. Comparison of the pattern of agenesis in the primary and permanent dentitions in a population characterized by agenesis in the primary dentition. *Int J Paediatr Dent* 1997;7:143–148.

Dermaut LR, Goeffers KR, De Smit AA. Prevalence of tooth agenesis correlated with jaw relationship and dental crowding. *Am J Orthod Dentofacial Orthop* 1986;90:204–210.

Dhanrajani PJ. Hypodontia: etiology, clinical features, and management. *Quintessence Int* 2002;33:294–320.

Ekim SL, Hatibovic-Kofman S. A treatment decision-making model for infra-occluded primary molars. *Int J Paediatr Dent* 2001;11:340–346.

Endo T, Ozoe R, Yoshino S, Shimooka S. Hypodontia patterns and variations in craniofacial morphology in Japanese orthodontic patients. *Angle Orthod* 2006;76:996–1003.

Endo T, Yoshino S, Ozoe R, Kojima K, Shimooka S. Association of advanced hypodontia and craniofacial morphology in Japanese orthodontic patients. *Odontology* 2004;92:48–53.

Flores-Mir C. More women in Europe and Australia have dental agenesis than their counterparts in North America. *Evid Based Dent* 2005;6:22–23.

Garn SM, Lewis AB. The gradient and the pattern of crown-size reduction in simple hypodontia. *Angle Orthod* 1970;40:51–58.

Gill DS, Jones S, Hobkirk J, *et al.* Counselling patients with hypodontia. *Dent Update* 2008;35:344–352.

Goodman JR, Jones SP, Hobkirk JA, King PA. Hypodontia:1. Clinical features and the management of mild to moderate hypodontia. *Dent Update* 1994;21:381–384.

Haselden K, Hobkirk JA, Goodman JR, Jones SP, Hemmings KW. Root resorption in deciduous canine and molar teeth without permanent successors in patients with severe hypodontia. *Int J Paediatr Dent* 2001;11:171–178.

He X, Shu W, Kang Y, *et al*. Esthetic and functional rehabilitation of a patient with nonsyndromic oligodontia: a case report from China. *J Esthet Restor Dent* 2007;19: 137–142.

Hobkirk JA, Brook AH. The management of patients with severe hypodontia. *J Oral Rehabil* 1980;7:289–298.

Hobkirk JA, Goodman JR, Jones SP. Presenting complaints and findings in a group of patients attending a hypodontia clinic. *Br Dent J* 1994;177:337–339.

Kaste SC, Hopkins KP. Micrognathia after radiation therapy for childhood facial tumors. Report of two cases with long-term follow-up. *Oral Surg Oral Med Oral Pathol* 1994;77:95–99.

Kokich VG. Maxillary lateral incisor implants: planning with the aid of orthodontics. *J Oral Maxillofac Surg* 2004;62:48–56.

Kotsiomiti E, Arapostathis K, Kapari D, Konstantinidis A. Removable prosthodontic treatment for the primary and mixed dentition. *J Clin Pediatr Dent* 2000;24:83–89.

Kotsiomiti E, Kassa D, Kapari D. Oligodontia and associated characteristics: assessment in view of prosthodontic rehabilitation. *Eur J Prosthodont Restor Dent* 2007; 15:55–60.

Kurol J. Impacted and ankylosed teeth: why, when, and how to intervene. *Am J Orthod Dentofacial Orthop* 2006;129(Suppl.4):S86–90.

Laing ER, Cunningham SJ, Jones SP, Moles D, Gill DS. The psychosocial impact of hypodontia in children. *J Orthod* 2008;35:225 (*abstract*).

Larmour CJ, Mossey PA, Thind BS, Forgie AH, Stirrups DR. Hypodontia – A retrospective review of prevalence and etiology. Part I. *Quintessence Int* 2005;36: 263–270.

Lucas J. The syndromic tooth–the aetiology, prevalence, presentation and evaluation of hypodontia in children with syndromes. *Ann R Australas Coll Dent Surg* 2000; 15:211–217.

Matalova E, Fleischmannova J, Sharpe PT, Tucker AS. Tooth agenesis: from molecular genetics to molecular dentistry. *J Dent Res* 2008;87:617–623.

Miller TE. Implications of congenitally missing teeth: orthodontic and restorative procedures in the adult patient. *J Prosthet Dent* 1995;73:115–122.

Nodal M, Kjaer I, Solow B. Craniofacial morphology in patients with multiple congenitally missing permanent teeth. *Eur J Orthod* 1994;16:104–109.

Nunn JH, Carter NE, Gillgrass TJ, *et al*. The interdisciplinary management of hypodontia: background and role of paediatric dentistry. *Br Dent J* 2003;194:245–251.

Øgaard B, Krogstad O. Craniofacial structure and soft tissue profile in patients with severe hypodontia. *Am J Orthod Dentofacial Orthop* 1995;108:472–477.

Oğuz A, Cetiner S, Karadeniz C, *et al*. Long-term effects of chemotherapy on orodental structures in children with non-Hodgkin's lymphoma. *Eur J Oral Sci* 2004; 112:8–11.

Ooshima T, Ishida R, Mishima K, Sobue S. The prevalence of developmental anomalies of teeth and their association with tooth size in the primary and permanent dentitions of 1650 Japanese children. *Int J Paediatr Dent* 1996;6:87–94.

Peck S, Peck L, Kataja M. Concomitant occurrence of canine malposition and tooth agenesis: evidence of orofacial genetic fields. *Am J Orthod Dentofacial Orthop* 2002;122:657–660.

Peck S, Peck L, Kataja M. Mandibular lateral incisor-canine transposition, concomitant dental anomalies, and genetic control. *Angle Orthod* 1998;68:455–466.

Pinho T, Tavares P, Maciel P, Pollmann C. Developmental absence of maxillary lateral incisors in the Portuguese population. *Eur J Orthod* 2005;27:443–449.

Pirinen S, Arte S, Apajalahti S. Palatal displacement of canine is genetic and related to congenital absence of teeth. *J Dent Res* 1996;75:1742–1746.

Polder BJ, Van't Hof MA, Van der Linden FP, Kuijpers-Jagtman AM. A meta-analysis of the prevalence of dental agenesis of permanent teeth. *Community Dent Oral Epidemiol* 2004;32:217–226.

Roald KL, Wisth PJ, Böe OE. Changes in craniofacial morphology of individuals with hypodontia between the ages of 9 and 16. *Acta Odontol Scand* 1982; 40:65–74.

Rune B, Sarnäs KV. Root resorption and submergence in retained deciduous second molars. A mixed-longitudinal study of 77 children with developmental absence of second premolars. *Eur J Orthod* 1984; 6:123–131.

Sarnäs KV, Rune B. The facial profile in advanced hypodontia: A mixed longitudinal study of 141 children. *Eur J Orthod* 1983;5:133–143.

Schalk-van der Weide Y, Bosman F. Tooth size in relatives of individuals with oligodontia. *Arch Oral Biol* 1996;41:469–472.

Schalk-van der Weide Y, Steen WH, Beemer FA, Bosman F. Reductions in size and left-right asymmetry of teeth in human oligodontia. *Arch Oral Biol* 1994; 39:935–939.

Schalk-van der Weide Y, Prahl-Andersen B, Bosman F. Tooth formation in patients with oligodontia. *Angle Orthod* 1993;63:31–37.

Shapira Y, Kuftinec MM. Maxillary tooth transpositions: characteristic features and accompanying dental anomalies. *Am J Orthod Dentofacial Orthop* 2001;119: 127–134.

Tarjan I, Gabris K, Rozsa N. Early prosthetic treatment of patients with ectodermal dysplasia: a clinical report. *J Prosthet Dent* 2005;93:419–424.

Tavajohi-Kermani H, Kapur R, Sciote JJ. Tooth agenesis and craniofacial morphology in an orthodontic population. *Am J Orthod Dentofacial Orthop* 2002;122:39–47.

Taylor RW. Eruptive abnormalities in orthodontic treatment. *Semin Orthod* 1998;4:79–86.

Walls AW, Steele JG, Sheiham A, Marcenes W, Moynihan PJ. Oral health and nutrition in older people. *J Public Health Dent* 2000;60:304–307.

Wisth PJ, Thunold K, Böe OE. The craniofacial morphology of individuals with hypodontia. *Acta Odontol Scand* 1974;32:281–290.

Wong AT, McMillan AS, McGrath C. Oral health-related quality of life and severe hypodontia. *J Oral Rehabil* 2006;33:869–873.

Woodworth DA, Sinclair PM, Alexander RG. Bilateral congenital absence of maxillary lateral incisors: a craniofacial and dental cast analysis. *Am J Orthod Dentofacial Orthop* 1985;87:280–293.

Zilberman Y, Cohen B, Becker A. Familial trends in palatal canines, anomalous lateral incisors, and related phenomena. *Eur J Orthod* 1990;12:135–139.

3 Providing Care

Introduction

The social, psychological and dental aspects of managing hypodontia are often difficult and complex, especially for patients who are severely affected (Nunn *et al.*, 2003; McNamara *et al.*, 2006; Worsaae *et al.*, 2007; Shafi *et al.*, 2008). The delivery of a suitably holistic care pathway for such patients requires the expertise of a number of specialists, which implies that such ideal care is difficult to provide through a single healthcare professional or specialty (Hobkirk *et al.*, 1994; Bergendal *et al.*, 1996; Shroff *et al.*, 1996; Nunn *et al.*, 2003; Duello, 2004; Kinzer and Kokich, 2005; Simeone *et al.*, 2007; Worsaae *et al.*, 2007; Nohl *et al.*, 2008).

For this reason, integrated care is best provided through an experienced team of clinicians from a range of specialties, preferably working in a dedicated hypodontia clinic or unit (Goodman *et al.*, 1994; Hobkirk *et al.*, 1994, 2006; Bergendal *et al.*, 1996; Hobson *et al.*, 2003; Nunn *et al.*, 2003; Bishop *et al.*, 2006, 2007a, 2007b; Worsaae *et al.*, 2007; Nohl *et al.*, 2008; Shafi *et al.*, 2008). However, although the multidisciplinary hypodontia clinic is considered to be the gold standard for the clinical care of patients, it has to be appreciated that other models might be more appropriate in situations where resources are restricted. It is also important to recognise that hypodontia is a lifetime problem, and frequently cannot be managed completely by early intervention. Treatment must be planned on a longitudinal basis to give optimised outcomes over a lifetime, and often requires phases both of active treatment and long-term clinical maintenance. The clinical team must therefore possess sufficient skills to plan treatment with a perspective on current and future needs.

Referral pathways to a hypodontia clinic

Figure 3.1 illustrates a typical referral pathway with possible management routes within, or coordinated through, a hypodontia clinic. Referral to a hypodontia team may be from the patient's primary care medical or dental practitioner or from a specialist practitioner, or a tertiary referral from another hospital-based medical or dental specialist.

Initial referral is usually from the general dental practitioner with whom the hypodontia team

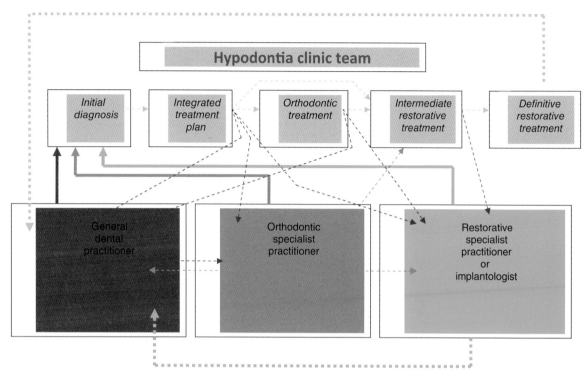

Figure 3.1   Referral pathways to and from the hypodontia clinic, showing initial referral (solid lines), treatment phase (dashed lines) and treatment complete/discharge (dotted lines).

should work closely. The referral may request a treatment plan only, or a treatment plan plus some or all elements of treatment, depending on the specific circumstances. If a treatment plan only is requested, then the multidisciplinary hypodontia team will devise a care pathway for treatment that can then be organised by the practitioner, who may arrange elements such as orthodontics through a local specialist practitioner. Alternatively, where requested, the hypodontia team may carry out the orthodontics before returning the patient to the general practitioner for intermediate and/or definitive restorative treatment. In other circumstances the practitioner may request that the hypodontia team provides all treatment phases.

An orthodontic specialist practitioner may refer some patients to the hypodontia clinic with a request for integrated treatment planning only. A plan can then be provided for which the orthodontist provides the orthodontic treatment, before returning the patient to either the patient's general dental practitioner or to a specialist practitioner in pros-

thodontics for restorative treatment. Alternatively the patient may be re-referred to the hypodontia clinic for specialist restorative care. Similarly, a specialist prosthodontic practitioner may refer the patient to a hypodontia clinic requesting provision of the orthodontic elements of integrated care before providing restorative treatment.

It is always important to maintain clarity as to where responsibility lies for the overall plan and its various elements, and to ensure that the treatment is provided in a flexible way that reflects each patient's individual needs. This enables the best use of resources and facilitates patient attendance.

Roles of a hypodontia team

In general, the roles of the team may encompass the following main areas:

1. Diagnosis and interdisciplinary treatment planning.

2. Patient and parent/carer counselling.
3. Provision of specific treatment plans for out-reach provision of care.
4. Provision of treatment by team members.
5. Education for students in training (including senior undergraduates, specialist trainees from associated specialties and development of successional staff), education of purchasers (including insurers and government agencies).
6. Data collection for local audit and clinic management.
7. Local and collaborative research at a national or international level.
8. Collaboration with national patient support groups.

Diagnosis and interdisciplinary treatment planning

Many patients are referred to a hypodontia team with some information about their condition provided by the referring practitioner. However, the extent of the hypodontia is often not made clear. In addition, some patients may be referred for management of the dental aspects of hypodontia, but present with a previously undiagnosed syndrome such as hypohidrotic ectodermal dysplasia (especially when this is mild and has been relatively asymptomatic). Although many patients have complaints relating to the hypodontia, such as poor appearance due to the spaces between teeth or functional problems with chewing or speaking, others have no complaints at the time of initial referral (Hobkirk et al., 1994). The extent of their complaints usually relates to the severity of their hypodontia and the number of missing permanent teeth, but the problems may be masked to some extent if there are any retained primary teeth (Hobkirk et al., 1994; Laing et al., 2010).

It is important that the dentition as a whole is examined and any primary disease managed at an early stage. The initial role of the team is to assess the patient fully in order to determine the extent of the hypodontia, the quality of the dentition, and the prognosis for the retention of primary teeth without successors. The use of a standard clinical assessment pro forma is recommended to ensure that the clinical assessment follows a consistent format.

Treatment planning should be provided on an interdisciplinary basis with an integrated structure. The team should agree with the patient (and, where relevant, with their carers) on a tentative long-term objective. This could, for example, be to provide an apparently complete natural dentition using fixed restorations. The plan might involve the optimised positioning of the permanent teeth and restoration of any spaces with implant-stabilised restorations. Establishing long-term objectives can help to define priorities but it should not be at the expense of meeting short-term goals. Depending on the patient's age, complaints and state of dental development, a treatment plan may be developed for immediate application or may be in a predictive format with short-, medium- and longer-term objectives. A sound principle is to begin active treatment *only* when there are good clinical indications for doing so, or when it is requested by the patient (Hobkirk et al., 1995; Carter et al., 2003; Nunn et al., 2003).

A major advantage of a hypodontia team is the availability of specialist opinions from different dental specialties. Various treatment modalities can be discussed and their feasibility ascertained. For example, in some circumstances it may not be possible to upright the roots of teeth adjacent to a potential implant site, thus precluding the use of such devices to replace missing teeth. If this is recognised and discussed with the patient at an early stage, it avoids giving unrealistic expectations about the treatment outcome. A restorative specialist is also ideally placed to assess if canines can be disguised as lateral incisors, which may impact on the complexity and length of orthodontic treatment.

Patient and family counselling

Many patients and their families arrive at the clinic with concerns about the possible causes of the condition and its lifetime implications. There may be a history of hypodontia within one or (less often) both sides of the family, which may be identified by questioning at the clinic, or discovered subsequently by the family once they become aware of the condition's genetic dimension.

Frequently there is an underlying feeling of guilt on the part of one or both parents, especially if they already suspect or understand the genetic basis of hypodontia. For this reason, counselling needs to be provided both to determine any familial hypodontia and to reassure patients and parents (Gill *et al.*, 2008). Where more complex family histories need to be investigated, or where patients with hypodontia associated with syndromes request genetic counselling (including implications for future pregnancies), referral to a clinical geneticist should be considered (Dahl, 1998; Gill *et al.*, 2008).

Counselling should also be provided at an early stage to outline the possible options for treatment in the short-, medium- and long-term. This can provide reassurance to patients, parents and carers that an integrated treatment plan can restore dentofacial aesthetics and dental function and improve psychosocial development (Gill *et al.*, 2008). In younger patients, if there are problems of poor self-esteem or reports of bullying because of the appearance of severe hypodontia, then early treatment can be initiated to address this (Nunn *et al.*, 2003). Where no such issues exist, counselling alone may be sufficient, with treatment deferred until a more developmentally suitable stage is reached.

Provision of specific treatment plans for outreach provision of care

Many patients are referred for integrated treatment within the unit housing the hypodontia clinic, but resource issues may often make it difficult to provide extensive, complex and expensive treatment for everyone without long waiting lists. For this reason, it can be helpful to involve dental care professionals who are external to the clinic, on an outreach basis, as part of a managed clinical network (Hobson *et al.*, 2003). Many patients favour local treatment based on geography and ease of access. Such arrangements can significantly reduce financial and organisational burdens on the family of a child who needs to attend the clinic often.

Many practitioners express the wish to maintain an active role in the management of their patients. They feel confident about providing discrete elements of the care pathway with advice and support from the hypodontia clinic team. To provide the most appropriate level of practitioner and patient

support, the team should be prepared to review the patient at any stage, at the practitioner's request, to provide on-going guidance.

Treatment can either be provided wholly through local practitioners or specialists to an integrated treatment plan developed by the hypodontia clinic team, or the hypodontia clinic team can provide discrete treatment elements, with other elements provided locally. Examples of this include specialist orthodontic treatment provided through the hypodontia clinic team, with restorative care (such as resin-retained bridges) provided by the patient's own dental practitioner. The use of dental implants may later require the involvement of the hypodontia team, or may be provided by a specialist locally. In this way, the hypodontia clinic can act both as a direct and an indirect provider of care.

Provision of treatment within the unit

Many referring practitioners request that the complex interdisciplinary management of patients with hypodontia is managed through the hypodontia clinic and provided directly by clinic members and their teams. This can produce well coordinated and streamlined care, with all specialties available on-site, and it is often highly successful due to the expertise offered by the hypodontia team gained through extensive experience of managing patients with these problems.

Single-site management particularly favours periodic joint reviews between specialists as individual phases of treatment such as orthodontics progress. It also facilitates the obtaining of *ad hoc* advice from a colleague, and provides the prosthodontist with the opportunity to approve final tooth positions and root paralleling prior to debonding of the fixed orthodontic appliances. Similarly, where there is microdontia in combination with hypodontia, the restorative dentist can plan build-ups using a diagnostic wax-up, discussing it with the orthodontist and patient before providing the treatment. One disadvantage is that clinical and financial resources can be problematical because of the potential numbers of patients needing treatment and the greater cost of treating them in a highly specialist centre. Where available resources are unable to match referrals, then inevitably long waiting lists are likely, which may lead to more protracted treatment times.

There may also be conflicting pressures from funding organisations, including healthcare insurance agencies and government healthcare purchasing bodies. These pressures may reflect a desire to control expenditure, or in some cases restricted knowledge of the potential lifetime benefits of advanced treatment. Consequently healthcare purchasers may seek to fund what they perceive as more routine restorative procedures, such as resin-retained bridges, through primary care practitioners rather than a secondary care hypodontia clinic. Such an approach can be difficult for the practitioner who may be reluctant to provide these aspects of care, favouring integrated treatment through a hypodontia clinic. Patient and family expectations of comprehensive care based on one site may also match this. This conflict of expectations and pressures often leads to the need for the hypodontia team to target resources by triaging patients based on the complexity of their treatment need. The team may also seek to arrange the treatment of less complex problems through the provision of detailed treatment plans for guided outreach management within the managed clinical network, with more complex problems being treated directly through the hypodontia clinic itself.

Teaching, research, and data collection

The clinical expertise of established hypodontia teams should be disseminated to other practitioners, not only to ensure the continuation of the clinic through clinician progression, but also to facilitate the development of other similar clinics nationally and internationally. More experienced hypodontia teams often attract colleagues as observers from other units with developing hypodontia clinics, to gain valuable insight into team-building and clinic dynamics. The lessons learned can later be translated into clinical successes for these developing clinics. Hypodontia clinics are also a valuable resource for the teaching and training of junior clinical staff or practitioners, who may then be more confident to take the acquired knowledge and skills into dental or specialist practice. In turn, these practitioners can become part of a managed clinical network for the provision of outreach care. Alternatively, trained staff can leave the clinic to establish new clinic teams themselves in other provider units.

Collaboration between clinics enables agreed treatment strategies to be developed and applied widely, such that specialist teams with access to traditional and evolving diagnostic and treatment technologies can continually work together to improve the management of patients with complex hypodontia (Bergendal et al., 1996; Hobkirk et al., 2006; Nohl et al., 2008). Hypodontia teams with extensive involvement in research will frequently employ a data manager or research assistant to collate data using an appropriate database system. Interaction between clinics at a national or international level is facilitated if common data are collected, so that clinical research or audit can be carried out on significantly larger samples through multicentre studies. To this end, an internationally agreed baseline data set can permit easy integration and exchange of information between groups (Hobkirk et al., 2006).

Collaboration with national patient support groups

Many countries now have patient support groups that have been established to help individuals and their families affected by ectodermal dysplasia (ED). Such groups have usually been established by members of affected families and have subsequently expanded into large fora, with access to expert lay and professional advice, personal experiences, counselling and family therapy (Hobkirk et al., 2006). Since the hypodontia associated with this condition is one of the most common manifestations, and one of particular concern to people with ectodermal dysplasia, the establishment of links between specialist hypodontia clinics and national support groups can be mutually beneficial. While such groups are not represented on individual hypodontia clinics, their contact details, advice leaflets and website addresses can be provided for patients and parents. These include:

- **UK Ectodermal Dysplasia Society:** www.ectodermaldysplasia.org
- **Canadian Dermatology Association:** www.ectodermadysplasia.ca
- **Australian Ectodermal Dysplasia Support Group:** www.ozed.org.au

- **Association Française des Dysplasies Ectoder-miques:** www.afde.net
- **National Foundation for Ectodermal Dyspla-sia:** www.nfed.org

In some countries, patient support groups also encourage and support research into hypodontia through grant funding.

Composition of the ideal hypodontia clinic team

Although several ideals have been proposed, funding pressures can influence access to some specialties and so representation of these in the hypodontia clinic may be limited. This decision is often linked to the size of the clinic and patient demographics and throughput. It is also influenced by the frequency with which specific conditions are encountered, and the effect on access needs for particular specialists. Individual hypodontia clinics vary in relation to the specialties represented (Carter *et al.*, 2003; Hobson *et al.*, 2003; Jepson *et al.*, 2003; Meechan *et al.*, 2003; Nunn *et al.*, 2003; Worsaae *et al.*, 2007; Gill *et al.*, 2008; Shafi *et al.*, 2008), but international conferences have developed consensus statements (Hobkirk *et al.*, 2006) that reflect international agreement. They recommend that particular specialties, as listed below, should either be represented directly on the hypodontia clinic, or should be available nearby:

- General dental practitioners
- Dental nurses
- Orthodontists
- Paediatric dentists
- Prosthodontists
- Oral and maxillofacial surgeons
- Specialist laboratory technicians
- Clinical psychologists
- Clinical geneticists
- Dermatologists
- Speech and language therapists

The general dental practitioner

Although the dental practitioners are rarely present on the hypodontia team, they form a vital component of the care pathway and need to be aware of the condition because they are responsible for the initial identification of the problem and subsequent referral to the clinic. The patient's standard of oral health, including caries control and oral hygiene status, will have been under the care of the practitioner, often over an extended period (Hobson *et al.*, 2003). The concept of shared care will require this to continue alongside any specialist treatment delivered through the hypodontia clinic team.

As a component of the orthodontic phase of treatment the practitioner may be asked to carry out any necessary primary or permanent (less frequently) tooth extractions. He or she may also be willing to carry out any necessary restorative treatment, including interim replacement of teeth with resin-bonded bridges or removable prostheses, together with re-contouring of microdont teeth with composite resin additions or veneers. Dental practitioners with special interests and additional skills may wish to provide necessary implant therapy. In the longer term, the practitioner will need to maintain the patient's restored dentition and replace worn or damaged prostheses (Hobson *et al.*, 2003; Shafi *et al.*, 2008).

Dental nurses

The dental nurse is usually the first team member that the patients and their families meet on arrival at the hypodontia clinic. They are the initial point of contact when arranging the appointment. This named contact will, throughout the patient's time, remain attached to the clinic, giving opportunities to raise any concerns.

There is often an element of apprehension for the family on arriving for the first visit, so the dental nurse should allay this when welcoming the patient. The large number of team members in an interdisciplinary hypodontia clinic can be intimidating for patients, but if the dental nurse prepares the family before they enter the clinic, by explaining who will be present and their roles, this can be of great comfort and benefit. Frequently, the patient or parents may raise issues and concerns with the dental nurse outside the clinic either before or after consultation, which they do not wish to bring up in discussion with the team. This gives the dental nurse a valuable role of patient advocate, and such concerns can be brought to the attention of the team.

The dental nurse also has the responsibility of ensuring that the clinic runs smoothly, by appropriate appointment scheduling, chair-side support and carrying out equipment decontamination processes. With larger clinics, where multiple dental chairs are used simultaneously, a team of dental nurses may be more appropriate than a single nurse. This is particularly useful if it enables one dental nurse to carry out the initial meeting with the family outside the clinical environment, while the remainder provide chair-side support. In some teams, this role may be filled by a designated clinic coordinator.

The orthodontist

The orthodontist's role is to provide knowledge of normal growth and development, and to assess any deviations from the normal associated with hypodontia (Bergendal et al., 1996; Chung et al., 2000; Carter et al., 2003; Thind et al., 2005). In addition, he or she may advise on any interceptive primary tooth extractions to guide the developing occlusion and provide appliance therapy to treat the malocclusion, including repositioning of ectopic permanent teeth and root paralleling of abutments (Bergendal et al., 1996; Herrero, 2003; Simeone et al., 2007). Where feasible, orthodontics should seek to close spaces completely, or reduce them to a more easily manageable size (Carter et al., 2003; Thind et al., 2005; Addy et al., 2006). If it is not possible to close the spaces, then the ultimate abutment sites and saddle lengths should be agreed with the prosthodontist before the orthodontist moves teeth to the agreed positions (Bergendal et al., 1996; Shroff et al., 1996; Richardson and Russell, 2001; Kinzer and Kokich, 2005; Jones, 2009). The use of dental implants in the treatment of hypodontia is increasing and can often be optimised, or even made feasible, by jointly planned tooth movement. In this way, the surgical envelope in implant sites can be improved, the size of spaces in the arch can be optimised, and potential occlusal issues can be managed.

The paediatric dentist

The paediatric dentist's role in the management of child and adolescent patients with hypodontia (Goodman et al., 1994; Bergendal et al., 1996; Nunn et al., 2003) may include behavioural management to encourage nervous children so that they accept dental care (both preventive and therapeutic forms). Treatment may involve restorative care of permanent and primary teeth to maximise their longevity, primary tooth extractions as required, dentoalveolar surgery for severely infra-occluded primary teeth, or the exposure and bonding of attachments to ectopic permanent teeth. In the intermediate restorative phase of treatment, the paediatric dentist may be asked to build up microdont permanent teeth with resin to improve aesthetics. Resin-retained bridges or removable prostheses may be required for more severe hypodontia. Patients with severe hypodontia and microdontia associated with ectodermal dysplasia may require more extensive overdentures at a very young age to improve self-esteem relating to dental and facial aesthetics, and function (Hobkirk et al., 1995; Nunn et al., 2003).

The prosthodontist

The prosthodontist's role is to plan and, where appropriate, agree with the orthodontist the ultimate sites and sizes of edentulous spaces, and the intended functional occlusion. Following orthodontic treatment the prosthodontist will provide a range of restorative treatment options, including fixed or removable prostheses, in order to restore aesthetics and function (Millar and Taylor, 1995; Francischone et al., 2003; Addy et al., 2006; Bishop et al., 2007a). Dental implants have become more widely used to restore single units or as supports for more extensive fixed prostheses (Bergendal et al., 1996; Guckes et al., 1998; Francischone et al., 2003; Herrero, 2003; Jepson et al., 2003; Forgie et al., 2005; Bishop et al., 2007b; Esposito et al., 2007). The potential use of implants requires that the roots of adjacent teeth are not converging into the intended implant zone, and root paralleling (or preferably root divergence) should have been agreed as an objective of the initial interdisciplinary treatment plan between the prosthodontist and orthodontist (Bergendal et al., 1996; Shroff et al., 1996; Richardson and Russell, 2001; Francischone et al., 2003; Kinzer and Kokich, 2005; Jones, 2009).

The oral and maxillofacial surgeon

The surgeon may be involved in dentoalveolar surgery on patients of all ages. It may include extractions, surgical removal of severely infra-occluded primary teeth, surgical exposure of ectopic permanent teeth, and the autotransplantation of permanent teeth from one site to another (Andreasen *et al.*, 1990a, 1990b, 1990c, 1990d; Meechan *et al.*, 2003; Mendes and Rocha, 2004; Bauss *et al.*, 2004, 2008; Amos *et al.*, 2009). Patients requiring dental implants for the definitive restorative phase may need bone grafting or sinus-floor lifts to increase available bone in the implant sites, using bone substitutes or bone harvested from the patient's hip (Wallace and Froum, 2003; Esposito *et al.*, 2008; Nkenke and Stelzle, 2009).

In some teams the surgeon may place dental implants, while in others this is something the prosthodontist carries out. In addition, patients with severe skeletal deformities may require orthognathic surgery to improve facial aesthetics and normalise jaw relationships prior to prosthodontic treatment (Bergendal *et al.*, 1996; Meechan *et al.*, 2003).

Specialist laboratory technicians

The complex nature of the treatment provided for patients with hypodontia requires high-quality laboratory support. Ideally the laboratory should be on site to enable the laboratory and clinical staff to discuss complex issues face-to-face and where necessary at the chair-side. However, where this is not feasible then an off-site service is acceptable, although this necessitates good communication.

The laboratory service is necessary to support the orthodontic phase of treatment, where fixed or removable auxiliary appliances may be required, and for the provision of orthodontic retainers. These often differ from routine retainers in that they include prosthetic teeth, which maintain spaces created during the active orthodontics and improve aesthetics during the retention phase.

The prosthodontic phases of treatment require high-quality fixed or removable prostheses and indirect restorations or veneers to be manufactured in the laboratory, to the clinician's prescription. The microdont or conical morphology of the teeth in many hypodontia patients may complicate such work and challenge the skills of the technician. Where dental implants are to be used, laboratory support is required for the manufacture of the positioning jigs or stents needed for accurate placement and the coronal superstructure. It goes without saying that high-quality clinical treatment can only be provided where supported by high-quality laboratory work.

The clinical psychologist

Patients with severe hypodontia may suffer from associated psychosocial problems (Wagenberg and Spitzer, 1998; Francischone *et al.*, 2003), and may benefit from a meeting with a clinical psychologist. Issues such as low self-esteem, social withdrawal and coping strategies (because of bullying) may be explored through discussions or group therapy (Nunn *et al.*, 2003; Gill *et al.*, 2008). In addition, the patient's parents sometimes benefit from discussing issues with the clinical psychologist, dissociating their own perceived problems from those of their child, and focusing on the developmental benefit to the child. This may lessen the risk of providing early treatment for a child with little or no personal concerns relating to their hypodontia, to allay what are actually parental concerns.

The clinical geneticist

The genetic basis of hypodontia is complex and was discussed fully in Chapter 1. Therefore the clinical geneticist may be involved both in the genetic testing of severe hypodontia patients and their parents and with their counselling. This may be especially useful where the hypodontia is associated with a familial genetic syndrome, and where parents are seeking advice about the risks for future planned pregnancies (Dahl, 1998). Similarly, patients with genetic syndromes may wish to discuss their own future family planning.

The dermatologist

Patients and families of patients with hypodontia-related syndromes with skin involvement, including the ectodermal dysplasias, may benefit from time with a dermatologist. They may discuss management strategies for hypohidrosis and subsequent skin dryness. Other syndromes (such as incontinentia pigmenti) cause patches of skin hyperpigmentation that may benefit from advice or treatment from a dermatologist.

The speech and language therapist

Young children with severe hypodontia may present with speech defects associated with large spaces. These defects may respond to speech and language therapy, and the integration of therapy both before and after treatment of the hypodontia can maximise the improvement in speech. The provision of extensive removable prostheses, or early implant therapy, in very young children to attempt to improve aesthetics, psychosocial development, and speech patterns is controversial (Bergendal et al., 1996; Wagenberg and Spitzer, 1998; Francischone et al., 2003). Where speech is perceived as the primary issue, improvement of speech processes through speech and language therapy may be less invasive, and more acceptable to the patient.

The hypodontia care pathway

The care pathway for patients with hypodontia frequently extends over many years, from initial presentation in early childhood through to completion of treatment as an adult. The key to such a long pathway is the provision of patient information. Initial counselling of patients and their parents or carers requires the hypodontia team to outline the nature and timescale of the care pathway, together with its key stages. These often comprise:

- Assessment
- Interceptive therapy (including early orthodontics or restorative treatment)
- Definitive orthodontics
- Intermediate restorative therapy
- Definitive restorative therapy (including implants)
- Long-term maintenance

It is psychologically important for patients and their parents or carers to understand that treatment will be in phases and will not be completed instantly. This is especially true for particularly young patients for whom the care pathway may seem to stretch over a very long period. In such cases, there will be times when the patient is simply under periodic review by the clinic in between active phases of care.

The principle of shared care must be explained to the family when elements of the pathway are likely to be provided as an outreach provision under the guidance of the team. In this way, the inclusive role of the general dental practitioner can be made clear at the outset in relation to routine dental care, the provision of agreed elements of the hypodontia treatment pathway, and long-term maintenance following discharge from the clinic (Hobson et al., 2003).

Once the nature of the care pathway has been explained, it is important to stress the flexibility of the plan, which may be modified as time progresses in the light of changes in growth and development, oral health, patient needs and motivation, including their education, and technological developments. Although the general principles of any treatment pathway can be discussed, there must be sufficient flexibility to enable modification of the specific plan over time in the light of individual patient needs (Shafi et al., 2008). For this reason, the proposed care pathway should not be seen as being cast in stone, particularly when discussed with a very young patient for whom many changes may occur over the time period. It is important that this flexibility is viewed from the outset as a significant and intended strategy, rather than indecision.

Informed consent will be required at each stage of the treatment pathway, but because changes may occur with time it is better to avoid a process that formalises decisions taken at an early stage and allows little flexibility. The information process and obtaining of informed consent can be markedly improved by the use of information leaflets. These may be developed locally or patients may be directed to appropriate websites on dental health issues or those of patient support groups. Families are becoming increasingly aware of the benefits of the internet for information relating to hypodontia, and its impact on dental and oral health (Chestnutt and Reynolds, 2006; Ní Ríordáin and McCreary, 2009).

Benefits of a multidisciplinary approach

A multidisciplinary approach to the management of hypodontia may be costly in terms of resources but it has many benefits. It ensures that there is an integrated and unified treatment plan, which has been agreed in advance by all specialties involved in the care pathway. The location and size of any edentulous saddles, together with the siting of abutments, can be agreed prior to orthodontic treatment, which eliminates surprises for the prosthodontist following the orthodontic phase. This in turn avoids possible disappointment for the patient should an intended mode of restorative care not be possible due to incorrect pre-restorative preparation by the orthodontist. This may be especially problematical when the space left for a prosthetic replacement is too narrow or too wide.

For the same reason, patients being prepared for implant therapy will require the orthodontist to ensure that the roots of adjacent teeth do not encroach into the implant site (Richardson and Russell, 2001). Unless the adjacent roots are parallel, or better still divergent, the risks associated with implant placement may mean that the patient loses the opportunity for an implant in favour of a bridge. This will have been discussed as part of the interdisciplinary planning.

An interdisciplinary approach with agreed and met objectives maximises the clinical outcomes for patients and is more likely to produce both satisfied patients and satisfied clinicians (Jones, 2009).

Computerised clinical databases

The database is a useful tool for collection and storage of information from a hypodontia clinic. It can be employed for clinical audit and research locally, and where a common database is used it can facilitate collaborative research both nationally and internationally (Hobkirk *et al.*, 2006). If direct electronic entry of data is not possible, a pro forma sheet can be used to ensure that all necessary information is gathered and recorded, and later entered

---

Key Points: Providing care

- The care pathway for patients with hypodontia is often complex, with the delivery of care best delivered through an integrated hypodontia clinic with access to the expertise of a range of dental and medical specialties
- The roles of a hypodontia clinic include the within-unit treatment of patients, the provision of treatment plans for outreach care, patient and family counselling, education and training, and research
- A number of patient support groups have been set up world-wide by affected families, providing a valuable service for patients through specialist advice, counselling and hypodontia research funding

---

into an electronic database. Figure 3.2 shows an example of a clinical data pro forma.

Computerised data storage is becoming more widespread alongside increasing use of digital imaging techniques for diagnosis and treatment planning. Software packages currently permit digital manipulation of clinical images, thus giving an opportunity to illustrate possible aesthetic outcomes for patients prior to commencing treatment. Prosthesis construction can also be facilitated by computer systems that use increasingly common CADCAM technology.

References

Addy L, Bishop K, Knox J. Modern restorative management of patients with congenitally missing teeth:2. Orthodontic and restorative considerations. *Dent Update* 2006;33:592–595.

Amos MJ, Day P, Littlewood SJ. Autotransplantation of teeth: An overview. *Dent Update* 2009;36:102–113.

Andreasen JO, Paulsen HU, Yu Z, *et al.* A long-term study of 370 autotransplanted premolars. Part I. Surgical procedures and standardized techniques for monitoring healing. *Eur J Orthod* 1990a;12:3–13.

Andreasen JO, Paulsen HU, Yu Z, Bayer T, Schwartz O. A long-term study of 370 autotransplanted premolars. Part II. Tooth survival and pulp healing subsequent to transplantation. *Eur J Orthod* 1990b;12:14–24.

Andreasen JO, Paulsen HU, Yu Z, Bayer T. A long-term study of 370 autotransplanted premolars. Part IV. Root development subsequent to transplantation. *Eur J Orthod* 1990c;12:38–50.

HYPODONTIA CLINIC

Hospital No:

Last name

1st Name

D.O.B.   M / F

Date: _____

Referred by: _____

Patient's complaint: _____

_____

Family history: Yes / No   **Medical history:**   Yes / No

If "Yes" provide details: _____

_____

_____

Skeletal pattern: I / II / III   **Incisor relationship:**   I / II$_1$ / II$_2$ / III

TEETH PRESENT

	8	7	6	5	4	3	2	1	1	2	3	4	5	6	7	8	
UR	□	□	□	□	□	□	□	□	□	□	□	□	□	□	□	□	UL
				E	D	C	B	A	A	B	C	D	E				
				□	□	□	□	□	□	□	□	□				
				□	□	□	□	□	□	□	□	□				
				E	D	C	B	A	A	B	C	D	E				
LR	□	□	□	□	□	□	□	□	□	□	□	□	□	□	□	□	LL
	8	7	6	5	4	3	2	1	1	2	3	4	5	6	7	8	

TEETH MISSING

	8	7	6	5	4	3	2	1	1	2	3	4	5	6	7	8	
UR	□	□	□	□	□	□	□	□	□	□	□	□	□	□	□	□	UL
				E	D	C	B	A	A	B	C	D	E				
				□	□	□	□	□	□	□	□	□				
				□	□	□	□	□	□	□	□	□				
				E	D	C	B	A	A	B	C	D	E				
LR	□	□	□	□	□	□	□	□	□	□	□	□	□	□	□	□	LL
	8	7	6	5	4	3	2	1	1	2	3	4	5	6	7	8	

PTO/ .....

Figure 3.2   Example of pro forma for recording clinical data.

Upper centreline | R ← | C | → L | Lower centreline | R ← | C | → L |

Overbite | ▲ | N | ▼ | Complete / Incomplete / AOB   Overjet: _____ mm

MOLAR RELATIONSHIP

Right: I / II$_h$ / II$_f$ / III$_h$ / III$_f$ Left: I / II$_h$ / II$_f$ / III$_h$ / III$_f$

ALIGNMENT

| | UPPER | Crowding ☐ | Spacing ☐ | Well aligned ☐ |
| | LOWER | Crowding ☐ | Spacing ☐ | Well aligned ☐ |

MICRODONTIA   Yes / No / Generalised

UR   8 7 6 5 4 3 2 1 | 1 2 3 4 5 6 7 8   UL
     ☐ ☐ ☐ ☐ ☐ ☐ ☐ ☐ | ☐ ☐ ☐ ☐ ☐ ☐ ☐ ☐

LR   ☐ ☐ ☐ ☐ ☐ ☐ ☐ ☐ | ☐ ☐ ☐ ☐ ☐ ☐ ☐ ☐   LL
     8 7 6 5 4 3 2 1 | 1 2 3 4 5 6 7 8

CROSSBITE: Yes / No | R | C | L |

INFRAOCCLUSION: Yes / No

UR   E D C B A | A B C D E   UL
     ☐ ☐ ☐ ☐ ☐ | ☐ ☐ ☐ ☐ ☐

LR   ☐ ☐ ☐ ☐ ☐ | ☐ ☐ ☐ ☐ ☐   LL
     E D C B A | A B C D E

BPE ──┼──┼──   Plaque   Decayed/   Freeway
                      index: ____   filled: ____%   space: ____ mm

ADDITIONAL FINDINGS: _____

_____

_____

RADIOGRAPHIC FINDINGS: _____

_____

_____

Signature: _____

Figure 3.2   (cont'd)

Andreasen JO, Paulsen HU, Yu Z, Schwartz O. A long-term study of 370 autotransplanted premolars. Part III. Periodontal healing subsequent to transplantation. *Eur J Orthod* 1990d;12:25–37.

Bauss O, Engelke W, Fenske C, Schilke R, Schwestka-Polly R. Autotransplantation of immature third molars into edentulous and atrophied jaw sections. *Int J Oral Maxillofac Surg* 2004;33:558–563.

Bauss O, Zonios I, Rahman A. Root development of immature third molars transplanted to surgically created sockets. *J Oral Maxillofac Surg* 2008;66:1200–1211.

Bergendal B, Bergendal T, Hallonsten AL, *et al.* A multidisciplinary approach to oral rehabilitation with osseointegrated implants in children and adolescents with multiple aplasia. *Eur J Orthod* 1996;18:119–129.

Bishop K, Addy L, Knox J. Modern restorative management of patients with congenitally missing teeth:1. Introduction, terminology and epidemiology. *Dent Update* 2006;33:531–537.

Bishop K, Addy L, Knox J. Modern restorative management of patients with congenitally missing teeth:3. Conventional restorative options and considerations. *Dent Update* 2007a;34:30–38.

Bishop K, Addy L, Knox J. Modern restorative management of patients with congenitally missing teeth:4. The role of implants. *Dent Update* 2007b;34:79–84.

Carter NE, Gillgrass TJ, Hobson RS, *et al.* The interdisciplinary management of hypodontia: orthodontics. *Br Dent J* 2003;194:361–366.

Chestnutt IG, Reynolds K. Perceptions of how the internet has impacted on dentistry. *Br Dent J* 2006;200:161–165.

Chung LK, Hobson RS, Nunn JH, Gordon PH, Carter NE. An analysis of the skeletal relationships in a group of young people with hypodontia. *J Orthod* 2000;27:315–318.

Dahl N. Genetics of ectodermal dysplasia syndromes. In: B Bergendal, G Koch, J Kurol, G Wänndahl (eds) *Consensus Conference on Ectodermal Dysplasia with Special Reference to Dental Treatment.* Gothia, Stockholm, 1998, pp. 22–31.

Duello GV. The utilization of an interdisciplinary team approach in esthetic, implant, and restorative dentistry. *Gen Dent* 2004;52:116–119.

Esposito M, Grusovin MG, Kwan S, Worthington HV, Coulthard P. Interventions for replacing missing teeth. Bone augmentation techniques for dental implant treatment. *Cochrane Database Syst Rev* 2008, July 16 (3), CD003607.

Esposito M, Murray-Curtis L, Grusovin MG, Coulthard P, Worthington HV. Interventions for replacing missing teeth. Different types of dental implants. *Cochrane Database Syst Rev* 2007, October17 (4), CD003815.

Forgie AH, Thind BS, Larmour CJ, Mossey PA, Stirrups DR. Management of hypodontia: restorative considerations. Part III. *Quintessence Int* 2005;36:437–445.

Francischone CE, Oltramari PV, Vasconcelos LW, *et al.* Treatment for predictable multidisciplinary implantology, orthodontics, and restorative dentistry. *Pract Proced Aesthet Dent* 2003;15:321–326.

Gill DS, Jones S, Hobkirk J, *et al.* Counselling patients with hypodontia. *Dent Update* 2008;35:344–352.

Goodman JR, Jones SP, Hobkirk JA, King PA. Hypodontia:1. Clinical features and the management of mild to moderate hypodontia. *Dent Update* 1994;21:381–384.

Guckes AD, Roberts MW, McCarthy GR. Pattern of permanent teeth present in individuals with ectodermal dysplasia and severe hypodontia suggests treatment with dental implants. *Pediatr Dent* 1998;20:278–280.

Herrero D. Orthodontics as a prerequisite to implant placement. *Dent Today* 2003;22:88–93.

Hobkirk JA, Goodman JR, Jones SP. Presenting complaints and findings in a group of patients attending a hypodontia clinic. *Br Dent J* 1994;177:337–339.

Hobkirk JA, King PA, Goodman JR, Jones SP. Hypodontia:2.The management of severe hypodontia. *Dent Update* 1995;22:8–11.

Hobkirk JA, Nohl F, Bergendal B, Storhaug K, Richter MK. The management of ectodermal dysplasia and severe hypodontia. International conference statements. *J Oral Rehabil* 2006;33:634–637.

Hobson RS, Carter NE, Gillgrass TJ, *et al.* The interdisciplinary management of hypodontia: the relationship between an interdisciplinary team and the general dental practitioner. *Br Dent J* 2003;194:479–482.

Jepson NJ, Nohl FS, Carter NE, *et al.* The interdisciplinary management of hypodontia: restorative dentistry. *Br Dent J* 2003;194:299–304.

Jones SP. The multidisciplinary management of hypodontia. *Dent Nurs* 2009;5:678–682.

Kinzer GA, Kokich VO Jr. Managing congenitally missing lateral incisors. Part III: Single-tooth implants. *J Esthet Restor Dent* 2005;17:202–210.

Laing E, Cunningham SJ, Jones S, Moles D, Gill D. Psychosocial impact of hypodontia in children. *Am J Orthod Dentofacial Orthop* 2010;137:35–41.

McNamara C, Foley T, McNamara CM. Multidisciplinary management of hypodontia in adolescents: case report. *J Can Dent Assoc* 2006;72:740–746.

Meechan JG, Carter NE, Gillgrass TJ, *et al.* The interdisciplinary management of hypodontia: oral surgery. *Br Dent J* 2003;194:423–427.

Mendes RA, Rocha G. Mandibular third molar autotransplantation – Literature review with clinical cases. *J Can Dent Assoc* 2004;70:761–766.

Millar BJ, Taylor NG. Lateral thinking: the management of missing upper lateral incisors. *Br Dent J* 1995;179:99–106.

Ní Ríordáin R, McCreary C. Dental patients' use of the internet. *Br Dent J* 2009;207:583–586.

Nkenke E, Stelzle F. Clinical outcomes of sinus floor augmentation for implant placement using autogenous bone or bone substitutes: A systematic review. *Clin Oral Implants Res* 2009;20(Suppl.4):124–133.

Nohl F, Cole B, Hobson R, *et al.* The management of hypodontia: present and future. *Dent Update* 2008;35: 79–88.

Nunn JH, Carter NE, Gillgrass TJ, *et al.* The interdisciplinary management of hypodontia: background and role of paediatric dentistry. *Br Dent J* 2003;194:245–251.

Richardson G, Russell KA. Congenitally missing maxillary lateral incisors and orthodontic treatment considerations for the single tooth implant. *J Can Dent Assoc* 2001;67:25–28.

Shafi I, Phillips JM, Dawson MP, Broad RD, Hosey MT. A study of patients attending a multidisciplinary hypodontia clinic over a five year period. *Br Dent J* 2008; 205:649–652.

Shroff B, Siegel SM, Feldman S, Siegel SC. Combined orthodontic and prosthetic therapy. Special considerations. *Dent Clin North Am* 1996;40:911–943.

Simeone P, De Paoli C, De Paoli S, Leofreddi G, Sgrò S. Interdisciplinary treatment planning for single-tooth restorations in the esthetic zone. *J Esthet Restor Dent* 2007;19:79–88.

Thind BS, Stirrups DR, Forgie AH, Larmour CJ, Mossey PA. Management of hypodontia: Orthodontic considerations (II). *Quintessence Int* 2005;36:345–353.

Wagenberg BD, Spitzer DA. A multidisciplinary approach to the treatment of oligodontia: A case report. *Periodontal Clin Investig* 1998;20:10–13.

Wallace SS, Froum SJ. Effect of maxillary sinus augmentation on the survival of endosseous dental implants. A systematic review. *Ann Periodontol* 2003; 8:328–343.

Worsaae N, Jensen BN, Holm B, Holsko J. Treatment of severe hypodontia-oligodontia – An interdisciplinary concept. *Int J Oral Maxillofac Surg* 2007;36:473–480.

Part 2

Key Issues

4 Space

Introduction

While the treatment of patients with hypodontia has important systemic and local dimensions, the latter can be thought of largely as a problem of space management both within and between the dental arches. To fully appreciate space issues, it is important that they are considered in three dimensions:

- Mesiodistally (between both the crowns *and* roots of adjacent teeth)
- Vertically (within and between the dental arches)
- Transversely (both within and between the dental arches)

The first of these effectively defines the mesiodistal dimension of the prosthetic envelope, and the third is important for restorative and orthodontic reasons. Restoratively, a minimal surgical envelope is required to enable implant placement, while orthodontically it is difficult to move teeth into an area of alveolar bone in which the ridge is insufficiently wide. This is often seen as a narrowing of the alveolar ridge below its crest and is sometimes referred to colloquially as 'necking' or 'waisting'.

A fourth dimension is time, and this can also be important particularly in growing individuals as it reflects both positive and negative changes in potentially available spaces as a result of normal or abnormal facial growth and development.

An understanding of space issues is fundamental to the management of hypodontia and the various skills that members of a multidisciplinary team can bring to its treatment.

Space issues within the dental arches

The underlying problem in many people affected by hypodontia is not only the excess of space but also the uneven distribution of that space within the dental arches (Figure 4.1). The space is often distributed in an uneven manner because the developing teeth tend to erupt and drift along the path of least resistance, often into areas where teeth are absent.

The maxillary and mandibular canines are particularly prone to this form of tooth movement

Hypodontia: A Team Approach to Management, First Edition
© J.A. Hobkirk, D.S. Gill, S.P. Jones, K.W. Hemmings, G.S. Bassi, A.L. O'Donnell and J.R. Goodman
Published 2011 by Blackwell Publishing Ltd

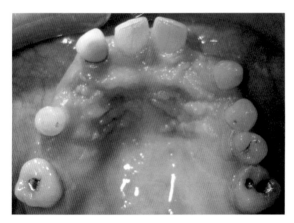

Figure 4.1   Uneven space distribution that often accompanies hypodontia that can complicate restorative treatment. (teeth UR7, UR5, UR3, UL2 and UL7 are missing).

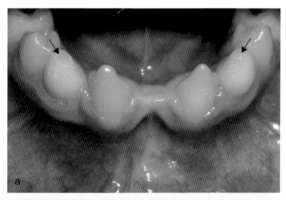

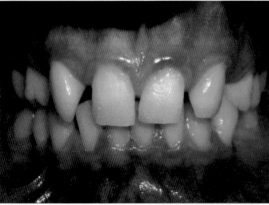

Figure 4.2   (a) The mandibular canines have erupted and migrated mesially in this patient with missing incisors. The primary canines (arrows) are retained. (b) The maxillary canines often erupt and migrate mesially when the lateral incisors are missing.

(Figure 4.2). The problem of uneven space distribution can be compounded by microdont teeth, which occupy less space than normal sized teeth, and tooth rotations, which are prevalent in the premolar region, as rotated (pre)molar teeth occupy more space in the line of the arch than their non-rotated equivalents.

Uneven space distribution may complicate prosthodontic tooth replacement and the restorative management of microdont teeth. This is because an optimal prosthodontic result can only be obtained when spaces are in an appropriate location for a replacement tooth, and their dimensions permit the placing of natural-looking and functioning restorations. A space that is too small or too large can be equally challenging and its static and dynamic relationships with opposing teeth must also be noted. A space which is excessive for restoration with a normal-sized tooth can be as challenging to manage as one which is inadequate. In both cases there may be aesthetic compromises with the restoration while in the latter situation implant treatment may be challenging – or impossible.

It is important when measuring space mesiodistally to consider not only the distance between the greatest bulbosities of the crowns of teeth adjacent to the space, but also the distance between their roots (Figure 4.3).

The dimensions of this space are crucial when planning implant-supported restorations. At least 1.5 mm of bone should lie between the implant fixture and the root of an adjacent tooth in order to minimise the risk of iatrogenic root damage during implant placement. The dimensions of the space between implants or between the implant and tooth significantly influences the generation of an interdental papilla (Gastaldo *et al.*, 2004). The available space around an implant applies not only to the horizontal dimension, for which 3 mm at the ridge crest is often recommended (Martin *et al.*, 2009), but also to the vertical distance between the bone and the contact point between restorations or restoration and natural crown.

Space issues within the dental arches are often multifactorial in origin. Factors influencing the amount of spacing present include:

- The severity of the hypodontia
- The presence of localised or generalised microdontia

- Retention of the primary teeth
- Abnormal eruptive paths and drifting of successional teeth

The severity of hypodontia

Both the severity of hypodontia and the distribution of missing teeth determine the degree and location of spacing present within the dental arches. In principle, spacing can be generalised or localised to particular regions depending on the teeth that are missing. Hypodontia may first become apparent and cause aesthetic concerns because spacing is noticed in the early mixed dentition stage, when the permanent maxillary incisors normally erupt. Occasionally primary teeth such as the lateral incisors are retained, and this will reduce the aesthetic impact of hypodontia (Laing *et al.*, 2010) and may result in it going unnoticed by the patient and family until pointed out by their general dental practitioner (Figure 4.4).

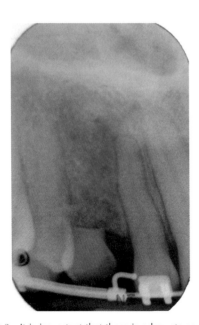

Figure 4.3   It is important that there is adequate space between the maximum bulbosity of the crowns and roots of teeth, as in this case with missing UR3, in order to facilitate future restorative treatment. This can be accurately demonstrated on a long-cone periapical radiograph taken perpendicular to the edentulous space. This is best carried out prior to removal of orthodontic appliances.

Spacing in the posterior region may be less visibly apparent and thus of minimal aesthetic concern, but it may have functional implications depending on its severity, particularly when the primary teeth are also absent. There is recent evidence to suggest that retention of primary molars may be important for functional reasons (Laing *et al.*, 2010).

Microdontia

There is an association between hypodontia and microdontia and the severity of microdontia appears to parallel that of hypodontia, particularly in more severely affected individuals (Garn and Lewis, 1970; Brook, 1984; Brook *et al.*, 2009). Interestingly there also appears to be a reduction in tooth size in *unaffected* relatives of patients affected by hypodontia (McKeown *et al.*, 2002), which suggests a possible genetic influence (Parkin *et al.*, 2009). Affected teeth are often smaller both mesiodistally and buccolingually with the effect on crown size being greatest in the buccolingual dimension (Brook *et al.*, 2009). A reduction in buccolingual width of the premolars and molars can influence the coordination between the maxillary and mandibular dental arches (see Chapter 8).

Microdontia may be localised or generalised. Any tooth within the dental arch can be affected, with studies suggesting that it occurs most commonly in the maxillary lateral incisors and mandibular

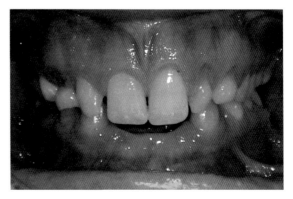

Figure 4.4   Patient with severe hypodontia with reduced aesthetic impact due to retention of several primary teeth in the upper arch.

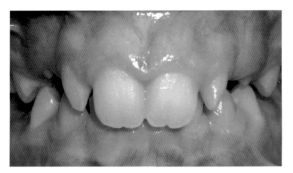

Figure 4.5   Peg-shaped maxillary lateral incisors (maxillary lateral incisors are often microdont).

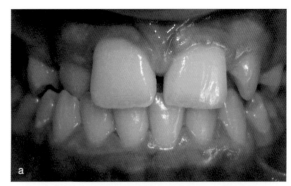

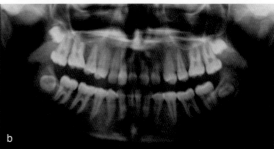

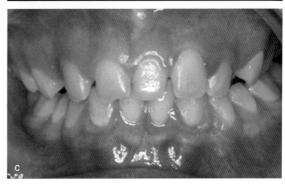

Figure 4.6   (a) Macrodontia of the maxillary central incisors in a patient with developmentally absent maxillary lateral incisors. (b) This patient with missing maxillary canines and lower central incisors has an upper supplemental incisor in the midline. (c) A clinical picture of the patient shown in (b).

central incisors (Brook *et al.*, 2009). Not only is tooth size altered, but tooth form also varies, as seen typically in the maxillary lateral incisors which can be peg-shaped (Figure 4.5) or a normal shape with slightly reduced dimensions (Peck *et al.*, 1996; Baidas and Hashim, 2005; Albashaireh and Khader, 2006).

Rarely, patients with hypodontia can be affected by localised macrodontia or even the presence of supernumerary teeth (Figure 4.6), and this association has been termed hypohyperodontia (Gibson, 1979; Varela *et al.*, 2009). The presence of macrodontia may help to reduce the size of potential spacing present within the arches.

Retention of primary teeth

The retention of a primary tooth can reduce the impact of hypodontia both aesthetically and functionally (Laing *et al.*, 2010). Little information exists in the literature about the long-term survival of retained primary teeth, although Haselden *et al.* (2001) have commented on root resorption of primary teeth lacking permanent successors. Bjerklin *et al.* (2008) followed a group of 99 patients between the mean ages of 12 and 25 years and found that less than 10% of retained primary mandibular second molars were lost during this period. Although there are several limitations to this research, it does suggest that a primary molar may be retained in some individuals until at least their mid-twenties when the majority of facial growth is complete. There are reports in the literature of primary molars surviving in people up to the age of 60 years, which highlights the large individual variability in the survival and retention of these teeth (Biggerstaff, 1992; Bjerklin and Bennett, 2000; Ith-Hansen and Kjaer, 2000; Sletten *et al.*, 2003) (Figure 4.7).

There are a number of benefits from retaining primary molars without underlying successors, including:

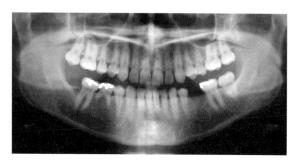

Figure 4.7 42-year-old patient with developmentally absent lower second premolars. The lower right second primary molar is retained and remains functional.

- The masking of the effects of hypodontia both functionally and aesthetically
- The maintenance of both vertical and buccolingual alveolar bone volume
- Space maintenance and the prevention of supra-eruption of opposing teeth

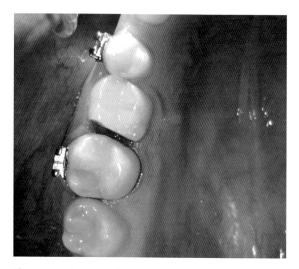

Figure 4.8 Patient with upper right second primary molar reduced distally to allow the upper first molar to move mesially into a better occlusal relationship. Exposed dentine has been protected with flowable composite material.

Although there are many advantages in retaining primary teeth, there are also some potential disadvantages in retaining full-sized primary molar teeth. These relate principally to the second primary molar, which is considerably larger than its permanent successor and, in particular, the lower second primary molar (which is also larger mesiodistally than its upper counterpart). The retention of these molars produces a tooth-size (Bolton) discrepancy that can make it difficult to achieve an ideal Class I molar relationship, although it should be pointed out that there is currently no published scientific evidence which supports the view that a Class I molar relationship is superior to any other arrangement.

Retention of a large primary molar can also complicate subsequent prosthodontic tooth replacement because the primary molar span is longer than that of its permanent successor, resulting in greater functional loads being exerted on any pontic that may be placed. To help overcome these potential disadvantages, reduction of the mesiodistal width of the primary molar, followed by orthodontic space closure, may be considered, thus helping to correct the tooth size discrepancy (Figure 4.8).

One concern often suggested as potentially limiting the degree of reduction that can be achieved is

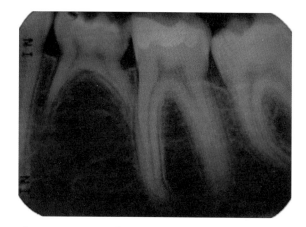

Figure 4.9 Periapical radiograph showing divergent roots of a retained primary molar tooth, which may limit the amount of space closure possible following interproximal tooth reduction.

the divergence of the mesial and distal roots of the primary molar teeth. It is often stated that if this is significant it will limit the degree of mesial movement of the first permanent molars that can be achieved before the adjacent roots begin to contact. It has therefore been recommended that a long-cone periapical radiograph is used to accurately assess the root morphology before considering tooth reduction (Figure 4.9). Kokich and Kokich

(2006) have however suggested that the divergence of the primary molar roots may not be as critical as previously thought because pressure from a mesially moving first permanent molar may preferentially induce resorption of the distal primary molar root, without causing damage to the first permanent molar root.

Another problem that can be faced when a primary molar is reduced interproximally is that of sensitivity of the exposed dentine. It is therefore recommended that any exposed dentine tubules are sealed with a flowable composite material to help protect the pulp–dentine complex. It is also very important that damage to the enamel of the adjacent tooth is minimised by placing a metal matrix band during reduction of the primary molar.

A number of factors can affect the long-term prognosis, and therefore the retention of primary teeth, such as:

- Dental caries
- Progressive root resorption
- Infra-occlusion
- Tooth wear
- Periodontal attachment loss

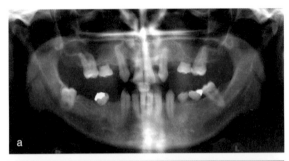

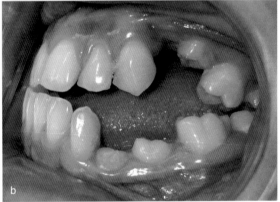

Figure 4.10 (a) Progressive root resorption (replacement resorption) of the retained primary molar teeth. (b) Severe example of infra-occlusion that can influence the long-term prognosis of retained primary teeth (affecting LLD, LLE and ULE).

Dental caries

Dental caries is a common cause of early loss of both retained primary teeth, and permanent teeth. Preventive advice that should be emphasised includes the benefits of topical fluoride application, good oral hygiene measures, and limiting the frequency of carbohydrate consumption. Fissure sealing may be considered to make tooth surfaces less plaque retentive and more caries resistant. This can be considered for molar surfaces (occlusal and buccal) and also deep palatal pits on incisors.

Root resorption

Progressive root resorption can affect the life expectancy of retained primary teeth (Figure 4.10a). The majority of teeth will undergo progressive root resorption, although there is considerable individual variation in the rate at which this progresses. Evidence suggests that it generally occurs at a slow rate and that roots showing small degrees of resorption at the ages of 11–12 years are likely to be retained at least until the completion of facial growth when implant-retained prostheses can be considered (Rune and Sarnäs, 1984; Bjerklin and Bennett, 2000; Ith-Hansen and Kjaer, 2000; Haselden et al., 2001).

Our understanding of individual variation in root resorption is currently incomplete, but both genetic and functional factors may be important. One benefit of retaining primary teeth affected by root resorption is that the resorbing roots are gradually replaced by alveolar bone, which helps to maintain bone volume and may simplify later restorative treatment.

Infra-occlusion

Ankylosis, an anatomical fusion between cementum and alveolar bone, prevents the normal compensatory eruptive mechanism that maintains the level of the occlusal plane during continued vertical skeletal development. Without compensatory eruption, an ankylosed tooth progressively becomes infra-occluded (Figure 4.10b). Evidence suggests a genetic role in the aetiology of infra-occlusion, since a high proportion of siblings of children with this condition are also affected (Kurol, 1981). The prevalence of infra-occlusion has been reported to be between 1.3% and 8.9%, with the mandibular first and second primary molars often cited as the most commonly affected teeth (Andlaw, 1974). The large variation in reported prevalence rates may also be related to age differences between the children investigated, differing definitions of infra-occlusion between studies, and racial variations. The prevalence of infra-occlusion appears to be higher in those affected by hypodontia, possibly suggesting a common aetiological mechanism (Bjerklin *et al.*, 1992).

A diagnosis of ankylosis cannot be made solely by the observation of a small step in the occlusal plane between the primary and adjacent permanent molar. This is because the crown of a primary molar is naturally shorter than that of an adjacent permanent tooth. Other tests can give uncertain results. Percussion is not necessarily a reliable indicator, since at least 20% of a root surface may have to be ankylosed before a definite metallic tone is elicited (Andersson *et al.*, 1984; Ne *et al.*, 1999). A lack of mobility is also unreliable because more than 10% of a root surface may need to be ankylosed before mobility is affected (Ne *et al.*, 1999). Obliteration of the periodontal membrane may not be identifiable on an intraoral radiograph since this only provides a two-dimensional view, and ankylosis on the buccolingual aspects of a tooth may be obscured. The most reliable indicator of ankylosis in a mildly infra-occluded tooth is the presence of a vertical step in the interproximal bone around the infra-occluded molar. This signifies a cessation of vertical bone formation normally associated with eruption (Kokich, 2002) (Figure 4.11).

Once a diagnosis of ankylosis has been made, it can be useful to quantify the degree of infra-occlusion using the following scale:

- *Mild:* The level of infra-occlusion is above the interproximal contact of the adjacent tooth
- *Moderate:* The level of infra-occlusion is within the interproximal contact area

- *Severe:* The level of infra-occlusion is below the interproximal contact of the adjacent tooth

A number of complications are associated with the presence of infra-occluded primary molar teeth and these are summarised in Table 4.1. Occlusal

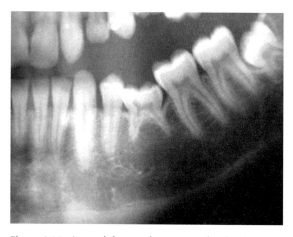

Figure 4.11   Lower left second primary molar showing signs of early infra-occlusion. An early reliable indicator of ankylosis is the presence of an angular alveolar defect between an ankylosed tooth and the adjacent teeth with normal eruptive mechanisms.

Table 4.1   Consequences of primary molar infra-occlusion.

Feature	Consequences
Infra-occluded primary molar	Delayed exfoliation Progressive infra-occlusion Difficulty with extractions
Permanent successor	Delayed eruption or impaction Abnormal eruption pattern Disturbed root development Rotation of successor Cyst formation
Developing occlusion	Potential site for developing malocclusion Centreline shift Overeruption of opposing tooth Tipping of adjacent teeth Localised open bite Reduced vertical alveolar bone development Impaired mastication The condition is also associated with a higher frequency of impacted maxillary canines, ectopic first permanent molars, hypodontia and taurodontism possibly due to a common genetic mechanism

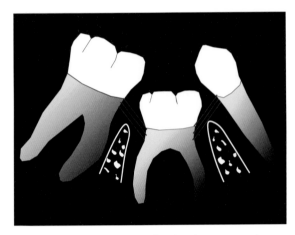

Figure 4.12 Tension generated within the trans-septal periodontal fibres (in red) may contribute to exaggerated tipping of teeth adjacent to an ankylosed primary tooth.

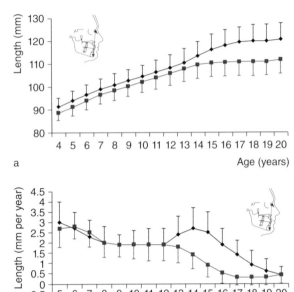

Figure 4.13 (a) A distance–growth curve for lower anterior face height in males (blue) and females (pink) (Nasion–Menton). Note that male growth is of greater magnitude and continues longer than female growth (Gill, 2008). (b) A velocity–growth curve for lower anterior face height (Nasion–Menton) in males (blue) and females (pink). Note the acceleration in facial growth in males associated with puberty (Gill, 2008).

disturbances such as exaggerated tipping of adjacent teeth, inhibition of vertical dental development and centreline shift are thought to be due to the tension generated within the trans-septal periodontal elastic fibres that interconnect adjacent teeth (Becker and Karnei-R'em, 1992a, 1992b; Becker et al., 1992) (Figure 4.12). The progression of infra-occlusion is correlated to the degree of remaining vertical skeletal facial growth.

The management of infra-occlusion is primarily dependent on its severity at the time of diagnosis and an estimation of the remaining vertical facial skeletal growth. This is crucial since any teeth with a normal eruptive mechanism will continue to erupt to compensate for vertical facial growth leading to progressive infra-occlusion of the adjacent ankylosed molar. Figure 4.13 shows the distance and velocity growth curves for vertical facial height in males and females. From this it can be appreciated that there is acceleration of vertical facial growth, and therefore tooth eruption, associated with puberty and that growth continues for a longer time in males than in females.

Orthodontists commonly use standing height measurements plotted on growth charts to estimate the remaining skeletal growth as there is some correlation between these measurements and skeletal facial growth (Van der Beek et al., 1996).

Treatment options for managing infra-occluded molars without permanent successors include:

- Monitoring if the infra-occlusion is mild (1–2 mm) and there is minimal remaining vertical facial growth
- Restoration of the occlusal surface to help prevent tipping of adjacent teeth and overeruption of opposing teeth
- Extraction of the ankylosed tooth if the adjacent teeth are significantly tipped with space loss and if there is a risk of the tooth becoming totally enveloped by bone

Because of ankylosis, infra-occluded teeth may require surgical removal, which can be destructive of surrounding bone and therefore complicate orthodontic space closure or future restorative treatment. The resorptive changes, which occur adjacent to a socket for a number of years following extraction, can also diminish alveolar bone levels (Ostler and Kokich, 1994). Surgical removal of an infra-occluded primary second molar may also risk damage to the mental nerve, which can result in permanent loss of sensation in its area of distribution.

Abnormal eruptive paths and drifting of successors

The presence of spacing within the dental arch can alter the normal eruptive pathway of a developing tooth. Normally, a permanent successor will resorb the roots of an overlying primary tooth, resulting in mobility, exfoliation and tooth emergence. In patients with hypodontia, the presence of space adjacent to a permanent successor may alter its eruptive pathway towards a direction of lesser resistance. This may result in the successor erupting into the surrounding space, rather than resorbing the roots of its primary predecessor, and reducing the immediate impact of hypodontia due to spacing. This situation is often seen when the permanent maxillary lateral incisor is developmentally absent, whereby the permanent canine often erupts into the lateral incisor position, leaving the primary canine retained. This can have the advantage of additional alveolar bone volume development in the lateral incisor position (as the canine erupts, bone develops adjacent to it). There is some evidence to suggest that if the canine is later retracted orthodontically, then the bone that remains in the lateral incisor position is extremely stable and does not undergo resorption as does bone surrounding an extraction site (Spear *et al.*, 1997). This technique has been termed 'orthodontic site development' and may help to facilitate future implant treatment.

It is also common for the maxillary canine to remain unerupted and palatally positioned when the maxillary lateral incisor is absent or diminutive (Brin *et al.*, 1986; Peck *et al.*, 1996). This is because the maxillary lateral incisor root may be important as a guide to the eruptive pathway of the permanent canine, so-called 'guidance theory', as proposed by Becker (1995). At the age of 9 years all patients should undergo a routine orthodontic examination in which the buccal sulcus should be palpated for the presence of a bulge indicating the correct position of the underlying canine. If the canine bulge is absent, radiographs should be used to accurately locate the position of the canine. If

this is demonstrated to be palatal, most orthodontists would advise extraction of the primary canine to help normalise the eruptive path of the permanent successor (Ericson and Kurol, 1988).

Space issues between the dental arches

The freeway space (FWS) or vertical difference between the separation of the jaws when the patient is at rest and when the mandible is in the intercuspal position may be affected in hypodontia.

Freeway space

Although poorly researched, partly due to the problems of determining the freeway space clinically, experience suggests that it tends to be increased in people affected by hypodontia. This is more likely to be the case as the severity of the hypodontia increases. Although the exact associations are poorly understood, a number of factors may contribute to an increased freeway space, as follows:

- Reduced vertical maxillary growth
- Reduced vertical dentoalveolar growth
- Microdontia in the vertical dimension
- Infra-occlusion of primary molars
- Tooth wear

Overbite

Overbite is the vertical overlap of opposing teeth in the intercuspal position with the occlusal plane orientated parallel to the true horizontal. A deep overbite may develop between the incisors and any other tooth when the opposing tooth is absent, and can complicate orthodontic management and prosthodontic tooth replacement in the incisor region. A number of factors may contribute to the development of a deep incisor overbite, namely:

- A reduced lower anterior facial height and/or abnormal counterclockwise mandibular growth rotation (Figure 4.14)

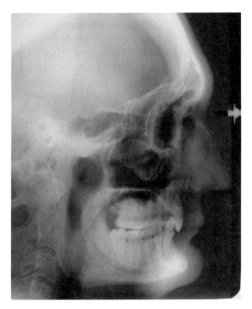

Figure 4.14   Lateral cephalogram showing the characteristic appearance of a patient with a counterclockwise (forward) mandibular growth rotation. Note the low mandibular plane angle. Such patients are prone to a deep overbite and successful overbite reduction can be problematic.

- A skeletal II pattern in which the lower incisors continue to erupt because of the lack of an occlusal stop (as a result of the increased overjet)
- Maxillary incisor overeruption due to the absence of the mandibular incisors
- Incisor retroclination

A deep overbite may also develop between teeth other than the incisors and can complicate treatment. For example, the permanent canines may overerupt, if unopposed, with a reduction in vertical space for prosthodontic tooth replacement in the opposing arch (Figure 4.15). In these circumstances orthodontic treatment can be beneficial for the management of overerupted teeth.

Principles of treatment planning

The principal issues in the management of spacing in hypodontia are:

- Multidisciplinary treatment planning
- Concerns of the patient

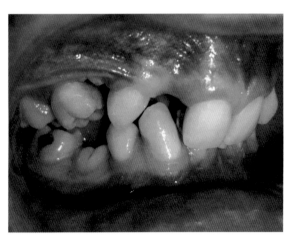

Figure 4.15   Overeruption of the lower canine can complicate prosthodontic tooth replacement in the opposing arch. This figure shows a multitude of other vertical problems including deep incisor overbite, infra-occlusion URE and severe tipping of UR6 leading to a lateral open-bite occlusion.

- Age of the patient
- Optimising the size and distribution of spaces in the dental arches

Multidisciplinary treatment planning

The management of excessive space in patients with hypodontia principally involves its alteration orthodontically either to remove its effects or to optimise their prosthodontic management. A vital principle of treatment planning is, therefore, that before commencing any active treatment all patients' care should be planned using a multidisciplinary approach (Hobson *et al.*, 2003; Hobkirk *et al.*, 2006), particularly before any form of orthodontic therapy is commenced (Carter *et al.*, 2003). The orthodontist must have a precise prescription for the space distribution and exact tooth positions required to achieve an ideal restorative outcome.

A diagnostic (Kesling) set-up is an excellent method for visualising and assessing the feasibility of a proposed treatment plan, and can also act as an invaluable aide memoire of the desired tooth positions to be achieved orthodontically. In cases where additional special investigations (such as cone-beam computerised tomography) or diagnostic set-ups are required, a series of appointments with the multidisciplinary team may be required. In other cases, only a single multidisciplinary visit is necessary for all the specialists to see the patient for diagnosis and treatment planning. The broader benefits of a multidisciplinary approach to treatment planning and care pathways have been discussed fully in Chapter 3.

Patient's concerns

Patient satisfaction at the end of treatment is best achieved with a treatment plan that addresses their concerns within the limitations of the clinical situation, available resources and the types of treatment that he or she is able or willing to undertake. All these issues must be explored with the patient and his or her carers as part of obtaining informed consent to an agreed plan. The most common complaints of patients with hypodontia appear to be missing teeth, spacing within the dental arches, and poor appearance (Hobkirk *et al.*, 1994). Although functional concerns can also occur, they are quite rare and mainly limited to chewing difficulties in people with large numbers of missing teeth (Laing *et al.*, 2010).

The patient's age

Age is an important factor in determining the treatment modalities available at any given time, reflecting both age-related effects on a patient's attitudes to dental problems and their management and their stage of dental development and the remaining degree of facial growth. Comprehensive orthodontic treatment is often not considered until all developing successional teeth have erupted, or until the completion of facial growth in people with skeletal discrepancies that require orthognathic surgery. Dental development is often delayed in individuals affected by hypodontia (Ruiz-Mealin *et al.*, 2009), which can delay the start of orthodontic treatment compared to their peers. As well as orthognathic treatment, dental implant therapy is rarely undertaken until completion of vertical facial growth so as to limit the risk of infraocclusion of the restored unit(s) which have no eruptive mechanism (Thilander *et al.*, 1999).

Optimisation of intra-arch spaces

Spacing within the dental arch can be principally managed in three ways:

1. Orthodontic redistribution (for idealisation of spaces for prosthodontic tooth replacement and/or tooth build-up where teeth are microdont).
2. Orthodontic space closure.
3. Acceptance of the space distribution with limited or no treatment.

The approach taken depends on a number of factors as outlined in Table 4.2.

Orthodontic space redistribution
The aim of space redistribution is to produce a space that is ideally sized and located for prosthodontic tooth replacement and/or for the build-up of microdont teeth or abnormally shaped teeth. It is most commonly done with fixed orthodontic appliances that allow for bodily tooth movement, helping to ensure that adequate root paralleling is achieved. This is particularly important if implant treatment is to be considered in the future. By contrast, the use of removable appliances, including clear aligner systems, does not achieve adequate control of root positions. While multidisciplinary decisions on space management can be complex, the key points are summarised in Table 4.2.

Space closure
Orthodontic space closure can help to avoid tooth replacement. It is particularly suited to patients in whom space is required for the management of a coexisting malocclusion, such as the relief of crowding or incisor retraction. The benefits of this approach include avoidance of future tooth replacement and the associated problems of cost, maintenance and plaque control around pontics. When deciding whether to open or close a maxillary lateral incisor space, it is important to have a prosthodontic opinion on the suitability of a canine for mimicking a lateral incisor. These issues are considered in detail in Chapter 9.

Figures 4.16 and 4.17 show situations that have been successfully managed by orthodontic space opening and space closure.

Table 4.2   Factors that may be taken into consideration when deciding to open or close intra-arch spaces.

Patient concerns and motivation for treatment	All treatment should attempt to address the patient's concerns. Complex treatment may be avoided if there are no concerns. It is important to ascertain the patient's motivation for treatment at an early stage as often the management of hypodontia involves numerous appointments that can be onerous for the patient with little motivation.
Oral health	The patient's dental health must be good before embarking on complex treatment.
Facial profile	A retrusive lip profile favours space opening to help improve lip support by incisor advancement. A protrusive profile favours space closure by incisor retraction.
Skeletal pattern	A mild to moderate skeletal II pattern favours upper arch space closure as the space can often be used for incisor retraction (orthodontic camouflage). If the skeletal II pattern is severe and orthognathic surgery is being considered, upper arch space opening maybe preferred to facilitate decompensation. A mild to moderate skeletal III pattern favours upper arch space opening to achieve maximum incisor advancement. This may camouflage the skeletal pattern as opening spaces in the upper arch facilitates advancement of the upper incisors. In the lower arch, space closure facilitates incisor retraction. A severe skeletal III pattern may favour upper arch space closure and lower arch space opening in order to facilitate decompensation before orthognathic surgery.
Incisor relationship	See skeletal pattern above.
Degree of spacing	Complete orthodontic space closure is less likely to be an option as the severity of hypodontia increases. Dental crowding favours orthodontic space closure.
Molar relationship	If at all possible an already well established molar relationship should be maintained when opening or closing intra-arch spaces.
Size, shape, colour and emergence levels and profiles of teeth	Such factors should be considered when deciding whether a tooth can be used to mimic a missing unit (e.g. a maxillary canine as a lateral incisor).

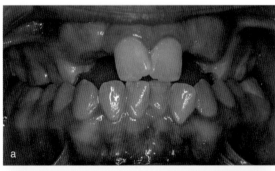

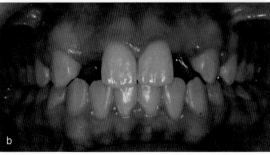

Figure 4.16   Patient treated by opening the missing maxillary lateral incisor spaces. The upper panel is pre-treatment, in which the canines are erupting into the position of the maxillary lateral incisors. Note the Class III incisor relationship which is one factor that supports the decision to open the lateral incisor spaces. The lower panel shows the final result after treatment with upper and lower pre-adjusted edgewise appliances and rapid maxillary expansion.

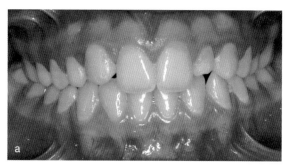

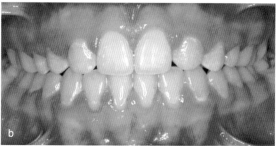

Figure 4.17   Patient treated by accepting closure of the upper right lateral incisor space and extraction of the microdont upper left lateral incisor followed by space closure. The upper panel is pre-treatment, in which the canines have a good colour match with the central incisors and a favourable size and form to mimic the lateral incisors aesthetically. Note the retained upper right primary canine. A Class II incisor relationship, although very mild in this case, favours space closure. The lower panel shows the final result, following treatment with upper and lower pre-adjusted edgewise appliances. The patient was satisfied with the appearance of the canines as lateral incisors without aesthetic enhancement.

Accepting the space distribution

Occasionally, the space distribution is acceptable for tooth replacement or build-up without orthodontic intervention. On other occasions the patient may be content to accept the treatment limitations imposed by not having the spaces ideally distributed. Such limitations may include the necessity for small pontics when available space is reduced, or acceptance of some residual spacing around normally sized pontics when space is excessive.

Inter-arch space

The muscles of mastication can operate effectively over a large range of occlusal vertical dimensions

(Kois and Phillips, 1997; Pepicelli *et al.*, 2005; Bloom and Padayachy, 2006; Ceneviz *et al.*, 2006; Yabushita *et al.*, 2006). This property can be useful when considering the restorative rehabilitation of a patient with hypodontia. If there is insufficient inter-arch space, the use of a 'Dahl appliance' or bite-plane can allow selective eruption of certain teeth and intrusion of others to create vertical space where it is needed. An excess of vertical space can be particularly helpful if cast cusp-covered restorations are being considered, as little reduction of the occlusal surface is required, thus maintaining as much sound tooth structure as possible. Adhesive onlay-type restorations with minimal preparation are especially useful for infra-occluded primary molar teeth that are being maintained for any significant length of time.

Key Points: Space issues in hypodontia

- Space should be considered in all three dimensions and may be influenced by continuing facial growth and development – the 'fourth dimension'
- Within the dental arches the degree of mesiodistal space is related to the severity of hypodontia, microdontia and the retention of primary teeth
- The long-term prognosis of primary teeth is related to root resorption, infra-occlusion, dental caries, tooth surface loss and periodontal disease
- Mesiodistal space is often poorly distributed for ideal tooth replacement, due to abnormal eruption paths and drifting of the permanent teeth
- Treatment options for mesiodistal space include:
  ○ Orthodontic space closure
  ○ Redistribution and idealisation of the space followed by prosthodontic restoration
  ○ Prosthodontic management within the limits of the existing spaces where orthodontic treatment is inappropriate
- Orthodontically optimised spaces should be assessed by a prosthodontist prior to the removal of fixed appliances.
- At least 1.5 mm of space should be present between an implant fixture and the adjacent root for safe placement. Space between the roots should be assessed with a long-cone periapical radiograph perpendicular to the edentulous space being restored before orthodontic appliances are removed.
- An increased overbite between the incisors or other teeth commonly occurs in patients with hypodontia and may complicate tooth replacement.

References

Albashaireh ZS, Khader YS. The prevalence and pattern of hypodontia of the permanent teeth and crown size and shape deformity affecting upper lateral incisors in a sample of Jordanian dental patients. *Community Dent Health* 2006;23:239–243.

Andersson L, Blomlöf L, Lindskog S, Feiglin B, Hammarström L. Tooth ankylosis. Clinical, radiographic and histological assessments. *Int J Oral Surg* 1984;13:423–431.

Andlaw RJ. Submerged deciduous molars. A review, with special reference to the rationale of treatment. *J Int Assoc Dent Child* 1974;5:59–66.

Baidas L, Hashim H. An anterior tooth size comparison in unilateral and bilateral congenitally absent maxillary lateral incisors. *J Contemp Dent Pract* 2005; 6:56–63.

Becker A, Karnei-R'em RM, Steigman S. The effects of infra-occlusion: Part 3. Dental arch length and the midline. *Am J Orthod Dentofacial Orthop* 1992;102:427–433.

Becker A, Karnei-R'em RM. The effects of infra-occlusion: Part 1. Tilting of the adjacent teeth and local space loss. *Am J Orthod Dentofacial Orthop* 1992a;102:256–264.

Becker A, Karnei-R'em RM. The effects of infra-occlusion: Part 2. The type of movement of the adjacent teeth and their vertical development. *Am J Orthod Dentofacial Orthop* 1992b;102:302–309.

Becker A. In defense of the guidance theory of palatal canine displacement. *Angle Orthod* 1995;65:95–98.

Biggerstaff RH. The orthodontic management of congenitally absent maxillary lateral incisors and second premolars: A case report. *Am J Orthod Dentofacial Orthop* 1992;102:537–545.

Bjerklin K, Al-Najjar M, Kårestedt H, Andrén A. Agenesis of mandibular second premolars with retained primary molars: A longitudinal radiographic study of 99 subjects from 12 years of age to adulthood. *Eur J Orthod* 2008;30:254–261.

Bjerklin K, Bennett J. The long-term survival of lower second primary molars in subjects with agenesis of the premolars. *Eur J Orthod* 2000;22:245–255.

Bjerklin K, Kurol J, Valentin J. Ectopic eruption of maxillary first molars and association with other tooth and developmental disturbances. *Eur J Orthod* 1992;14:369–375.

Bloom DR, Padayachy JN. Increasing Occlusal vertical dimension – Why, when and how? *Br Dent J* 2006;200: 251–256.

Brin I, Becker A, Shalhav M. Position of the maxillary permanent canine in relation to anomalous or missing lateral incisors: A population study. *Eur J Orthod* 1986; 8:12–16.

Brook AH. A unifying aetiological explanation for anomalies of human tooth number and size. *Arch Oral Biol* 1984;29:373–378.

Brook AH, Griffin RC, Smith RN, Townsend GC, Kaur G, Davis GR, Fearne J. Tooth size patterns in patients with hypodontia and supernumerary teeth. *Arch Oral Biol* 2009;54(Suppl.1):S63–70.

Carter NE, Gillgrass TJ, Hobson RS, *et al.* The interdisciplinary management of hypodontia: Orthodontics. *Br Dent J* 2003;194:361–366.

Ceneviz C, Mehta NR, Forgione A, *et al.* The immediate effect of changing mandibular position on the EMG activity of the masseter, temporalis, sternocleidomastoid, and trapezius muscles. *Cranio* 2006;24:237–244.

Ericson S, Kurol J. Early treatment of palatally erupting maxillary canines by extraction of the primary canines. *Eur J Orthod* 1988;10:283–295.

Garn S, Lewis A. The gradient and the pattern of crown-size reduction in simple hypodontia. *Angle Orthod* 1970;40:51–58.

Gastaldo JF, Cury PR, Sendyk WR. Effect of the vertical and horizontal distances between adjacent implants and between a tooth and an implant on the incidence of interproximal papilla. *J Periodontol* 2004;75:1242–1246.

Gibson AC. Concomitant hypo-hyperodontia. *Br J Orthod* 1979;6:101–105.

Gill D (2008) *Orthodontics at a Glance.* Blackwell Publishing, Oxford.

Haselden K, Hobkirk JA, Goodman JR, Jones SP, Hemmings KW. Root resorption in retained deciduous canine and molar teeth without permanent successors in patients with severe hypodontia. *Int J Paediatr Dent* 2001;11:171–178.

Hobkirk JA, Goodman JR, Jones SP. Presenting complaints and findings in a group of patients attending a hypodontia clinic. *Br Dent J* 1994;177:337–339.

Hobkirk JA, Nohl F, Bergendal B, Storhaug K, Richter MK. The management of ectodermal dysplasia and severe hypodontia. International conference statements. *J Oral Rehabil* 2006;33:634–637.

Hobson RS, Carter NE, Gillgrass TJ, *et al.* The interdisciplinary management of hypodontia: the relationship between an interdisciplinary team and the general dental practitioner. *Br Dent J* 2003;194:479–482.

Ith-Hansen K, Kjaer I. Persistence of deciduous molars in subjects with agenesis of the second premolars. *Eur J Orthod* 2000;22:239–243.

Kois JC, Phillips KM. Occlusal vertical dimension: Alteration concerns. *Compend Contin Educ Dent* 1997;18:1169–1177.

Kokich VG, Kokich VO. Congenitally missing mandibular second premolars: Clinical options. *Am J Orthod Dentofacial Orthop* 2006;130:437–444.

Kokich VO Jr. Congenitally missing teeth: Orthodontic management in the adolescent patient. *Am J Orthod Dentofacial Orthop* 2002;121:594–595.

Kurol J. Infra-occlusion of primary molars: An epidemiologic and familial study. *Community Dent Oral Epidemiol* 1981;9:94–102.

Laing E, Cunningham SJ, Jones S, Moles D, Gill DS. Psychosocial impact of hypodontia in children. *Am J Orthod Dentofacial Orthop* 2010;137:35–41.

Martin W, Lewis E, Nicol A. Local risk factors for implant therapy. *Int J Oral Maxillofac Implants* 2009;24(Suppl.):28–38.

McKeown HF, Robinson DL, Elcock C, Al-Sharood M, Brook AH. Tooth dimensions in hypodontia patients, their unaffected relatives and a control group measured by a new image analysis system. *Eur J Orthod* 2002;24:131–141.

Ne RF, Witherspoon DE, Gutmann JL. Tooth resorption. *Quintessence Int* 1999;30:9–25.

Ostler MS, Kokich VG. Alveolar ridge changes in patients congenitally missing mandibular second premolars. *J Prosthet Dent* 1994;71:144–149.

Parkin N, Elcock C, Smith RN, Griffin RC, Brook AH. The aetiology of hypodontia: The prevalence, severity and location of hypodontia within families. *Arch Oral Biol* 2009;54(Suppl.1):S52–56.

Peck S, Peck L, Kataja M. Prevalence of tooth agenesis and peg-shaped maxillary lateral incisor associated with palatally displaced canine (PDC) anomaly. *Am J Orthod Dentofacial Orthop* 1996;110:441–443.

Pepicelli A, Woods M, Briggs C. The mandibular muscles and their importance in orthodontics: A contemporary review. *Am J Orthod Dentofacial Orthop* 2005;128:774–780.

Ruiz-Mealin EV, Gill DS, Parekh S, Jones SP, Moles DR. A radiographic study of tooth development in hypodontia. *J Orthod* 2009;36:291.

Rune B, Sarnäs KV. Root resorption and submergence in retained deciduous second molars. A mixed-longitudinal study of 77 children with developmental absence of second premolars. *Eur J Orthod* 1984;6:123–131.

Sletten DW, Smith BM, Southard KA, Casko JS, Southard TE. Retained deciduous mandibular molars in adults: A radiographic study of long-term changes. *Am J Orthod Dentofacial Orthop* 2003;124:625–630.

Spear FM, Mathews DM, Kokich VG. Interdisciplinary management of single-tooth implants. *Semin Orthod* 1997;3:45–72.

Thilander B, Odman J, Jemt T. Single implants in the upper incisor region and their relationship to the adjacent teeth. An 8-year follow-up study. *Clin Oral Implants Res* 1999;10:346–355.

Van der Beek MC, Hoeksma JB, Prahl-Andersen B. Vertical facial growth and statural growth in girls: A longitudinal comparison. *Eur J Orthod* 1996;18:549–555.

Varela M, Arrieta P, Ventureira C. Non-syndromic concomitant hypodontia and supernumerary teeth in an orthodontic population. *Eur J Orthod* 2009;31:632–637.

Yabushita T, Zeredo JL, Fujita K, Toda K, Soma K. Functional adaptability of jaw-muscle spindles after bite-raising. *J Dent Res* 2006;85:849–853.

5 Occlusion

Introduction

The study of occlusion in humans has produced extensive contributions to the dental literature. Clinicians often have their own opinions on occlusal philosophies, yet while there is a scientific basis behind much of the work on occlusion there are many areas where controversy continues to exist. Kahn (1964) stated that the controversy surrounding occlusion cannot be resolved for three reasons. Firstly, because much of the knowledge is based on empirical rather than scientific information. Secondly, because the tolerance of the oral organ is great or its upper and lower physiologic limits are so broad that because a certain concept fails in one specific mouth does not mean it will fail in all mouths. Thirdly, because there is great variability between individual dentists and the standards by which they evaluate completed restorations. Kahn suggested that because 'there is no one answer to occlusal problems, the dentist should use the philosophy that works best in his own hands and at the same time does the most good, or better yet, the least harm to the patient' (Kahn, 1964).

The study of occlusion and occlusal pathology on natural teeth is complex, and when the management of fixed and removable restorations is also considered then the controversies become greater (Pameijer, 1983; Henderson, 2004). Over the last 20 years the introduction of dental implants has further complicated discussions (Taylor et al., 2005).

For many patients with mild hypodontia, occlusal principles may be simple to apply. As the severity of hypodontia increases, depending on the type of restoration placed to re-contour or replace teeth, some compromise of occlusal principles is inevitable. Some patients may present with deranged occlusions with an absence of anterior guidance, a lack of posterior support, or open bites. Treatment aims to provide an aesthetic and durable occlusion, and the goal of orthodontics is the 'creation of the best possible occlusal relationships within the framework of acceptable facial aesthetics and stability of result' (Proffit et al., 2007). For patients with hypodontia this invariably requires a multi-disciplinary approach and some ingenuity on behalf of clinicians (Goodman et al., 1994; Hobkirk

Hypodontia: A Team Approach to Management, First Edition
© J.A. Hobkirk, D.S. Gill, S.P. Jones, K.W. Hemmings, G.S. Bassi, A.L. O'Donnell and J.R. Goodman
Published 2011 by Blackwell Publishing Ltd

et al., 1994, 2006; Bergendal et al., 1996; Hobson et al., 2003; Nunn et al., 2003; Bishop et al., 2006, 2007a, 2007b; Worsaae et al., 2007; Nohl et al., 2008; Shafi et al., 2008).

Principles of occlusion (occlusal philosophies)

Ideal occlusion or normal occlusion

Orthodontists and prosthodontists have different concepts of the nature of an ideal occlusion. Orthodontists contrast an ideal occlusion with a normal occlusion and malocclusions, while prosthodontists tend to consider an ideal occlusion in relation to a balanced occlusion. In orthodontic terms, an ideal occlusion is a theoretical concept based on the morphology of the teeth. It can be precisely described and used as a standard by which other occlusions can be judged. The definition of 'normal occlusion' allows for minor variations from the ideal, which are aesthetically and functionally acceptable. Therefore, a malocclusion represents a range of conditions, which may deviate from the ideal.

As early as 1802, Duval (cited in Dewey and Anderson, 1948) stated that the lower teeth should be properly arranged adjacent to one another and with those of the upper jaw. White developed this principle further in 1850, when he considered that the first permanent molar was the most important tooth in the arch to be arranged within a full complement of the teeth in the dental arches (cited in Dewey and Anderson, 1948). In 1899, Angle produced his classification of malocclusion, stating that for an ideal occlusion to exist, the mesiobuccal cusp of the maxillary first molar should occlude with the buccal groove of the mandibular first molar. The anterior and posterior teeth had to conform to this arrangement in a similar manner and, furthermore, the upper incisors needed to 'overhang' the lower incisors by about one third of the crown length. This arrangement was termed Angle's Class I occlusion. When the mandibular molar teeth had a more distal arrangement than the maxillary arch this malocclusion was termed as post-normal, or Class II, and if a more mesial relationship existed the occlusion was termed pre-normal, or Class III. Angle later recognised the

relevance of occlusal factors to orthodontic post-treatment stability (Angle, 1907).

Hellman (1921) described a more prescriptive ideal occlusion whereby the arrangement of the teeth would provide 138 occlusal contacts in the full adult dentition of 32 teeth. It was also important that there were accurate proximal contacts in each dental arch. He felt that only if all of these contacts were present would full masticatory efficiency exist (Hellman, 1921). Beyron (1964) studied occlusions among Aborigines and, in contrast to current thinking, observed that there was no occlusal contact between the incisors in the intercuspal position in this population. Andrews studied the occlusions of non-orthodontic patients with the aid of study casts to finally develop his 'six keys to a normal occlusion' (Andrews, 1972). The six keys were:

- Inter-arch relationships
- Crown angulation (tooth tip)
- Crown inclination (tooth torque)
- Rotations
- Tight contacts
- Curve of Spee

Inter-arch relationships

- The mesiobuccal cusp of the maxillary first permanent molar should occlude in the groove between the mesial and middle buccal cusps of the mandibular first permanent molar.
- The distal marginal ridge of the maxillary first permanent molar should occlude with the mesial marginal ridge of the mandibular second permanent molar.
- The mesiopalatal cusp of the maxillary first molar should occlude in the central fossa of the mandibular first molar.
- The buccal cusps of the maxillary premolars should have a cusp to embrasure relationship with the mandibular premolars.
- The palatal cusps of the maxillary premolars should have a cusp to fossa relationship with the mandibular premolars.
- The maxillary canine should have a cusp to embrasure relationship with the mandibular canine and first premolar. The tip of its cusp should be slightly mesial to the embrasure.

- The maxillary incisors should overlap the mandibular incisors.
- The midlines of the arches should be coincident.

Crown angulation (tooth tip)

- The gingival portion of the long axis of all crowns should be more distal than the incisal portion.
- The degree of crown tip varies with each tooth but is consistent within each type.

Crown inclination (tooth torque)

- For upper incisors, the occlusal portion of the crowns and labial surface should be labial to the gingival portion. For all other crowns the occlusal portion of the labial buccal surface is palatal or lingual to the gingival portion.
- Lingual crown inclination should be slightly more pronounced in the molars than in the canines and premolars.
- Lingual inclination of mandibular posterior crowns should progressively increase.

Rotations

- All teeth should be free of rotations.

Tight contacts

- In the absence of tooth-size discrepancies all contact points should be tight, with no spaces.

Curve of Spee

- The plane of occlusion should be flat or have a very slight curve of Spee (less than 1.5 mm deep).

With the six keys in mind, it was felt that an ideal static occlusion should result in ideal function (Andrews, 1976; Roth, 1976a) (Figures 5.1–5.3). Roth (1976a) used a pantograph to record and mount the models of a large number of post-treatment orthodontic patients on a semi-adjustable articulator. He concluded that the concept of producing an ideal orthodontic occlusion to achieve centric relation closure and a mutually protected occlusion with the elimination of interferences

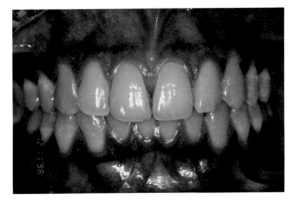

Figure 5.1   Ideal Class I occlusion of anterior teeth.

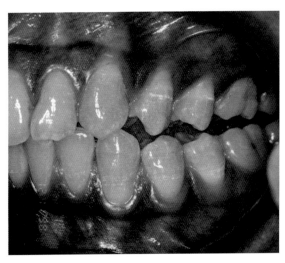

Figure 5.2   Ideal occlusion, showing left working-side excursion showing canine guidance and posterior disclusion.

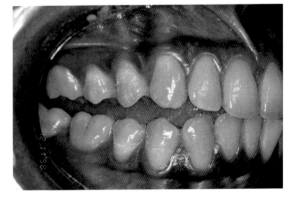

Figure 5.3   Ideal occlusion, showing right posterior disclusion during left working-side excursion.

came very close to the concept of Andrews' six keys of static occlusion (Roth, 1976a). In contrast to this, others have suggested that there is no relationship between a static and functional occlusion (Tipton and Rinchuse, 1991; Lauret and Le Gall, 1996; Al-Nimri *et al.*, 2010). These authors thought that there was a trend for the occlusion to be balanced, rather than the desired mutually protected and functional occlusion. It has been suggested that the goal of achieving a perfect occlusion is unrealistic (Howat, 1993; Clark and Evans, 2001) and it is generally accepted that satisfactory function is possible with a less than ideal static occlusion (Rinchuse and Sassouni, 1982; Vlachos, 1995) (Figures 5.1–5.3).

Balanced occlusion and ideal occlusion

To assist the reader the definitions of various occlusal terms, many of which have changed with time, are included in the Glossary).

In restorative dentistry and prosthodontics, greater emphasis had been placed on dynamic occlusion. An ideal or normal static occlusion is recognised as being important for occlusal stability, whereby occlusal and interproximal contacts will prevent adverse tooth movements, leaving the teeth in more stable positions. The terms centric occlusion (CO) or intercuspal position (ICP) have often been used interchangeably. Proffit *et al.* (2007) described ICP as 'the occlusal position with the teeth in maximum intercuspation irrespective of condylar position' (Crawford, 1999). It has been suggested that the dental occlusion should be in harmony with the optimal condylar position, known as the retruded contact position (RCP) or centric relation (CR) (Shillingburg *et al.*, 1997).

The retruded contact position (RCP) has been defined as 'the relationship of the mandible to the maxilla when the condyles are in their most posterior position in the glenoid fossa from which unstrained lateral movement can be made at the occluding vertical dimensions normal to the individual'. However, this definition has been amended by a number of authors. Lauritzen (1974) felt that the retruded contact position occurred on the 'terminal hinge relation' and that the terminal hinge interocclusal position represented maximum intercuspation with the mandible in its rear most posi-

tion. In contrast, Celenza and Nasedkin (1978) suggested that RCP was 'the most anterior, superior physiological position of the condyles against the slopes of the articular eminence, permitted by the limiting structures of the temporomandibular joints (TMJs) at the given level of vertical dimension'. Dawson (1974) proposed that RCP should coincide with the maximum intercuspation of the teeth (ICP). He felt that this occlusal scheme would promote optimum neuromuscular function, although later he changed his point of view, stating that RCP was not a position commonly associated with maximum intercuspation (Dawson, 1979). This was more in keeping with the work of Posselt (1952) who had shown that in 96% of individuals there was a discrepancy between RCP and ICP.

Occlusal philosophies have developed over the last 100 years as a result of investigation into the subject, but also the need to treat patients with removable or fixed prostheses. Details of these philosophies can be found both in a number of texts on occlusion as well as papers on the subject (Pameijer, 1983; Becker and Kaiser, 1993). Prior to the 1930s there was a general belief that a bilateral balanced occlusion in eccentric movements was essential for most dental treatment, based mainly on the concepts employed when treating patients with complete dentures. The subsequent 30–40 years saw a considerable amount of research into mandibular movements, condylar positions and occlusal contacts, as the use of dental articulators became more sophisticated. Pantographic tracings permitted the accurate measurement of condylar positions and mandibular border movements. From this work, three recognised concepts of occlusion were developed:

1. *Bilateral balanced occlusion:* During excursive jaw movements the posterior teeth on both the working side and the non-working side are in contact. This type of occlusion is strived for with complete dentures (Figure 5.4) and built on the early work of Monson (1921) who attempted to achieve contact of all the opposing teeth in all positions of the mandible. The concept behind this belief was that all the occlusal forces would be evenly distributed around the dental arch. However, this is now recognised as an abnormal state for the natural dentition as it would produce excessive

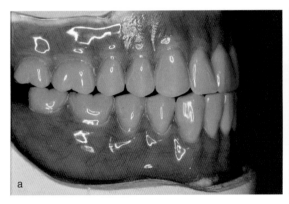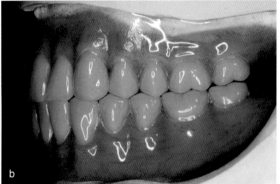

Figure 5.4   (a) Balanced occlusion with complete dentures with left working-side excursion showing bilaterally balanced occlusion on non-working side. (b) Balanced occlusion with complete dentures showing right working side.

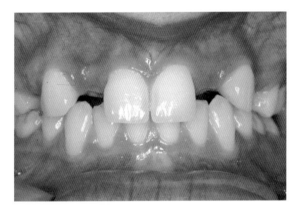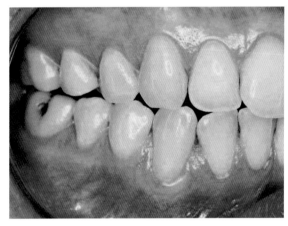

Figure 5.5   Canine guidance in an ideal occlusion following orthodontics to idealise space for upper lateral incisors.

Figure 5.6   Group function shown on a right lateral excursion. The canine cusp tip has worn, allowing simultaneous contact between the lateral incisor, canine and first premolar.

frictional wear on the teeth (McCollum and Evans, 1970).

2. *Canine protected occlusion (mutually protected occlusion):* During excursive movements of the mandible there are no contacts between the posterior teeth on either side (disclusion). This type of occlusion was popularised by D'Amico (1958) and followed by others (McCollum and Evans, 1970; Lucia, 1979; McHorris, 1979a, 1979b). The term 'mutually protected occlusion' represents canine-guided occlusion in lateral excursions protecting the posterior teeth (Figure 5.5). In the intercuspal position the pos-

terior teeth would contact leaving the anterior teeth out of contact.

3. *Group function occlusion:* During lateral excursions teeth other than the canine teeth are involved in contacts on the working side. Ultimately, the buccal cusps of the posterior teeth on the working side would all be in contact. This type of occlusion was shown to be relatively common by Beyron (1964) (Figure 5.6).

There appears to be no consensus on what an ideal occlusal scheme should be, and it is acknowledged that there is a difference in occlusions

- The ICP and the RCP should be coincident, meaning there should be good cuspal interdigitation of the posterior teeth in the intercuspal position with light or no contact on the anterior teeth (this is rare in the natural dentition but may be achievable if full-arch restorative or prosthodontic dental treatment is carried out)
- There should be no non-working side interferences
- In lateral excursions, there should be canine guidance or group function concentrated on anterior teeth (incisors, canine and premolars)
- In protrusive jaw movements, contact should be on the anterior teeth only with no posterior teeth contacting
- There should be good contact points between each tooth
- There should be multiple tooth contacts in the intercuspal position between opposing premolar and molar teeth

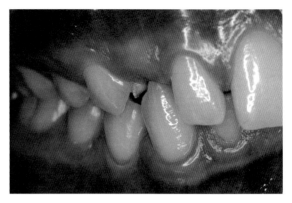

Figure 5.7   Excessive wear of the right maxillary primary canine opposing a permanent canine.

between individuals. Occlusal schemes may be more applicable to the provision of complete and partial dentures or fixed restorations. Nevertheless there appear to be a number of desirable features for a dynamic occlusion as set out in Box 5.1. If these features can be incorporated into a natural or restored dentition it is likely that the occlusion will be stable (Roth, 1976b; Timm *et al.*, 1976; Aubrey, 1978).

Age changes

As patients age, they undergo degenerative changes in the soft and hard tissues. These can affect any aspect of the masticatory system including the teeth and periodontium, the muscles, ligaments, temporomandibular joint, nerves and bone. The most significant effect on the occlusion will be tooth wear, which is believed to be multifactorial in nature, although in approximately 30% of cases the precise aetiology is unknown (Smith and Knight, 1984a). A minimal amount of tooth wear on the occlusal and interproximal areas is normal and is termed physiological (Berry and Poole, 1974,

1976). Pathological tooth wear is defined as 'tissue loss likely to prejudice the survival of the teeth' and clearly requires active intervention (Smith and Knight, 1984b). It has been observed in Scandinavia that there is dentine exposure from tooth wear in approximately 20% of adults aged between 20 and 29 years of age (Ekfeldt, 1989). Tooth wear appears to be more common in males than in females but the severity increases with age (Salonen, 1990). Johannson *et al.* (1993) suggested that tooth wear varies with time, occurring 'as bursts of activity', although it is likely that some individuals experience slow progressive continuous tooth wear throughout their lives. Alveolar bone growth often occurs to compensate for tooth wear and helps to maintain the occlusal vertical dimension (OVD) (Berry and Poole, 1974, 1976). However, where tooth wear has been rapid this may be accompanied by a reduction in the OVD and an increase in the interocclusal (or freeway) space. If overeruption of unopposed teeth occurs then disruption of the occlusal plane can ensue.

In patients with hypodontia the situation is complicated, as often they have retained primary teeth. It is clear that primary teeth wear less favourably than permanent teeth, although this has not been quantified. Primary teeth are usually lost through root resorption (Haselden *et al.*, 2001), but if retained for a long time they can eventually be lost through tooth wear. Occlusal discrepancies can occur when permanent teeth oppose primary teeth, which are slowly worn away with time (Figure 5.7).

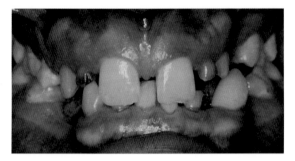

Figure 5.8 Occlusal disruption in a patient with severe hypodontia.

Features of occlusion in hypodontia patients

Patients with hypodontia seek a dentition with a good appearance and normal occlusion that is in keeping with their peers in society. There are a number of features that patients with hypodontia have which complicate the attainment of a normal occlusion (Figure 5.8). These are:

- Missing teeth
- Microdontia
- Retained primary teeth
- Delayed eruption of permanent teeth
- Deep overbite
- Reduced OVD
- Lack of anterior guidance and/or posterior stability if multiple teeth are missing

Occlusal variations depending on the severity of hypodontia

Patients with hypodontia may have single or multiple teeth missing. The need for extensive orthodontic treatment is likely to be greater when there are few teeth missing. More severe forms of hypodontia are associated with the absence of multiple permanent teeth with effects on the soft and hard tissues; the need for restorative treatment becomes greater in these situations. The occlusal aims of treatment are to provide an ideal occlusion with good anterior guidance and posterior stability. Whether spaces can be closed, re-created or improved on will depend on the severity of hypodontia and the degree of inherent crowding in the particular case. It is generally preferable to close spaces where aesthetics and function can be acceptable, eliminating the need for restorative work, which needs a lifetime of maintenance once provided. In patients with mild hypodontia there is likely to be little effect on the occlusion whether spaces are closed or maintained, although when upper lateral incisors are missing considerable planning and decision-making are required in relation to aesthetics. Where canine teeth are missing, the ability to provide good anterior or canine guidance is lost and group function occlusion would then be the aim of treatment.

Absent maxillary lateral incisor teeth

When maxillary lateral incisors are absent a decision has to be made whether to approximate the canine tooth next to the central incisor or to maintain the lateral incisor space. The aesthetic result is often determined by the contour and shade of the canine tooth. There is some evidence to suggest that there is better periodontal health after lateral incisor space closure than after space opening (Robertsson and Mohlin, 2000). However, from an occlusal point of view the preferred arrangement would be to maintain canine guidance. Unfortunately, the eruption of permanent canine teeth can be aberrant as a result of missing upper lateral incisors (Brin et al., 1986; Zilberman et al., 1990).

If space closure is carried out and the canine is placed in the upper lateral incisor position, the preferred occlusal outcome is a group function between the canine and the first premolar against the lower opposing teeth. It has been shown that the upper first premolar can act as a guidance tooth as long as it is organised in group function with adjacent teeth in excursions (Nordquist and McNeill, 1975). If possible the premolar should be rotated mesiopalatally to improve the aesthetics by hiding the palatal cusp and to improve contacts with the lower teeth. Also, to allow alignment of the both upper and lower arches it may be necessary to consider some reduction of the palatal cingulum of the canine tooth and palatal cusp of the first premolar (Rosa and Zachrisson, 2001). One long-term concern is tooth wear of the lower anterior teeth. The larger canine tooth opposes the incisor teeth, which are less able to cope with occlusal forces in the long term. The situation is worsened with time, or if the

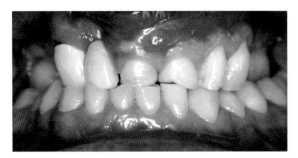

Figure 5.9 An unfavourable occlusion showing severe wear worsened by the conventional cantilever bridge UR2.

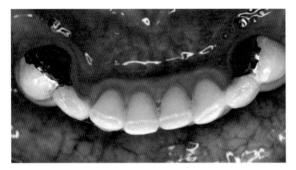

Figure 5.10 Cantilever resin-bonded bridges. The occlusion should be organised to avoid contacts on the pontics in excursions.

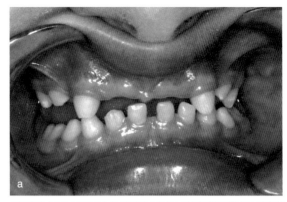

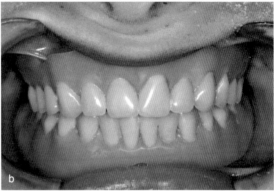

Figure 5.11 (a) Severe hypodontia in a young patient suitable for treatment with overdentures. (b) Complete overdentures restoring appearance, OVD and balanced occlusion.

canine tooth is restored with a porcelain or metal restoration (Figure 5.9).

If the space for the upper lateral incisor is preserved, conformative tooth replacement should be carried out. This could be achieved using a partial denture, resin-retained bridge or a single dental implant (Millar and Taylor, 1995). The occlusion must be arranged to protect the restoration, which is viewed as weaker than the natural teeth (Figure 5.10).

Occlusal variations as a result of microdontia

The management of the occlusion will vary depending on whether the microdontia is localised or generalised. If the microdontia is localised orthodontic treatment aims to equalise tooth spaces, and assuming that the tooth has a good prognosis it should be moved to the optimal position for restoration. The provision of the restoration should be in a conformative manner to achieve an ideal or canine-guided occlusion. As the severity of the microdontia increases, or is generalised, a decision has to be made whether all the teeth should be restored by a full-mouth reconstruction or whether sufficient improvement can be made with localised treatment to groups of teeth. Limited treatment should be carried out in a conformative manner. Significant disruptions to the occlusion and facial profile may involve a reorganised approach with removable overdentures (Figure 5.11).

Rotations, tilting, cross bites and abutment alignment

When space closure is contemplated, treatment of the malaligned teeth forms an integral part of the orthodontic treatment. Similarly if space maintenance is carried out it is important to provide ideal tooth positioning for potential abutment teeth for fixed or removable prostheses. For the best appearance and function, restorations require sufficient interdental, buccolingual and vertical space for ideal tooth replacement. The space required will be determined by whether or not the tooth to be replaced is a molar, premolar, canine or incisor. Where dental implants may be used, an imaginary cylinder of space of 6–7 mm diameter is required to accommodate the necessary components. If sufficient space is not available, inevitably the appearance and health of the gingival tissues are compromised.

When there is extreme shortage of space, the method of tooth replacement may need to be reconsidered since the restorations are unlikely to be durable in the long term. It is useful to plan for an ideal path of insertion for a fixed or removable prosthesis (Bowden and Harrison, 1994). The orthodontic uprighting of tilted molar teeth can also improve the occlusion in order to provide better intercuspation in the ICP (Ceen and Rubler, 1985). Sufficient interdental clearance is required to accommodate adequately thick restorations so as to improve their durability. Orthodontics can often reduce deep overbites in this respect and correct supra-erupted teeth (Thind et al., 2005).

Rotations are more common in patients with hypodontia (Baccetti, 1998) and when corrected orthodontically the aesthetics and occlusion are improved. Rotational correction can result in an increase or decrease in the availability of intra-arch space, depending on the tooth involved (Andrews, 1972). If a premolar is de-rotated, space will be generated (Figure 5.12); in contrast, additional space will be required if a lower incisor is de-rotated. Orthodontically de-rotated teeth frequently exhibit a high tendency to relapse, and may require extended or permanent retention (Littlewood et al., 2006a, 2006b).

Deep overbite

As the severity of hypodontia increases, there is an increased frequency of deep overbites (Øgaard and Krogstad, 1995; Chung et al., 2000). Overbite reduction is helpful in improving the aesthetics and occlusion and it has been reported that over time

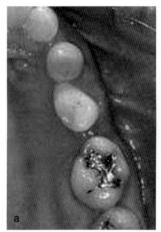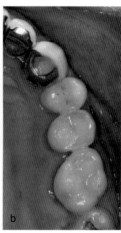

Figure 5.12   (a) Rotated premolar and molar preventing optimal occlusion and appearance. (b) Teeth de-rotated permitting conformative premolar replacement.

patients with a deep overbite appear to be more prone to severe tooth wear (Bauer et al., 1997; Mizrahi, 2006). In addition to reducing the potential for tooth wear in the future, if any anterior restorative work is required, an improved interocclusal space simplifies treatment. Overbite reduction is best carried out in younger patients, particularly during the pubertal growth spurt (Lawton and Selwyn-Barnett, 1975a, 1975b; McDowell and Baker, 1991).

A variety of orthodontic appliances can be used to reduce overbites, including removable appliances with bite planes or functional appliances (Lawton and Selwyn-Barnett, 1975a, 1975b; Sandler and DiBiase, 1996) (Figure 5.13). Bite planes are designed to reduce a deep overbite by relative intrusion of the lower anterior teeth. This is brought about by permitting the posterior teeth, which are held out of occlusion by the contact of the lower incisors with the bite plane, to continue to erupt, thus levelling the curve of Spee (Lawton and Selwyn-Barnett, 1975a, 1975b). Because this requires growth adaptation to a new OVD, bite planes are less effective in non-growing or adult patients.

Functional appliances can similarly provide overbite reduction in patients who also require correction of a Class II malocclusion, but this tends to be more associated with incisor tipping and molar overeruption (Ball and Hunt, 1991). Overbite reduc-

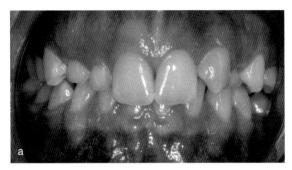

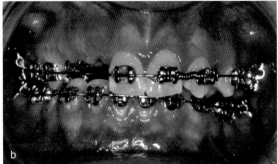

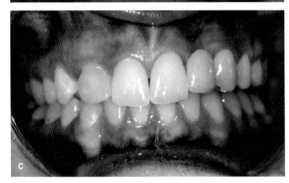

Figure 5.13 (a) Class II division 2 incisal relationship with increased overbite. (b) Overbite correction as part of fixed appliance therapy. (c) Overbite reduction complete after orthodontic treatment.

tion is more difficult when the hypodontia is more severe, since there are fewer posterior teeth to erupt.

Although overbite reduction is more difficult in adults, it can be more effectively carried out with metal bite planes (Dahl et al., 1975; Briggs et al., 1997; Gough and Setchell, 1999; Saha and Summerwill, 2004; Poyser et al., 2005; Mizrahi, 2006) (Figure 5.14). The original Dahl appliance was a removable device (Dahl et al., 1975) but these

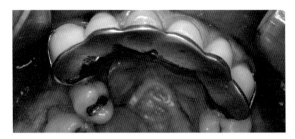

Figure 5.14 Incisal view of a removable metal bite plane (Dahl appliance) in a patient with a cleft lip and palate, and hypodontia.

appliances are now more frequently cemented to the teeth to improve compliance and effectiveness. A variation on this method is the bonding of composite resin to teeth to provide bite planes, a technique that has been shown to be effective in patients with tooth wear (Darbar and Hemmings, 1997; Redman et al., 2003) (Figure 5.15).

The use of fixed appliances with utility arches to produce intrusion of anterior teeth is a technique often favoured by orthodontists (Dake and Sinclair, 1989; Weiland et al., 1996). However, orthodontics for adults may be more complex because of the lack of growth potential, the presence of large restorations or bone loss due to periodontal disease (Shroff et al., 1996). These problems may occasionally necessitate the acceptance of an increased level of compromise in the final result.

Reduced occlusal vertical dimension (OVD)

A reduced OVD is common in patients who have severe hypodontia, generalised microdontia or a combination of the two conditions. The lower face height is reduced with the teeth in occlusion and the freeway space (FWS) is typically increased to 5–10 mm (Goodman et al., 1994; Hobkirk et al., 1995). The occlusion may also be deranged and there may be poor lip support. Invariably the restoration of the occlusion involves a reorganised approach whereby a new OVD is selected and a completely new occlusal scheme developed, determined by the type of prosthesis used.

As a diagnostic procedure, and often as a definitive treatment option, an overdenture can be

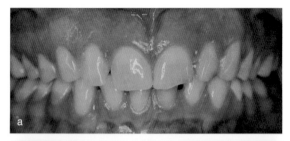

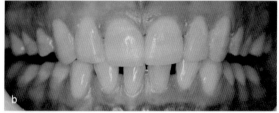

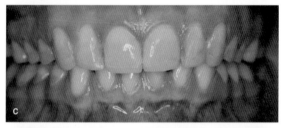

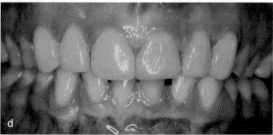

Figure 5.15 (a) Microdontia of maxillary lateral incisor teeth with localised anterior tooth wear. (b) Composite resin palatal and incisal restorations placed at an increased OVD (Dahl appliance) showing posterior disclusion. (c) Posterior occlusion re-established in 4 months. (d) Labial porcelain veneers placed on the anterior maxillary teeth.

employed. Overdentures may be complete or partial and may include overlay or onlay components (Hemmings *et al.*, 1995) (Figure 5.16). There are also variant components, which may be onlay or overlay in nature. The construction of such appliances and the factors influencing the final decision on the appropriate vertical dimension to select is well described in the prosthodontic litera-

ture (Hemmings *et al.*, 1995; Faigenblum, 1999). If the planned changes are not extensive it may be that the patient's original arch form is largely followed. If a more complex prosthesis is required in order to significantly expand the dental arch perimeter, similar complete denture techniques to those used for edentulous patients should be employed. When extreme changes in OVD are contemplated it is wise to use a diagnostic appliance in the first instance. This may be a simple occlusal splint appliance (Capp, 1999), although it is often more useful to have some form of partial denture which gives the patient an idea of the appearance of the final prosthesis. Some patients may be able to adapt to the new occlusion in a matter of weeks but others may need up to 6 months (Hemmings *et al.*, 1995). If it is possible to restore the dentition with fixed appliances an ideal occlusion should be aimed for (Hemmings and Harrington, 2004). If removable appliances are used, a bilaterally balanced occlusion would be more suitable.

Shortened dental arch

A shortened dental arch was first suggested by Käyser (1981) as a treatment option for the partially dentate elderly patient. Depending on the patient's age, eight to twelve occlusal units were considered acceptable for appearance and function (Allen *et al.*, 1996; Witter *et al.*, 1990, 1997, 1999). An occlusal unit comprises of two opposing teeth, and so a premolar occlusion would comprise ten occlusal units. This approach was considered acceptable as long as there was no significant dental pathology such as tooth wear, temperomandibular joint (TMJ) dysfunction or periodontal drifting of teeth (Witter *et al.*, 1990, 1991). Patients with severe hypodontia that includes absent molar teeth may find it acceptable to have a shortened dental arch with their remaining teeth (Kalk *et al.*, 1993) (Figure 5.17). Orthodontics may be able to close spaces and optimise occlusal contacts in the intercuspal position, while restorative treatment may be able to replace a small number of missing units or restore microdont teeth to provide a functional shortened dental arch (Kalk *et al.*, 1993). The occlusion for the fixed restorations would be organised as an ideal occlusion.

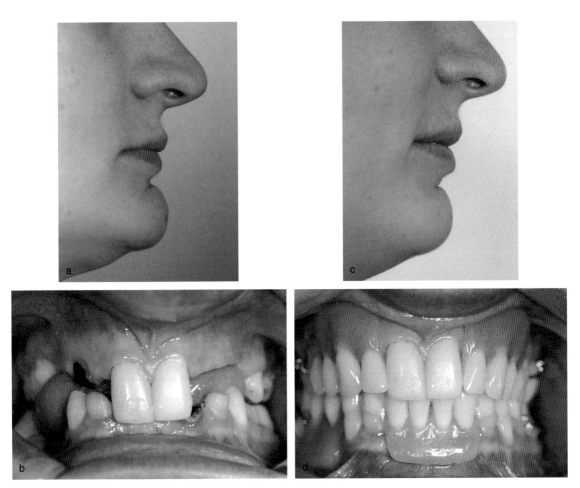

Figure 5.16   (a) Profile view of a patient with severe hypodontia showing over-closed appearance. (b) Anterior occlusion with deep overbite and reduced OVD. The URC[/] and LLB[/] are deteriorating as overdenture abutments. (c) Improved appearance following provision of partial overdentures. (d) Occlusion with partial overdentures in place.

Retained primary teeth

The prognosis for retained primary teeth is variable. Previous work has suggested that primary canine teeth show the least tendency to root resorption in the long term, while primary first molar teeth have a poor long-term prognosis, and primary second molar teeth have an unpredictable prognosis (Haselden et al., 2001). During growth, some primary teeth may become infra-occluded (Rune and Sarnäs, 1984; Kurol and Olson, 1991; Noble et al., 2007). If the dentition remains healthy these teeth can be restored to bring them back to a normal function and appearance (Kurol, 2006), although placing large occlusal loads on primary teeth should be avoided since it is likely to increase the rate of root resorption (Brezniak and Wasserstein, 1993; Davies et al., 2001; Rudzki-Janson et al., 2001; Nunn et al., 2003). The avoidance of lateral excursive tooth contacts on such restored primary teeth is prudent, and if the infra-occlusions are localised, then this is relatively easy to provide. If the infra-occlusions are present in a depleted dentition, however, then avoidance of occlusal loading on these teeth can be challenging. It is not uncommon to see primary canine teeth being retained into the third or fourth decade of life. Even if root resorption is not severe, it is likely that these teeth will be affected by tooth wear, and as this wear increases so the amount of canine guidance will

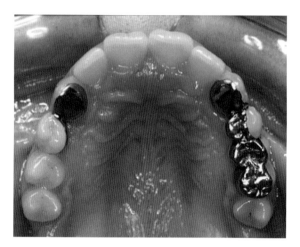

Figure 5.17 Shortened dental arch in a patient with hypodontia.

decrease. Such wear can sometimes be so severe that replacement of the primary canine teeth is extremely difficult because of overeruption of the opposing permanent canine tooth (Figure 5.7). In these cases interocclusal space needs to be generated by restorations or orthodontic treatment – in hindsight, earlier intervention may have permitted simpler treatment. Primary canines are smaller than their permanent successors and if retained there will be some aesthetic compromise, which will be less obvious if there is associated microdontia.

Restoration of the occlusion

The repair and restoration of individual teeth has been extensively documented in the dental literature. It is not the remit of this chapter to cover standard procedures for operative or restorative care. However, there are some aspects where occlusal principles need to be applied in the re-contouring or replacement of teeth for patients with hypodontia. The usual aim is not only to provide an ideal and stable occlusion but also to facilitate the provision of durable restorations or prostheses. For restorations to be successful in the long term it is important to control occlusal forces exerted on them and provide sufficient bulk of material to withstand such forces over a long period of time.

When teeth are to be repaired or replaced the dentist can either use a conformative or reorganised approach. With a conformative approach, restorations are provided in harmony with the existing jaw relationships (Celenza and Litvak, 1976). In this situation the intercuspal position is not altered and the restorations or prosthesis can conform to the current intercuspal position.

There are two possibilities when using a conformative approach:

1. The occlusion is untouched prior to operative treatment.
2. The occlusion is modified prior to treatment by minor occlusal adjustment. This may involve shortening of opposing tooth cusps, eliminating interferences or deflective tooth contacts (Wise, 1986).

When using a reorganised approach the entire occlusal scheme is modified such that the restorations or prosthesis are provided in harmony with the new jaw relationships. The main features of such an approach would be:

*   The retruded contact position is chosen as a reproducible occlusal position
*   An even stable occlusion is provided with posterior stability and anterior guidance
*   The occlusion is provided in harmony with border movements
*   Interferences or deflective contacts are avoided

A reorganised approach is indicated in the following circumstances:

*   If multiple posterior restorations or replacement of teeth is planned
*   If the tooth or teeth involved are initial contacts in retruded contact position, or a significant slide from the retruded contact position to the intercuspal position is present
*   If a planned change to the OVD is indicated
*   If there are signs and symptoms of occlusal pathology

If few teeth need to be replaced or small re-contouring restorations are indicated in patients with mild hypodontia it is likely that a conformative approach will be used. As the severity of hypodontia increases it is more likely that a reorganised approach to the restoration of the dentition is undertaken.

Plastic restorations, veneers and crowns

Patients with mild or severe hypodontia exhibit a higher prevalence of hypoplastic or microdont permanent teeth. They may also have retained primary teeth, which may require re-contouring to improve the appearance and durability. Composite resin or porcelain can function well in providing durable and aesthetic restorations for patients. Both these materials may be considered to be brittle or liable to fracture and wear, if not provided in sufficient bulk or insufficiently supported by tooth structure. Therefore tooth preparation and the manipulation of materials are important for long-term success (Mount and Hume, 2005). In the majority of circumstances such restorations are placed to conform to the existing occlusion. Occlusal contacts in lateral and protrusive excursions should be avoided as far as possible, however if contact is unavoidable the aim should be to provide a good thickness of material to maximise the strength of the restoration.

It may be that in some circumstances a heavy occlusal load is inevitable on restorations if the teeth involved are guidance teeth, or there is a reduced number of occluding teeth as is found in severe hypodontia. If there were doubts whether the material could withstand these occlusal forces the only option would be to provide a group function in an attempt to share the occlusal loads, or consider alternative restorations. If porcelain is used as a veneering material for a crown it should be supported by a good coping design, which is made of metal or strengthened porcelain. In extreme circumstances metal occlusal surfaces may be indicated (Figure 5.18). The metal may need to be extended to the incisal edge of the crown to avoid occlusal contacts on the weaker veneering material.

Occlusion on dentures

It is clear that many dentists achieve success with removable dentures by using varying occlusal phi-

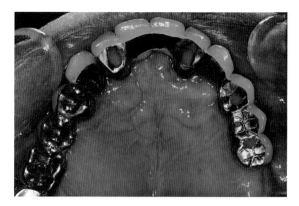

Figure 5.18   Metal palatal and occlusal surfaces to protect porcelain in a full-arch reconstruction supported by implants and teeth.

losophies. Although many observations and techniques in the past were scientifically unproven, they remain largely unchanged in clinical practice as accepted methods of care (Jacob, 1998). In cases of mild hypodontia, small numbers of teeth on a removable prosthesis should be provided in a conformative nature. Only intercuspal contacts should be arranged on the denture teeth, while guidance should be organised on the natural teeth. As the size of the denture increases it becomes impossible to avoid contact on denture teeth in excursions, and in these circumstances it is more successful to arrange a group function, sharing loads across multiple denture teeth (Winstanley, 1984). As the severity of the hypodontia increases, it may be that a complete denture or overdenture is made. These usually function best with a bilaterally balanced occlusion (Henderson, 2004) (Figure 5.19).

Resin-retained bridges

Resin-retained bridges are usually provided in a conformative manner, replacing a small number of missing teeth. They are rarely used to provide replacement of multiple missing teeth or for full-arch treatment. Originally, when new restorations were first provided in the 1980s, it was customary to reduce the opposing teeth to accommodate the retaining wing of the bridge. This concept has now been superseded by the use of the 'Dahl principle' whereby the bridges are cemented in 'high'. In young patients, intrusion of contacting teeth and

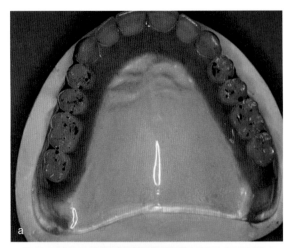

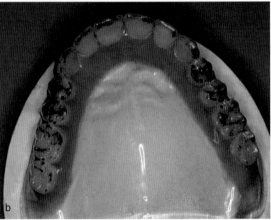

Figure 5.19 (a) Palatal ICP contacts on a complete overdenture. (b) Balancing occlusal contacts on a complete overdenture in left and right excursions.

overeruption of non-contacting teeth occurs within three to 6 months. In older patients this may take a little longer, between 6 and 12 months, but it is rare for these tooth movements not to occur (Hobkirk *et al.*, 1995; Djemal *et al.*, 1999; Gough and Setchell, 1999; St George *et al.*, 2002a, 2002b). Resin-retained bridges demonstrate the best survival when a small number of units are being replaced and cantilever designs are used (Djemal *et al.*, 1999). However, for enhanced orthodontic stability it is often requested that the resin-retained bridge design splints adjacent teeth that have been involved in significant tooth movements. Occasionally splinting can offer some extra benefit in that the anterior guidance can be organised across the retaining wings and the

pontics (Figure 5.11). It is useful to avoid heavy contacts on pontics particularly if cantilever designs are used. Any occlusal contact on the cantilever will be transmitted as a high occlusal force to the materials and supporting teeth (Taylor *et al.*, 2005). The use of aesthetic facings with a reduced occlusal table does not have a functional advantage unless there is an absence of occlusal contacts on the pontic.

Conventional bridges

The use of conventional bridges has been the mainstay of tooth replacement for over a 100 years. It is only in the last 25 years that their use has been largely supplanted by the successful utilisation of resin-retained bridges, and later dental implants. There are many standard protocols to help the clinician obtain a successful result from an occlusal point of view (Wise, 1995; Shillingburg *et al.*, 1997). When a small number of teeth are to be replaced, a conformative approach is employed. Occlusal adjustments may be minimal to optimise the interocclusal space and occlusal relationships. A reorganised approach would be used when the OVD needs to be increased or a full-mouth reconstruction is contemplated. In these cases an ideal occlusion would be prescribed, with ICP and RCP coincident, guidance on the anterior teeth in excursions, posterior disclusion, and even contacts in the intercuspal position.

Caution should be exercised when combining the 'Dahl principle' and conventional crowns on bridges. Most clinicians would employ the use of a Dahl appliance to create planned occlusal changes before providing definitive restorations. It is thought, but not proven, that the pulpal insult created by tooth preparation and occlusal adjustment at the same time may lead to an irreversible pulpitis. There is also some concern about the survival of temporary restorations if used in this way.

Dental implants

Single tooth and small-span dental implant restorations are usually provided in a conformative manner (Kim *et al.*, 2005; Gross, 2008), with the restorations provided with a slight infra-occlusion

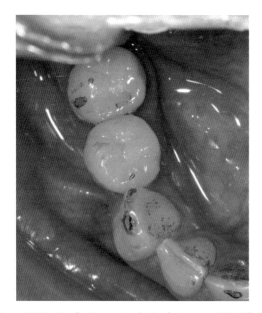

Figure 5.20 Occlusion on single implant crown LR4. The light contact on the implant crown should be removed so that a shimstock foil can be withdrawn when the teeth are in occlusion. This would leave contacts on the natural teeth and the conventional crown in light occlusion.

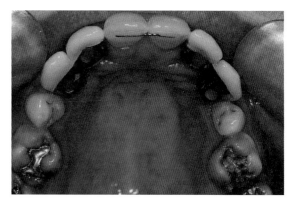

Figure 5.21 Implant-splinted crowns used to replace lateral incisors and canines. The occlusion in lateral excursions should be a group function, sharing load over the implants and natural teeth if possible.

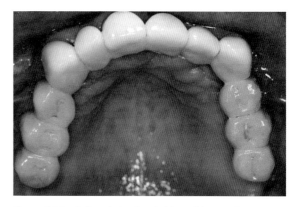

Figure 5.22 Full-arch implant bridge with posterior cantilevers replacing the first molars with premolar pontics. The occlusal contacts on the cantilevered pontics were minimal in ICP in order to reduce torquing forces.

of approximately 30 microns. This permits the withdrawal of a shimstock foil with a thickness of 10–12 microns, and it usually allows optimum patient comfort, taking into account the differential mobility between natural teeth and dental implants. It is important to avoid occlusal overload on dental implants (Misch *et al.*, 2005) (Figure 5.20). If heavy occlusal loads or guidance cannot be avoided on a long-span implant prosthesis it is important to space the implants out as far as possible to reduce bending moments. There is a definite biomechanical advantage to providing fixed implant bridges as fixed–fixed or splinted designs, since cantilever designs produce unfavourable stresses (Figure 5.21).

When a full-arch restoration is considered it is impossible to avoid occlusal contacts in the intercuspal position and all excursions. When a full-arch implant prosthesis opposes natural teeth or dental implants an ideal occlusion should be obtained so as to reduce wear of materials and the risk of occlusal pathology; such an arrangement is also prosthetically convenient during construction (Figure 5.22). When a full-arch implant bridge

opposes a complete denture then a bilateral balanced occlusion should be achieved. In this situation the occlusal forces are lower and the stability of the denture is more important.

Relapse, splinting and retainers

The risk of orthodontic relapse is significantly reduced if good anterior guidance and posterior stability are provided. It is also important to maintain interdental tooth contacts, which will frequently require the post-orthodontic replacement of absent teeth by fixed or removable methods. If complex orthodontic treatment has been carried out to redistribute space without restoring arch continuity, relapse should be expected. Orthodontic relapse is more common in hypodontia patients if space closure has been carried out in the absence of crowding (Carter *et al.*, 2003). A particularly common form of post-orthodontic relapse is the reopening of a median diastema between the upper central incisor teeth where appropriate splinting has not been carried out. Similarly rotations are prone to relapse. The reduction of a deep overbite is also likely to be unstable unless there is positive occlusal stop on the incisor teeth, and an appropriate lower incisal edge to upper incisor intercuspal relationship (Houston, 1989; Selwyn-Barnett, 1991, 1996).

For all these reasons, it is sensible to consider some form of splinting of one or both arches following orthodontic and restorative treatment, and prolonged retention in excess of 10 years or even as permanent retention in cases of space closure have been recommended (Rosa and Zachrisson, 2001). The long-term use of removable orthodontic retainers has been recommended particularly for patients requiring anterior tooth replacement, where any relapse is readily apparent (Vanarsdall, 1989). Immediately after orthodontic treatment, many patients will have a removable retainer fitted, either of a conventional acrylic plate design or a vacuum formed (Essix) retainer (Littlewood *et al.*, 2006a, 2006b). If sufficient tooth structure exists on teeth to be splinted, a fixed retainer could be provided in the form of a spiral wire and composite resin splint (Zachrisson, 1977, 2007; Littlewood *et al.*, 2006a, 2006b). If restorative treatment is required after orthodontic treatment it may be that a splinted bridge or implant prosthesis can be provided. In general terms there is no doubt that effective splinting is best provided by fixed splints, and most patients find it easier to maintain good oral hygiene and dental health by using fixed splints. However, the long-term maintenance is likely to be more frequent and costly when fixed splinting is involved. When restorative treatment is required after orthodontic treatment it should ideally be carried out after at least 3 months of use of an orthodontic retainer, with some centres preferring to carry out treatment 6 months after the completion of orthodontic treatment (Jepson *et al.*, 2003).

There is a higher mechanical failure rate with cantilever-design resin-retained bridgework (Hussey *et al.*, 1991), while there is also a higher failure rate if conventional bridgework is not maintained appropriately, with patients observing excellent oral hygiene (Walton *et al.*, 1986). However, it has been shown that long-span or cross-arch conventional bridges can be successful if stringent treatment planning has been carried out and excellent periodontal support is provided in the long term (Nyman and Lindhe, 1979; Laurell *et al.*, 1991; Kourkouta *et al.*, 2007).

Occlusal pathology

If occlusal forces overload the masticatory system pathology may ensue and the following clinical conditions may be observed:

- Temperomandibular joint dysfunction
- Tooth wear
- Periodontal bone loss and tooth mobility
- Fracture of teeth
- Fracture or failure of restorations
- Implant failure

There does not appear to be a high incidence of TMJ dysfunction in patients with hypodontia (Gesch *et al.*, 2004), although in adults a link has been suggested where there are more than five posterior teeth missing (McNamara *et al.*, 1995). There may be an increased tendency for tooth wear affecting the retained primary teeth. If the hypodontia is mild it is likely that the teeth and restorations will survive in the long term. As the severity increases higher maintenance must be expected. It is usually sensible to provide patients with an occlusal splint for long term use to protect their restored teeth or restorations. Careful review of the occlusion is important, as it will change with wear over time.

Conclusions

Treatment for patients with hypodontia aims to provide them with a functional occlusion with good aesthetics. Occlusal relationships can be considerably improved with orthodontics, however as the severity of hypodontia increases so the need for restorative treatment also increases. It is desirable to provide an ideal occlusion with canine guidance and posterior support in most circumstances. When complete dentures or overdentures are required it may be that a bilaterally balanced occlusion provides most comfort for the patient. In many circumstances, some element of compromise has to be accepted, although survival of the teeth or restorations will not be ideal if this is the case. An ideal occlusion for a treated hypodontia patient should provide the following:

- Class I incisal relationship
- Canine guidance
- Posterior stability
- No spacing and tight interproximal contacts
- Good tooth and gingival aesthetics
- Sufficient interocclusal space for appropriate thickness of restorative materials

Key Points: Managing the occlusion in hypodontia

- The occlusal aims of treatment are to provide an ideal occlusion with anterior guidance and posterior stability; orthodontics aims to provide ideal tooth spaces and optimise occlusal relationships.
- As the severity of hypodontia increases, the occlusion has to be shared between natural teeth and prosthetic replacements with a progression from an ideal occlusion to a group function, and finally a bilaterally balanced occlusion on complete or overdentures.
- With mild hypodontia, tooth replacement will usually be occlusally conformative. As the severity increases there will be an increasing need to consider a reorganised approach with a probable increase in the OVD.
- Single or small-span implant replacements are best placed in infra-occlusion of about 30 microns. Long-span or full-arch restorations have to accept full occlusal loads and perform best biomechanically if implants are splinted.
- Lifelong orthodontic stability can only be maintained if removable or fixed retainers are used.

References

Allen PF, Witter DF, Wilson NH, Käyser AF. Shortened dental arch therapy: Views of consultants in restorative dentistry in the United Kingdom. *J Oral Rehabil* 1996;23:481–485.

Al-Nimri KS, Bataineh AB, Abo-Farha S. Functional Occlusal patterns and their relationship to static occlusion. *Angle Orthod* 2010;80:65–71.

Andrews LF. The six keys to normal occlusion. *Am J Orthod* 1972;62:296–309.

Andrews LF. The diagnostic system: Occlusal analysis. *Dent Clin North Am* 1976;20:671–690.

Angle EH. Classification of malocclusion. *Dent Cosmos* 1899;41:248–64.

Angle EH. *Treatment of the Malocclusion of Teeth*, 7th edn. SS White Manufacturing, Philadelphia, 1907.

Aubrey RB. Occlusal objectives in orthodontic treatment. *Am J Orthod* 1978;74:162–175.

Baccetti T. Tooth rotation associated with aplasia of non-adjacent teeth. *Angle Orthod* 1998;68:471–474.

Ball JV, Hunt NP. The effect of Andresen, Harvold and Begg treatment on overbite and molar eruption. *Eur J Orthod* 1991;13:53–58.

Bauer W, van den Hoven F, Diedrich P. Wear in the upper and lower incisors in relation to incisal and condylar guidance. *J Orofac Orthop* 1997;58:306–319.

Becker CM, Kaiser DA. Evolution of occlusion and occlusal instruments. *J Prosthodont* 1993;2:33–43.

Bergendal B, Bergendal T, Hallonsten AL, *et al.* A multidisciplinary approach to oral rehabilitation with osseointegrated implants in children and adolescents with multiple aplasia. *Eur J Orthod* 1996;18:119–129.

Berry DC, Poole DF. Masticatory function and oral rehabilitation. *J Oral Rehabil* 1974;1:191–205.

Berry DC, Poole DF. Attrition: Possible mechanisms of compensation. *J Oral Rehabil* 1976;3:201–206.

Beyron HL. Occlusal relations and mastication in Australian aborigines. *Acta Odontol Scand* 1964;22:597–678.

Bishop K, Addy L, Knox J. Modern restorative management of patients with congenitally missing teeth: 1. Introduction, terminology and epidemiology. *Dent Update* 2006;33:531–537.

Bishop K, Addy L, Knox J. Modern restorative management of patients with congenitally missing teeth: 3. Conventional restorative options and considerations. *Dent Update* 2007a;34:30–38.

Bishop K, Addy L, Knox J. Modern restorative management of patients with congenitally missing teeth: 4. The role of implants. *Dent Update* 2007b;34:79–84.

Bowden DEJ, Harrison JE. Missing anterior teeth: Treatment options and their orthodontic implications. *Dent Update* 1994;21:428–434.

Brezniak N, Wasserstein A. Root resorption after ortho-dontic treatment: Part 2. Literature review. *Am J Orthod Dentofacial Orthop* 1993;103:138–146.

Briggs PF, Bishop K, Djemal S. The clinical evolution of the 'Dahl Principle'. *Br Dent J* 1997;183:171–176.

Brin I, Becker A, Shalhav M. Position of the maxillary permanent canine in relation to anomalous or missing lateral incisors: a population study. *Eur J Orthod* 1986; 8:12–16.

Capp NJ. Occlusion and splint therapy. *Br Dent J* 1999;186: 217–222.

Carter NE, Gillgrass TJ, Hobson RS, *et al.* The interdisci-plinary management of hypodontia: orthodontics. *Br Dent J* 2003;194:361–366.

Ceen RF, Rubler CG. Orthodontic intervention as an aid in restorative dentistry. *Dent Clin North Am* 1985;29: 279–291.

Celenza FV, Litvak H. Occlusal management in con-formative dentistry. *J Prosthet Dent* 1976;36:164–170.

Celenza FV, Nasedkin JN. *Position Paper in Occlusion. The State of the Art*. Quintessence Publishing, Chicago, 1978.

Chung LK, Hobson RS, Nunn JH, Gordon PH, Carter NE. An analysis of skeletal relationships in a group of young people with hypodontia. *J Orthod* 2000;27:315–318.

Clark JR, Evans RD. Functional occlusion: I. A review. *J Orthod* 2001;28:76–81.

Crawford SD. Condylar axis position, as determined by the occlusion and measured by the CPI instrument, and signs and symptoms of temporomandibular dys-function. *Angle Orthod* 1999;69:103–116.

D'Amico A. The canine teeth-normal functional relation of the natural teeth in man. *J South Calif Dent Assoc* 1958;26:6–23, 49–60, 127–142, 175–182, 194–208, 239–241.

Dahl KL, Krogstad O, Karlsen K. An alternative treat-ment in cases with advanced localized attrition. *J Oral Rehabil* 1975;2:209–214.

Dake ML, Sinclair PM. A comparison of Ricketts and Tweed-type arch levelling techniques. *Am J Orthod Dentofacial Orthop* 1989;95:72–78.

Darbar UR, Hemmings KW. Treatment of localized anterior toothwear with composite restorations at an increased OVD. *Dent Update* 1997;24:72–75.

Davies KR, Schneider GB, Southard TE, *et al.* Deciduous canine and permanent lateral incisor differential root resorption. *Am J Orthod Dentofacial Orthop* 2001;120: 339–347.

Dawson PE. *Evaluation, Diagnosis and Treatment of Occlusal Problems*. CV Mosby, St Louis, 1974.

Dawson PE. Centric relation: Its effect on occluso-muscle harmony. *Dent Clin North Am* 1979;23:169–180.

Djemal S, Setchell D, King P, Wickens J. Long-term sur-vival characteristics of 832 resin-retained bridges and splints provided in a post-graduate teaching hospital between 1978 and 1993. *J Oral Rehabil* 1999;26:302–320.

Dewey M, Anderson GM. *Practical Orthodontics*, 7th edn. CV Mosby, St Louis, 1948.

Ekfeldt A. Incisal and occlusal tooth wear and wear of some prosthodontic materials. An epidemiological and clinical study. *Swed Dent J Suppl* 1989;65:1–62.

Faigenblum M. Removable prostheses. *Br Dent J* 1999; 186:273–276.

Gesch D, Bernhardt O, Kirbschus A. Association of malocclusion and functional occlusion with temporo-mandibular disorders (TMD) in adults: A systematic review of population-based studies. *Quintessence Int* 2004;35:211–221.

Goodman JR, Jones SP, Hobkirk JA, King PA. Hypodontia: 1. Clinical features and the management of mild to moderate hypodontia. *Dent Update* 1994;21:381–384.

Gough MB, Setchell DJ. A retrospective study of 50 treat-ments using an appliance to produce localised occlusal space by relative axial tooth movement. *Br Dent J* 1999;187:134–139.

Gross MD. Occlusion in implant dentistry. A review of the literature of prosthetic determinants and current concepts. *Aust Dent J* 2008;53(Suppl.1):S60–68.

Haselden K, Hobkirk JA, Goodman JR, Jones SP, Hemmings KW. Root resorption in retained decidu-ous canine and molar teeth without permanent succes-sors in patients with severe hypodontia. *Int J Paediatr Dent* 2001:11:171–178.

Hellman M. Variation in occlusion. *Dent Cosmos* 1921;63: 608–619.

Hemmings K, Harrington Z. Replacement of missing teeth with fixed prostheses. *Dent Update* 2004;31:137–141.

Hemmings KW, Howlett JA, Woodley NJ, Griffiths BM. Partial dentures for patients with advanced tooth wear. *Dent Update* 1995;22:52–59.

Henderson D. Occlusion in removable partial prostho-dontics. *J Prosthet Dent* 2004;91:1–5.

Hobkirk JA, Goodman JR, Jones SP. Presenting com-plaints and findings in a group of patients attending a hypodontia clinic. *Br Dent J* 1994;177:337–339.

Hobkirk JA, King PA, Goodman JR, Jones SP. Hypodontia: 2. The management of severe hypodontia. *Dent Update* 1995;22:8–11.

Hobkirk JA, Nohl F, Bergendal B, Storhaug K, Richter MK. The management of ectodermal dysplasia and severe hypodontia. International conference state-ments. *J Oral Rehabil* 2006;33:634–637.

Hobson RS, Carter NE, Gillgrass TJ, *et al.* The interdisci-plinary management of hypodontia: the relationship between an interdisciplinary team and the general dental practitioner. *Br Dent J* 2003;194:479–482.

Houston WJ. Incisor edge-centroid relationships and overbite depth. *Eur J Orthod* 1989;11:139–143.

Howat AP. Orthodontics and health: Have we wid-ened our perspectives? *Community Dent Health* 1993;2: 29–37.

Hussey DL, Pagni C, Linden GJ. Performance of 400 adhesive bridges fitted in a restorative dentistry department. *J Dent* 1991;19:221–225.

Jacob RF. The traditional therapeutic paradigm: Complete denture therapy. *J Prosthet Dent* 1998;79:6–13.

Jepson NJ, Nohl FS, Carter NE, Gillgrass TJ, *et al.* The interdisciplinary management of hypodontia: restorative dentistry. *Br Dent J* 2003;194:299–304.

Johannson A, Haraldson T, Omar R, Kiliaridis S, Carlsson GE. A system for assessing the severity and progression of occlusal tooth wear. *J Oral Rehabil* 1993;20:125–131.

Kahn AE. Unbalanced occlusion in occlusal rehabilitation. *J Prosthet Dent* 1964;14:725–738.

Kalk W, Käyser AF, Witter DJ. Needs for tooth replacement. *Int Dent J* 1993;43:41–49.

Käyser AF. Shortened dental arches and oral function. *J Oral Rehabil* 1981;8:457–462.

Kim Y, Oh TJ, Misch CE, Wang HL. Occlusal considerations in implant therapy: Clinical guidelines with biomechanical rationale. *Clin Oral Implants Res* 2005;16: 26–35.

Kourkouta S, Hemmings KW, Laurell L. Restoration of periodontally compromised dentitions using cross-arch bridges. Principles of perio-prosthetic patient management. *Br Dent J* 2007;203:189–195.

Kurol J. Impacted and ankylosed teeth: why, when, and how to intervene. *Am J Orthod Dentofacial Orthop* 2006;129 (Suppl.4):S86–90.

Kurol J, Olson L. Ankylosis of primary molars–a future periodontal threat to the first permanent molars? *Eur J Orthod* 1991;13:404–409.

Laurell L, Lundgren D, Falk H, Hugoson A. Long-term prognosis of extensive polyunit cantilevered fixed partial dentures. *J Prosthet Dent* 1991;66:545–552.

Lauret JF, Le Gall MG. The function of mastication: A key determinant of dental occlusion. *Pract Periodontics Aesthet Dent* 1996;8:807–817.

Lauritzen AG. *Atlas of Occlusal Analyses.* HAH Publications, Colorado Springs, CO, 1974.

Lawton DB, Selwyn-Barnett B. Overbite: Variations and management: 1. *Dent Update* 1975a;2:183–190.

Lawton DB, Selwyn-Barnett B. Overbite: Variations and management: 2. *Dent Update* 1975b;2:238–245.

Littlewood SJ, Millett DT, Doubleday B, Bearn DR, Worthington HV. Orthodontic retention: A systematic review. *J Orthod* 2006a;33:205–212.

Littlewood SJ, Millett DT, Doubleday B, Bearn DR, Worthington HV. Retention procedures for stabilising tooth position after treatment with orthodontic braces. *Cochrane Database Syst Rev* 2006b; CD002283.

Lucia VO. Principles of articulation. *Dent Clin North Am* 1979;23:199–211.

McCollum BB, Evans RL. The gnathological concepts of Charles E. Stuart, Beverly B. McCollum and Harvery Stallard. *Georgetown Dent J* 1970;36:12–20.

McDowell EH, Baker IM. The skeletodental adaptations in deep bite correction. *Am J Orthod Dentofacial Orthop* 1991;100:370–375.

McHorris WH. Occlusion with particular emphasis on the functional and parafunctional role of anterior teeth. Part 1. *J Clin Orthod* 1979a;13:606–620.

McHorris WH. Occlusion with particular emphasis on the functional and parafunctional role of anterior teeth. Part 2. *J Clin Orthod* 1979b;13:684–701.

McNamara JA Jr, Seligman DA, Okeson JP. Occlusion, orthodontic treatment, and temporomandibular disorders: A review. *J Orofac Pain* 1995;9:73–90.

Millar BJ, Taylor NG. Lateral thinking: the management of missing upper lateral incisors. *Br Dent J* 1995;179: 99–106.

Misch CE, Suzuki JB, Misch-Dietsh FM, Bidez MW. A positive correlation between occlusal trauma and peri-implant bone loss: Literature support. *Implant Dent* 2005;14:108–116.

Mizrahi B. The Dahl principle: Creating space and improving the biomechanical prognosis of anterior crowns. *Quintessence Int* 2006;37:245–251.

Monson GS. Impaired function as a result of a closed bite. *J Am Dent Assoc* 1921;8:833–839.

Mount GJ, Hume WR. *Preservation and Restoration of Tooth Structure*, 2nd edn. Knowledge Books and Software, Queensland, 2005.

Noble J, Karaiskos N, Wiltshire WA. Diagnosis and management of the infraerupted primary molar. *Br Dent J* 2007;203:632–634.

Nohl F, Cole B, Hobson R, *et al.* The management of hypodontia: present and future. *Dent Update* 2008;35: 79–88.

Nordquist GG, McNeill RW. Orthodontic vs. restorative treatment of the congenitally absent lateral incisor: Long-term periodontal and occlusal evaluation. *J Periodontol* 1975;46:139–143.

Nunn JH, Carter NE, Gillgrass TJ, *et al.* The interdisciplinary management of hypodontia: background and role of paediatric dentistry. *Br Dent J* 2003;194:245–251.

Nyman S, Lindhe J. A longitudinal study of combined periodontal and prosthetic treatment of patients with advanced periodontal disease. *J Periodontol* 1979;50: 163–169.

Øgaard B, Krogstad O. Craniofacial structure and soft tissue profile in patients with severe hypodontia. *Am J Orthod Dentofacial Orthop* 1995;108:472–477.

Pameijer JHN. *Periodontal and occlusal factors in crown and bridge procedures.* Amsterdam Dental Centre for Postgraduate CourseS, 1983.

Posselt U. Studies in the mobility of the human mandible. *Acta Odontol Scand Suppl* 1952;10:1–160.

Poyser NJ, Porter RW, Briggs PF, Chana HS, Kelleher MG. The Dahl Concept: Past, present and future. *Br Dent J* 2005;198:669–676.

Proffit WR, Fields HW Jr, Sarver DM. *Contemporary Orthodontics*, 4th edn. Mosby Elsevier, St Louis, 2007.

Redman CD, Hemmings KW, Good JA. The survival and clinical performance of resin-based composite restorations used to treat localised anterior tooth wear. *Br Dent J* 2003;194:566–572.

Rinchuse DJ, Sassouni V. An evaluation of eccentric occlusal contacts in orthodontically treated subjects. *Am J Orthod* 1982;82:251–256.

Robertsson S, Mohlin B. The congenitally missing upper lateral incisor. A retrospective study of orthodontic space closure versus restorative treatment. *Eur J Orthod* 2000;22:697–710.

Rosa M, Zachrisson BU. Integrating esthetic dentistry and space closure in patients with missing maxillary lateral incisors. *J Clin Orthod* 2001;35:221–234.

Roth RH. Five year clinical evaluation of the Andrews straight-wire appliance. *J Clin Orthod* 1976a;10:836–850.

Roth RH. The maintenance system and occlusal dynamics. *Dent Clin North Am* 1976b;20:761–788.

Rudzki-Janson I, Paschos E, Diedrich P. Orthodontic tooth movement in the mixed dentition. Histological study of a human specimen. *J Orofac Orthop* 2001;62:177–190.

Rune B, Sarnäs KV. Root resorption and submergence in retained deciduous second molars. A mixed-longitudinal study of 77 children with developmental absence of second premolars. *Eur J Orthod* 1984;6:123–131.

Saha S, Summerwill AJ. Reviewing the concept of Dahl. *Dent Update* 2004;31:442–447.

Salonen L. Oral health status in an adult Swedish population. A cross-sectional epidemiological study of the northern Alvsborg county. *Swed Dent J Suppl* 1990;70:1–49.

Sandler J, DiBiase D. The inclined biteplane – A useful tool. *Am J Orthod Dentofacial Orthop* 1996;110:339–350.

Selwyn-Barnett BJ. Rationale of treatment for Class II division 2 malocclusion. *Br J Orthod* 1991;18:173–181.

Selwyn-Barnett BJ. Class II/Division 2 malocclusion: A method of planning and treatment. *Br J Orthod* 1996;23:29–36.

Shafi I, Phillips JM, Dawson MP, Broad RD, Hosey MT. A study of patients attending a multidisciplinary hypodontia clinic over a five year period. *Br Dent J* 2008;205:649–652.

Shillingburg HT Jr, Hobo S, Whitsett LD, Jacobi R, Brackett SE. *Fundamentals of Fixed Prosthodontics*, 3rd edn. Quintessence Publishing, Carol Stream, IL, 1997.

Shroff B, Siegel SM, Feldman S, Siegel SC. Combined orthodontic and prosthetic therapy. Special considerations. *Dent Clin North Am* 1996;40:911–943.

Smith BGN, Knight JK. A comparison of patterns of tooth wear with aetiological factors. *Br Dent J* 1984a:157:16–19.

Smith BGN, Knight JK. An index for measuring the wear of teeth. *Br Dent J* 1984b;156:435–438.

St George G, Hemmings K, Patel K. Resin-retained bridges re-visited. Part 1: History and indications. *Prim Dent Care* 2002a;9:87–91.

St George G, Hemmings K, Patel K. Resin-retained bridges re-visited. Part 2: Clinical considerations. *Prim Dent Care* 2002b;9:139–144.

Taylor TD, Wiens J, Carr A. *Evidence-based considerations for removable prosthodontic and dental implant occlusion: A literature review.* University of Connecticut School of Dental Medicine, University of Detroit Mercy, Mayo College of Medicine, 2005.

Thind BS, Stirrups DR, Forgie AH, Larmour CJ, Mossey PA. Management of hypodontia: Orthodontic considerations (II). *Quintessence Int* 2005;36:345–353.

Timm TA, Herremans EL, Ash MM Jr. Occlusion and orthodontics. *Am J Orthod* 1976;70:138–145.

Tipton RT, Rinchuse DJ. The relationship between static occlusion and functional occlusion in a dental school population. *Angle Orthod* 1991;61:57–66.

Vanarsdall RL. Orthodontics: Provisional restorations and appliances. *Dent Clin North Am* 1989;33:479–496.

Vlachos CC. Occlusal principles in orthodontics. *Dent Clin North Am* 1995;39:363–378.

Walton JN, Gardner FM, Agar JR. A survey of crown and fixed partial denture failures: Length of service and reason for replacement. *J Prosthet Dent* 1986;56:416–421.

Weiland FJ, Bantleon HP, Droschl H. Evaluation of continuous arch and segmented arch leveling techniques in adult patients – A clinical study. *Am J Orthod Dentofacial Orthop* 1996;110:647–652.

Winstanley RB. Prosthodontic treatment of patients with hypodontia. *J Prosthet Dent* 1984;52:687–691.

Wise MD. *Failure in the Restored Dentition: Management and Treatment.* Quintessence Publishing, Chicago, 1995.

Wise MD. *Occlusal and Restorative Dentistry for the General Practitioner*, 2nd edn. British Dental Association, London, 1986.

Witter DJ, Allen PF, Wilson NH, Käyser AF. Dentists' attitudes to the shortened dental arch concept. *J Oral Rehabil* 1997;24:143–147.

Witter DJ, Cramwinckel AB, van Rossum GM, Käyser AF. Shortened dental arches and masticatory ability. *J Dent* 1990;18:185–189.

Witter DJ, De Haan AF, Käyser AF, Van Rossum GM. Shortened dental arches and periodontal support. *J Oral Rehabil* 1991;18:203–212.

Witter DJ, van Palenstein Helderman WH, Creugers NH, Käyser AF. *Community Dent Oral Epidemiol* 1999;27: 249–258.

Worsaae N, Jensen BN, Holm B, Holsko J. Treatment of severe hypodontia-oligodontia–an interdisciplinary concept. *Int J Oral Maxillofac Surg* 2007;36:473–480.

Zachrisson BU. Clinical experience with direct-bonded orthodontic retainers. *Am J Orthod* 1977;71:440–448.

Zachrisson BU. Long-term experience with direct-bonded retainers: update and clinical advice. *J Clin Orthod* 2007;41:728–737.

Zilberman Y, Cohen B, Becker A. Familial trends in palatal canines, anomalous lateral incisors, and related phenomena. *Eur J Orthod.* 1990;12:135–139.

6 Supporting Tissues

Introduction

Hypodontia by definition involves the absence of teeth, and may be associated with other changes in the structure and dimensions of the tissues in the orofacial region as described in Chapter 4. These commonly detract from the appearance and function of the mouth and may consequently reduce the quality of a patient's life. Although such problems are often amenable to treatment, this may be challenging due to their severity, the involvement of several structures and the need to provide care for a young patient. Treatment is often influenced by the form and function of the perioral tissues. For example, a decision to orthodontically reposition a tooth will be related not only to the desired outcome but also to the contours and activity of the related soft tissues and the shape and volume of adjacent alveolar bone. Similarly the replacement of multiple missing teeth using dental implants may be compromised by the shape and size of the potential maxillary and mandibular surgical envelopes and their vertical and horizontal relationships.

While it is convenient to examine issues relating to the various supporting tissues individually, in practice they should be considered collectively when exploring potential treatment options.

The oral cavity

The management of hypodontia should be based on the effects of the condition on the patient as an individual, and their wishes as to its management. The treatment plan should therefore take account of the patient's general health and any social, cultural and educational impacts of the condition. Nevertheless, important as these systemic considerations are, any dental treatment will be significantly influenced by changes in the oral tissues as a result of the patient's hypodontia, and the local effects of any associated systemic disorders such as one of the ectodermal dysplasias.

The oral cavity is delineated laterally by the cheeks, anteriorly by the lips, inferiorly by the floor of the mouth and mandible, and superiorly

Hypodontia: A Team Approach to Management, First Edition
© J.A. Hobkirk, D.S. Gill, S.P. Jones, K.W. Hemmings, G.S. Bassi, A.L. O'Donnell and J.R. Goodman
Published 2011 by Blackwell Publishing Ltd

by the maxilla. Posteriorly lies the oropharynx, from which it may be separated partially or totally by the actions of the tongue, the fauces and the soft palate. The space is also markedly influenced internally by the morphology and functions of the tongue. The vertical dimension of the envelope with the teeth, if any, in occlusion is determined by their eruption and occlusal contacts, and the vertical growth of alveolar bone, while at rest the freeway space (FWS) influences the rest vertical dimension (RVD).

Within the oral cavity and perioral tissues lie two three-dimensional spaces of crucial importance to the clinician – the surgical and prosthetic envelopes. The former lies predominantly within the jaw bones and defines the space potentially available for the placement of dental implants. The latter lies within the oral cavity where it demarcates the spaces available for the positioning of prosthetic restorations used to replace missing teeth and their supporting tissues. The interrelationships of these two spaces are critical in planning treatment, while their boundaries are often amenable to adjustment by surgical, orthodontic or prosthodontic techniques.

The prosthetic envelope in each dental arch has its occlusal surface determined by its static and dynamic relationships with the opposing teeth, whether they are natural or artificial, while the shape of the alveolar processes and adjacent soft tissues determine the envelope's lingual, buccal, alveolar and sometimes distal boundaries. Teeth adjacent to an edentulous area similarly demarcate the mesial and distal aspects of the envelope within the dental arch.

It is important to recognise that where the contours of the prosthetic envelope are determined by soft tissues, and especially muscles, then its shape is very variable and may at rest be only potential. This is particularly the case where patients have few teeth or are edentulous. In these situations the cheeks will tend to collapse lingually while the tongue spreads laterally. As a result there may be little or no space physically present when the patient is at rest, although the insertion of a prosthesis, which in effect creates a space, may provide the patient with improved function and appearance. The provision of support in this way requires the estimation of an optimal boundary for the envelope which is obtained by tissue displacement when recording

impressions and jaw relationships, and when determining the positions of the artificial teeth.

The cheeks, lips and tongue

The cheeks are formed by the buccinator muscles, which are inserted superiorly and inferiorly into the mandible and maxilla, and distally into the pterygomandibular raphae, which lie on the lingual aspect of the mandible. Anteriorly their fibres decussate to form the corners of the mouth. This arrangement enables the buccinator muscle to work with the tongue in keeping a food bolus between the posterior teeth during mastication, acting from the buccal aspect of the dental arch, while the tongue retains the food bolus between the teeth from the lingual aspect. Anteriorly the modiolus touches the tongue, preventing escape of the bolus in this direction, while a similar effect occurs distally where the fibres of buccinator sweep behind the last molar teeth to be inserted into the pterygomandibular raphe. Where teeth are missing, the muscles tend to adapt to control the bolus despite the spaces in the arch.

The contours of the cheeks are influenced by the support provided by the teeth and are also related to the rest and occlusal vertical dimensions. The lack of posterior teeth results in the cheeks tending to collapse lingually due to inadequate support, resulting in an unsatisfactory appearance similar to that of an edentulous individual. A comparable effect occurs when the freeway space is large, allowing the patient to approximate the mandible more closely to the maxilla than normal. While it has been found that the majority of individuals with hypodontia have a freeway space within the normal range in some this is greatly increased (Hobkirk et al., 1994) especially where there is a lack of occluding posterior teeth, tooth surface loss especially of primary teeth, or reduced alveolar development (Figure 6.1). These effects become more evident with increasing age and loss of tissue elasticity.

The lips are formed by the orbicularis oris and buccinator muscles, of which those fibres closest to the labial margins decussate, thus facilitating the production of a labial seal. These muscles are capable of a wide range of movements by virtue of their intrinsic structure and the muscles inserted

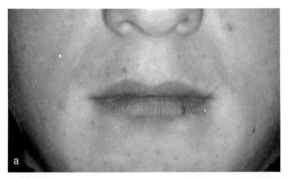

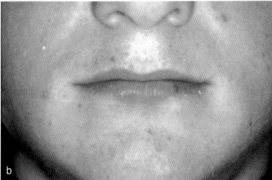

Figure 6.1   An increased freeway space is often evident when viewing a patient in (a) repose and (b) the intercuspal position.

into them, which can make local modifications to their shape. These comprise the quadratus labii superioris and inferioris, caninus, zygomaticus, mentalis, triangularis (also known as the depressor anguli oris) and risorius.

The shape and activity of the lips are of considerable importance in the management of hypodontia. In repose, while they may not expose the dentition, their contours hint at the positions of the underlying teeth, frequently in the case of people with hypodontia suggesting either their absence or diminutive size. Where the patient has a longer or shorter lip than usual then this will influence the visibility of the anterior teeth when the lip is at rest.

In function the lips form a dynamic frame for the dentition within which the patient, and all with whom they come into contact, view their teeth, and sometimes their surrounding structures, especially in the anterior maxilla. The extent to which the clinical crowns of the upper anterior teeth are evident when smiling is affected by lip length and

activity, the level of the maxillary occlusal plane, and the anteroposterior positions of the teeth, as well as by delayed tooth eruption and by gingival height. A low occlusal plane will tend to make the teeth more evident, and vice versa, while teeth that are more labially positioned will tend to effectively shorten the lip, making them appear more prominent. The length of the lips and the extent to which they move in function also affects the visibility of the teeth, a high lip-line when smiling making them more apparent. These matters are of importance when planning treatment in patients with hypodontia, as any procedure that effectively moves the anterior teeth labially will apparently shorten the lips and make the crowns of the teeth more evident. This can occur for example by orthodontic procedures or prosthodontic techniques such as crown re-contouring with adhesive restorations, veneers or conventional crowns, or the provision of an overdenture. Often it is necessary to alter the appearance of microdont teeth or those moved orthodontically into a substitute location, or to replace missing teeth with fixed or removable restorations, all of which are challenging in the anterior segment, especially if the lip-line is high when it is at rest or active. Where implant treatment is being planned this situation can be especially difficult to manage as the point of emergence of the implant superstructure through the soft tissues may be visible. If the alveolar bone is not optimally shaped for this procedure then the dictates of the bony contours may require compromise in the location of the implant body, which can be difficult to disguise. Often in these circumstances the associated soft tissues also tend to have an unnatural appearance.

The tongue is a highly active and muscular organ with important functions in mastication, deglutition and speech. Its great mobility is derived from three groups of intrinsic muscles, inferior and superior longitudinal, transverse and vertical, together with four paired extrinsic muscles: the genioglossus, styloglossus, palatoglossus and hyoglossus. It is capable of subtle movement with low forces as well as generating much higher loads. These can influence the buccolingual and labiolingual positions of the natural teeth and exert destabilising forces on removable prostheses. In addition, a habitual positioning of the tongue between opposing teeth is thought to be associated with their

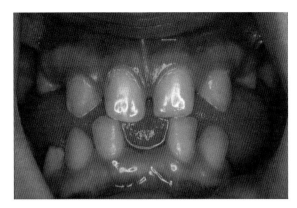

Figure 6.2 Failure of jaw growth and eruption of posterior teeth creating a large vertical occlusal deficiency and allowing the tongue to spread laterally.

impeded eruption, and can also arise where these fail to erupt fully or there is a failure of jaw growth (Figure 6.2).

Mucosa

While there is little evidence of oral mucosal changes in patients with hypodontia it is recognised that those with an ectodermal dysplasia may have a reduced salivary flow (Bergendal *et al.*, 2006), which may make the oral mucosa and periodontal tissues more prone to infection, create problems in the use of removable prostheses and place the teeth at increased risk of caries. It has been reported that such individuals may have a reduced production of mucus in the respiratory tract with associated mucosal symptoms (Siegel and Potsic, 1990), as well as symptoms of dry eyes related to a reduced lachrymal flow (Kaercher, 2004).

Intraoral forces

The dental arches are subject to forces generated during mastication, deglutition and speech, although the latter two are significantly smaller.

In Western populations the average maximum occlusally directed force has been reported to be in the range of 600–750N between the molar teeth (Hagberg, 1987), 120–350N between the canine

teeth (Lyons and Baxendale, 1990), and 140–200N between the incisors (Hellsing, 1980). Typical chewing forces are however rather lower, being in the order of 100–150N on natural teeth and implant-supported fixed prostheses (Richter, 1995). They also appear to vary considerably from individual to individual, an effect which is often greater than that of the food being chewed (Hobkirk and Psarros, 1992). Masticatory forces are exerted not only down the long axes of the teeth but also horizontally as a result of the effects of the non-linear path of the mandible during mastication, the forces resulting from the viscosity of the food bolus during the lateral movements of chewing, and the angulation of the cusps of posterior teeth and guiding contacts on anterior teeth. Horizontally acting forces are also generated by the actions of the cheeks, lips and tongue during mastication, deglutition and speech. These forces can influence the buccolingual and labiolingual positions of the natural teeth, however they are much lower than the vertically directed forces, being reported by Richter (1998) as approximately 11N (±1.5N) for the oral forces and 21N (±6N) for the buccal forces acting on dental implants at the level of the ridge crest.

The lips also generate forces on the anterior teeth which are important in relation to the stability of their positions, whether they are natural or artificial. Full lips which do not contract markedly in function will allow for the positioning of prosthetic anterior teeth, which are relatively labial to the alveolar ridges, or natural teeth, which are proclined in a normal fashion, while lips which are tense exert higher labial forces that will tend to unstabilise removable prostheses or retrocline natural anterior teeth. These anatomical and functional features are of importance when planning orthodontic tooth movement as they can influence the feasibility of the procedure and the stability of the final outcome. Equally they are of significance when preparing for prosthodontic care as restorations should equally be in a harmonious functional relationship with the surrounding soft tissues.

It has been shown that increasing the horizontal bulk of a prosthesis which restores a mandibular free-end saddle will result in it being subjected to greater lingually and buccally directed forces in function. While these reduce over time as a result of adaptation, the effect is somewhat restricted (Yazdanie and Hobkirk, 1997).

The development of patterns of activity in the perioral tissues and the tongue is related to the development of the dentition. Where teeth are missing it has been suggested that speech development in particular may be adversely affected, although the evidence for this is based only on a small numbers of cases (Tarjan *et al.*, 2005) and the reported views of parents of children with hypodontia.

Intraoral space

Horizontal dimension

In an edentulous patient or one with few remaining posterior teeth the cheeks tend to collapse lingually and the tongue to spread laterally. As a result the space that would normally be occupied by the teeth and their supporting structures becomes much reduced or almost non-existent due to the activity of the soft tissues. When replacing the missing teeth and their supporting structures with a prosthesis it is necessary to reclaim this space so as to provide a more natural appearance. This necessitates the recording of impressions that displace the soft tissues in order to record the optimum shape for the restoration, and requires techniques, impression trays and materials that will produce this in a controlled manner. The procedure is therefore fundamentally different to that involved when recording impressions for the fabrication of fixed restorations, in which accurate replication of the existing clinical situation is vital. In the former situation, the clinician needs to exercise judgement as to which soft tissue contours are to be created and their relevance to the intended outcome.

Vertical dimension

The vertical dimension of the space, like its horizontal counterpart, is infinitely variable within physiological limits. It is conventionally considered in terms of the rest and occlusal vertical dimensions (the RVD and OVD, respectively), and the vertical separation between the two, or freeway space (FWS). While it is technically possible to measure these dimensions, there are currently no

simple and accurate clinical methods of doing so (Baba *et al.*, 2000). Indeed they are considered as being measured between points on the maxilla and mandible, which in prosthodontic practice are not precisely defined. As a result, assessment of OVD and RVD requires a largely subjective interpretation by the clinician, supplemented by the use of a number of measuring techniques of dubious accuracy and repeatability. Consequently it has been recommended that a range of methods should be employed (Walther, 2003).

The OVD is determined by maxillary and mandibular growth, eruption of the dentition, and alveolar bone formation (Lux *et al.*, 2004). It is also influenced by tooth wear and it has been suggested, on the basis of studies in older individuals, that where there is a balancing correction of the effects of this wear on OVD due to tooth eruption and growth of the mandible and alveolar bone then the OVD will remain largely unchanged. However, when these mechanisms over- or undercompensate, it has been proposed that the OVD will increase or decrease (decreasing with a corresponding increase in the freeway space) (Berry and Poole, 1976).

In the case of individuals with hypodontia, tooth wear is often seen as a result of fewer occluding pairs of teeth and the retention of primary teeth, which are less resistant to wear than the permanent teeth (Correr *et al.*, 2007), beyond an age when they would normally be shed.

Tooth wear, sometimes referred to as tooth surface loss (TSL), is a normal process unless it prejudices tooth survival or is of concern to the patient (when it is classified as pathological). Its causes are multifactorial and include erosion, attrition and abrasion (Table 6.1) although erosion is a

Table 6.1   The principal causes of tooth surface loss.

Type	Definition
Erosion	The progressive loss of hard dental tissues by chemical processes (acids) not involving bacterial action
Attrition	The loss by wear of tooth substance or a restoration caused by mastication or contact between occluding or approximal surfaces
Abrasion	The loss by wear of tooth substance or a restoration caused by factors other than tooth contact

significant factor in most cases of tooth surface loss (Smith and Knight, 1984).

Erosion is caused principally by diet, although there are other factors such as regurgitation of gastric contents, medication and occupational hazards. A major factor is the consumption of carbonated drinks, which have a low pH and in some formulations are perceived as a 'healthy' dietary item. This problem is obviously of particular concern to people with hypodontia who are already suffering from a dental deficit. Where a patient has hypohidrotic ectodermal dysplasia then there may be a reduced salivary flow, with the resultant problems of delayed clearance of food from the mouth and less effective buffering capacity. Such patients may also choose to drink more carbonated drinks to lubricate their mouths.

Excessive attrition can occur as a result of a tooth-grinding habit, or where only a small number of occluding teeth are available for mastication, while undue abrasion is also typically associated with incorrect tooth brushing or occasionally an excessively abrasive diet.

The rest position of the mandible, and hence the RVD, varies within each person. It may be influenced by many factors including:

- Speech
- Emotion
- The jaw relationship
- Alveolar resorption
- Head position
- Loss of natural tooth contacts
- Some types of medication, whether prescription or recreational

The assessment of its adequacy is usually based on estimates of the freeway space and an assessment of the patient's appearance at the OVD where this is possible (Toolson and Smith, 1982).

The OVD may be increased readily using both removable and fixed prostheses, as discussed in Chapters 5 and 9. Conversely there are occasions where it is desirable to intrude teeth to facilitate prosthodontic procedures, for example to provide space for a connector on a removable partial denture (RPD) or an implant crown or a pontic. Intrusion may be carried out using temporary fixed onlays (Poyser *et al.*, 2005) or as part of orthodontic mechanotherapy.

The teeth

Hypodontia, by definition, involves the congenital absence of teeth, as discussed in detail in Chapter 1. The principal complaints relating to missing teeth found in patients attending a multidisciplinary hypodontia clinic are the absence of the teeth and the spacing between the reduced number present (Hobkirk *et al.*, 1994).

Tooth eruption

Delayed eruption and failure to erupt fully are features of hypodontia that can have significant effects on the appearance of the mouth and any treatment procedures (Figures 6.3–6.5).

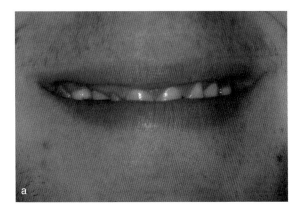

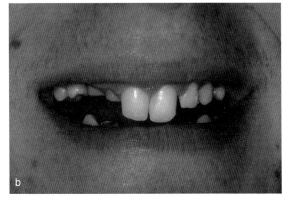

Figure 6.3 (a) Patient who has developed a habit of covering his maxillary teeth when smiling in an attempt to disguise their appearance. This is evident in (b) when the patient smiles in a more relaxed fashion.

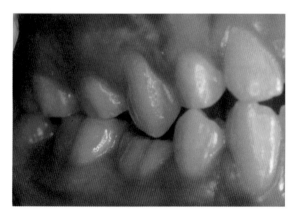

Figure 6.4   Overeruption of UR3 opposed by an infra-occluded LRE, resulting in a reduced prosthetic envelope in the second premolar region.

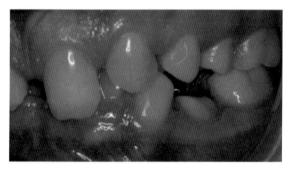

Figure 6.5   Overeruption of the teeth opposing the infra-occluded LLE has been prevented by their occlusal contacts. The angulations of the roots of LL2 and LL3, however, may encroach on the surgical envelope in the anterior mandible, while the relationships of UR1 and UL1 to the mandible in the intercuspal position similarly challenge the prosthetic envelope.

Appearance

The location of the teeth can significantly influence the effects of hypodontia both directly, by detracting from the appearance of the mouth (especially where the upper jaw is affected), and indirectly by its effects on treatment requirements and any potential restorative and orthodontic procedures needed to meet them.

If the remaining teeth are in the inter-canine area and have normal contact points then the effects on the patient's appearance are likely to be significantly less than if there were spaces in the first premolar region. Complaints about oral appear-

ance may relate not only to missing teeth but also to microdontia and severely tapered teeth. These give them an unappealing appearance as well as often resulting in spacing, which has a similar effect.

The number of missing teeth is thus partly related to the most common complaints (Figure 2.13) in this group of patients (Hobkirk *et al.*, 1994), although the locations of those that are present are also important in terms of the effects of the hypodontia on appearance and the number of occluding pairs of teeth.

From the viewpoint of treatment, the numbers and locations of the missing teeth partly define the extent of any potential restorations as well as placing restrictions on their design. Other key factors are the size and shape of the teeth and the presence or absence of any crowding in the arches. This is unusual in hypodontia, but may be manifested as a lack of space to replace all the missing teeth. In itself this is rarely a problem, provided there is room for the six anterior teeth and one premolar on either side of the arch. Since a natural appearance is best obtained with teeth of normal dimensions it is often necessary to orthodontically move teeth to optimise the final outcome by permitting the re-contouring of microdont teeth to a more appropriate size and the replacement of missing teeth on a similar basis.

Masticatory problems

Patients with hypodontia rarely complain about masticatory difficulties, possibly because they lack personal experience of eating with a complete dentition. While there is little evidence that such individuals tend to limit their diets by avoiding foods that are difficult to chew, it has been shown that the edentulous elderly, or those with very few occluding pairs of teeth do restrict their food choice (Walls *et al.*, 2000; Nowjack-Raymer and Sheiham, 2007). It is probable that patients with anodontia or severe hypodontia may be similarly affected.

Speech

Speech problems are thought to be more common when there are many teeth missing. There have

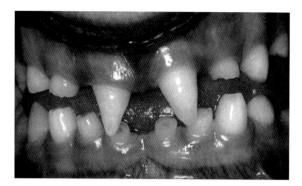

Figure 6.6   Conical permanent teeth, spacing as a result of microdontia and tooth surface loss all detract from the appearance of the anterior teeth.

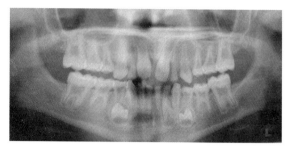

Figure 6.7   Taurodont teeth are more commonly seen in patients with hypodontia, as in this patient in whom the maxillary first and second primary molars and first permanent molars have been affected.

been allegorical reports of the speech development of affected children being significantly improved following provision of partial or complete overdentures.

Form and size

Microdontia and tapering-crown forms are common features of hypodontia, which can detract from the appearance of the dental arches (Figure 6.6). They can also make it more difficult to place adhesive orthodontic brackets and restorations. In addition the placing of a restoration on a microdont tooth to provide the illusion of a normal crown size can result in a restoration with a very narrow profile as it emerges at the gingival margin. This detracts from the patient's appearance and the area can be difficult to clean, resulting in an increased risk of periodontal disease. Such restorations can also create an unfavourable crown to root ratio. Where a tooth has a crown form that is suboptimal for the placing of a restoration or treatment with a removable partial denture then orthodontic realignment can sometimes be beneficial and should be considered as part of the preliminary treatment plan.

Taurodontism, although not rare in the general population, occurs in syndromes, particularly in those that have an ectodermal defect. It has been reported as being more common in patients with hypodontia (Seow and Lai, 1989) and it is therefore important to be aware of this association when

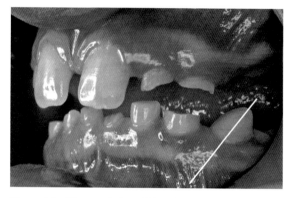

Figure 6.8   The angulation of LL3 places restrictions on the placement of implants in the jaw immediately mesial to this tooth.

assessing an individual with hypodontia (Figure 6.7).

Tooth angulation

The angulations of the teeth are important in relation to the appearance of the dental arch, occlusal contacts, and the shape of the interdental contact areas, as well as their effects on the space available within the jaw for the insertion of dental implants. Teeth are often tipped around their long axes in patients with hypodontia as a result of spacing, or the presence of infra-occluded retained primary teeth (Figure 6.8). Such teeth may adversely affect the appearance of the dentition, result in occlusal interferences, or place restrictions on the design of the occlusal surfaces of restorations They also occupy a disproportionate length of the dental arch, and the interdental spaces in these situations may either be excessively narrow or broad, leading potentially to periodontal problems as well as an unnatural appearance. Uprighting of tipped teeth often results in projection above the occlusal plane, necessitating their intrusion or crown reduction.

The widespread use of dental implants in the treatment of patients with hypodontia has brought into focus the need to consider carefully the surgical envelope into which they may be placed. This is not only important in terms of its ability to accommodate the implant with an acceptable margin of bone, but also to do so in osseous material of optimal quality. Furthermore the location of a dental implant cannot be divorced from the emergence point of the connecting components through the mucosa and the angulation of the subsequent restoration (Figure 6.9). All these factors need to be considered during patient assessment, even though the restorative approach to be adopted may not have been finally decided (in the case of potential implant treatment this could be many years in the future). Considerations of this nature underline the importance of multidisciplinary treat-

ment planning (Hobkirk *et al.*, 2006) and the need to do so within a long-projected time frame.

Root resorption of retained primary teeth

Tables 6.2 and 6.3 show typical ages at which the primary and permanent dentitions erupt, and Tables 6.4 and 6.5 list the average tooth sizes.

As delayed eruption is a feature of hypodontia, the retention of a primary tooth beyond the normal time for eruption of its permanent successor is not diagnostic of the absence of that tooth (which should be confirmed radiographically as part of the initial assessment). Where a primary tooth does not have a permanent successor then it is likely to be retained and can remain a functional unit for many years.

Retained primary teeth are prone to occlusal tooth surface loss which may require treatment with adhesive restorations or stainless steel crowns

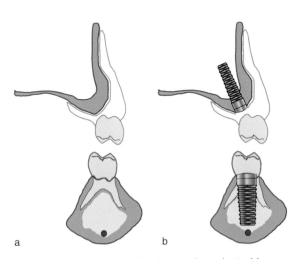

a   b

Figure 6.9 (a) Surgical (red outline) and prosthetic (blue outline) envelopes delineating potential spaces for placement of prostheses and dental implants, where appropriate. (b) The superimposition of implants demonstrates the compromised surgical envelopes due to lack of bone in the maxilla and the location of the mandibular canal. The relationship of the surgical and prosthetic envelopes in the maxilla is also unfavourable.

Table 6.2   Average ages at which primary teeth erupt and are shed.

	Tooth	Age at eruption	Age when shed
Mandible	I1	6–10 months	6–7 years
	I2	10–16 months	7–8 years
	C	17–23 months	9–12 years
	M1	14–18 months	9–11 years
	M2	23–31 months	10–12 years
Maxilla	I1	8–12 months	6–7 years
	I2	9–13 months	7–8 years
	C	16–22 months	10–12 years
	M1	13–19 months	9–11 years
	M2	25–33 months	10–12 years

Table 6.3   Average ages at which permanent teeth erupt.

Tooth	Age at eruption (years)	
	Mandible	Maxilla
I1	6–7	7–8
I2	7–8	8–9
C	9–10	11–12
P1	10–12	10–11
P2	11–12	10–12
M1	6–7	6–7
M2	11–13	12–13
M3	17–21	17–21

Table 6.4   Average sizes in mm of primary teeth (data from Sicher, 1960).

Tooth	Overall length (mm)	Crown length	Maximum crown width	Labio/buccolingual cervical diameter
MAXILLA				
Central incisor	17.0–19.0	6.0–7.3	6.0–7.15	
Lateral incisor	14.5–17.0	5.5–6.8	4.2–6.6	
Canine	17.5–22.0	6.5–7.8	6.2–8.0	
First molar	14.0–17.0	5.8–6.5	6.6–9.8	
Second molar	17.5–19.5	6.0–6.7	8.3–9.3	9.0–10.2*
MANDIBLE				
Central incisor	15.0–19.0	5.0–6.6	3.6–5.5	
Lateral incisor	15.0–19.0	5.6–7.0	3.8–5.9	
Canine	17.5–22.0	6.5–8.1	5.2–7.0	
First molar	14.0–17.0	6.6–7.0	7.5–8.5	
Second molar	17.5–19.5	6.5–7.2	10.0–11.5	8.5–9.2*

*Maximum diameter of crown in this dimension.

Table 6.5   Average sizes in mm of permanent teeth (data from Sicher 1960).

Tooth	Overall length	Crown length	Max. crown width	M–D cervical diameter	Labio/buccolingual cervical diameter	Height of buccal surface	Height of lingual surface (mm)
MAXILLA							
Central incisor	24.0	11.6	8.4	6.7	7.3	–	–
Lateral Incisor	22.5	9.0–10.2	6.5	5.1	6.0	–	–
Canine	27.0	10.9	7.6	5.6	8.1	–	–
First premolar	21.7	–	6.8	4.8–5.3	8.5–9.3	8.7	7.5
Second premolar	21.5	–	6.5	–	–	7.9	7.5
First molar	21.3	–	10.1	–	11.7*	7.7	–
Second molar	21.1	7.7	9.8	–	11.5*	–	–
MANDIBLE							
Central incisor	21.4	9.4	5.4	3.9	5.9	–	–
Lateral Incisor	23.2	9.9	5.9	4.2	6.2	–	–
Canine	25.4	11.4	6.7	5.3	7.8	–	–
First premolar	18.5–27.0	–	6.0–8.0	–	–	7.5–11.0	5.0–5.8
Second premolar	23.2	8.5	7.3	5.5	8.3	–	–
First molar	22.8	8.3	11.5	–	10.4*	–	–
Second molar	22.8	8.1	10.7	–	9.8*	–	–

*Maximum diameter of crown in this dimension.

if they are to remain functional. They may also become ankylosed and thus cease to erupt in harmony with any adjacent teeth. As a result they become infra-occluded, sometimes described incorrectly as submerged (an inappropriate term since the tooth does not move apically but ceases to move occlusally). Infra-occluded teeth can be prone to caries where their location makes oral hygiene difficult. They may become increasingly less evident and can become lodged below the mesial or distal convexity of an adjacent permanent tooth. This can result in the initiation of a periodontal pocket or carious lesion in the adjacent tooth.

While the roots of infra-occluded primary teeth are eventually resorbed this process can take many years, thus there are instances when they are better removed. Removal is indicated when they are carious or associated with disease in adjacent permanent teeth or causing these to tip. The extraction of teeth like these can be challenging as they are usually brittle with fine roots which are prone to fracture due to the lack of a periodontal ligament and fusion of the roots to the alveolar bone. When removing them it is important to minimise the destruction of the bone, which is usually at a premium in patients with hypodontia and can be crucial in orthodontic and implant treatment. This topic is discussed in detail in Chapter 7.

For retained primary teeth without permanent successors that are not infra-occluded, a decision must be made as to the appropriateness of their continued retention. This is based on systemic and local factors, including the status of the tooth, its functional role, and the overall treatment plan, all of which are inter-related.

Systemic factors

When a primary tooth has a poor prognosis there is usually little option but to extract it and manage the resultant space within the context of the patient's wishes and oral needs. However, where elective extraction of these teeth is considered then it is usually to facilitate other procedures, typically repositioning of adjacent teeth as a result of normal growth and development of the dental arches by orthodontic mechanotherapy. The retention of primary teeth in these circumstances can simplify treatment at this stage, but usually at the cost of restricted, more complex or time-consuming treatment at a later stage, possibly at a time when the patient finds this impacts negatively on his or her education, social activities or employment. When retained primary teeth eventually fail, the resultant space may be inadequate or excessive for the placement of an optimally sized restoration or insertion of a dental implant, dictating a restricted or compromised range of treatment options. Their retention may also preclude orthodontic treatment at a later stage or make it more complex or lengthy, so these issues need to be explored fully with patients and their carers.

If a patient has a systemic condition that reduces their ability to cooperate with treatment, or provide high levels of home care, then this argues for a less complex treatment plan. Similarly patients with

medical disorders that make dental extractions more hazardous or challenging may be better served by the retention of primary teeth that lack permanent successors.

Local factors
Presence of a permanent successor

Where a primary tooth has a permanent successor then sometimes the extraction of the primary tooth can be of benefit. It potentially reduces the interval before the permanent tooth erupts and encourages an improvement in the path of eruption. If the extraction is carried out too early then there may be space loss, leading to impaction of the permanent tooth.

Caries status

Extensive caries or large restorations reduce the prognosis of the tooth; however when its retention is important for space maintenance then restoration with a preformed stainless-steel crown can be effective as an interim measure (Randall, 2002).

Periodontal disease

Significant loss of periodontal tissue and ongoing periodontal disease can result in a poor prognosis for the affected tooth and has implications for the status of the other teeth. In addition it may lead to loss of alveolar bone which can impact on potential future treatment with dental implants.

Root resorption

A major consideration when assessing the prognosis of a retained primary tooth lacking a permanent successor is that of root resorption. This tends to occur at a considerably slower rate than where there is a permanent successor tooth and it is common to observe primary teeth that have been retained into the second and third decades of life (on occasions even into the fourth and fifth decades). Haselden et al. (2001) have shown that for primary canine and molar teeth without successors, regardless of gender or radiographic age, the lower deciduous canines appear to show the least amount of resorption and the upper first deciduous molars the most. Their findings are discussed in Chapter 2 and summarised in Tables 6.6 and 6.7.

Primary teeth can remain functional even when they have undergone significant root resorption. While treatment plans should be predicated on their eventual loss, this may be significantly delayed so careful consideration should be given to their retention (provided that it does not compromise the eventual outcome). Primary teeth may be used to provide support for partial or complete overdentures and some have proposed their use as abutments for fixed restorations. However, there is little published evidence to support this view, and there have been suggestions that high occlusal loads can hasten root resorption.

Dental implants – the third dentition?

There is currently considerable debate as to the appropriateness of placing dental implants in young patients with hypodontia (Yap and Klineberg, 2009). While this treatment modality has in general proved very effective in the management of the condition in carefully selected cases, doubts have been expressed about its use in the growing child. Such doubts arise because there is some evidence that the implants, once integrated, remain where they are placed and subsequent growth of the jaws results in a suboptimal positioning that may jeopardise further treatment. Concerns

have also been expressed about elective surgery in young patients when the potential benefits are uncertain, their understanding of the procedure may be restricted and it usually remains possible to carry out implant treatment when they are older. For these reasons most clinicians working in this field currently advise that implant treatment is deferred until skeletal maturity. There have been suggestions that primary teeth lacking permanent successors should be routinely replaced with dental implants, however Bergendal (2008) did not find any robust evidence in the literature to support this view.

Bone

The bone of the facial skeleton is a vital tissue when treating hypodontia as it influences the contours of the facial tissues, reflects the apical base relationship of the jaws, limits the space for the dental arches, and provides locations into which teeth may be moved orthodontically or dental implants inserted. Where it is lacking or shaped unfavourably then it may impose limits on the restoration of the dental arches, restricting their relationships and limiting the potential to use orthodontic mechanotherapy and dental implant procedures (unless the bone can be reshaped or supplemented).

None of these issues is unique to patients with hypodontia, however they often need treatment that is extensive and employs clinical procedures to their full potential. In these circumstances any limitations may have an undue effect on treatment outcomes.

Hypodontia is associated with defects in tissues derived from epithelium and any changes in the jaw bones are usually secondary to the absence of teeth – in which case the lack of alveolar bone will

Table 6.6 Guidelines for root resorption of retained primary teeth lacking permanent successors.

1	Individual variation is very large.
2	Root resorption for a given tooth tends to be more rapid in the maxilla than the mandible.
3	The canine is least affected.
4	The first molar is most affected.
5	The second molar is less affected than the first molar.

Table 6.7 The degree of root resorption of primary, canine and molar teeth without permanent successors at different ages (data from Haselden et al., 2001).

Primary tooth	12 years	24 years	35 years
Canine	–	–	60–89% minimal resorption Balance <50% resorption
First molar	20% minimal resorption Balance <50% resorption	–	–
Second molar	–	40–60% minimal resorption Balance resorption 25–50%	–

be similar to that in jaws that have been edentulous for a considerable period. This arises where teeth are absent or subsequent to the loss of primary teeth that have no permanent successors. There are some unusual situations in which the hypodontia has been caused by factors that have also influenced the connective tissues, such as irradiation, or the influence of a local tumour (Friedrich *et al.*, 2003).

Several studies have been conducted into the relationship between hypodontia and craniofacial structure. Øgaard and Krogstad (1995) concluded that the typical dentofacial structure in patients with 'advanced hypodontia', defined by Endo *et al.* (2004) as a congenital absence of four or more permanent teeth, may be due to dental and functional compensation, rather than to a different growth pattern. In a study of Japanese patients, Endo *et al.* (2006) reported that every hypodontia group showed shorter anterior and overall cranial base lengths, shorter maxillary length, greater retroclination and elongation of mandibular incisors, and a larger inter-incisal angle than the control group. In a study that analysed skeletal relationships in a group of young people with hypodontia attending a clinic in the UK, Chung *et al.* (2000) reported that the mean values for the whole sample were within the normal range and did not demonstrate any feature specific to the group. They did nevertheless note that patients with more severe hypodontia showed tendencies to a Class III skeletal relationship and a reduced maxillary–mandibular planes angle.

The principal effects of hypodontia on the jaws are thus:

- Reduced alveolar development
- The effects of retained primary teeth
- Narrowing of the alveolar ridge

Reduced alveolar development

Alveolar bone forms in response to the presence of teeth and a healthy periodontal ligament, and is remodelled in response to loads on the bone, probably as a result of internal strain. Where a tooth erupts actively then the shape of the alveolar bone is modified so as to maintain its relationship with the tooth. Similarly orthodontic mechanotherapy

can result in remodelling of the alveolar bone. Loss of a tooth will result in the exponentially reducing resorption of the associated bone, producing the all too familiar effects of a resorbed jaw, often with a subsequent unfavourable impact on the facial appearance. In addition the loss of alveolar bone brings with it challenges in providing prosthetic restorations, whether they are mucosa-, tooth- or implant-stabilised. Where teeth are congenitally absent then the alveolar bone will grow to a very limited extent producing similar effects. A further effect of reduced alveolar growth, which may be exacerbated by a lack of occluding posterior teeth and tooth surface loss, especially of primary teeth, may be an increase in the freeway space.

The effects of retained primary teeth

Retention of primary teeth beyond the age at which they are normally shed can be beneficial where there is no permanent successor as they can provide a substitute for many years and also preserve bone. Where, however, such teeth become ankylosed then they lose their eruptive potential and will become infra-occluded. This causes a discontinuity in the contours of the jaw that may require restoration and place limitations on treatment.

Ridge narrowing

A common finding in patients with hypodontia is that the alveolar ridge in edentate areas is not only low, but also significantly narrowed labiolingually below its crest (Figures 6.10 and 6.11) which may be deceptively wide. This is more common in the mandible, and can make it difficult to achieve a

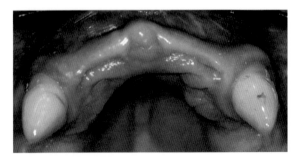

Figure 6.10 Sub-crestal narrowing of the alveolar ridge associated with absence of the permanent incisor teeth.

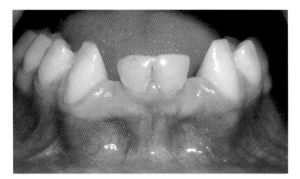

Figure 6.11   Narrowing of the alveolar ridge below the crest making placement of dental implants challenging both in the lower and upper jaws (Figure 6.10).

natural appearance with a fixed bridge. It also presents problems in the insertion of dental implants since in these situations they are at risk of penetrating the jaw labially or lingually. Sometimes this can be overcome by increasing the thickness of the ridge below its crest using a particulate graft either before or at the time of surgery (Figures 6.12). Where this is difficult to contain then a membrane may be used to restrict the relatively mobile particulate material until it has been infiltrated with connective tissue.

Bone grafting

Graft materials

The lack of alveolar bone in patients with hypodontia often creates aesthetic problems as well as difficulties with implant placement, which requires a suitable surgical envelope if treatment is to be optimised – or indeed even be possible. As a result there are occasions where augmentation of the jaws is necessary. This may be carried out using grafting procedures, with or without a guiding membrane, or surgical reconstruction of the bone itself (Costantino *et al.*, 2002). A wide range of techniques and materials are available for this (Eppley *et al.*, 2005; Kao and Scott, 2007). A bone graft should ideally heal by induction, become incorporated within the surrounding tissues, and be remodelled to resemble native bone (Habal and Reddi, 1994). Bone grafts can be classified as autografts (where the graft is obtained from the patient them-

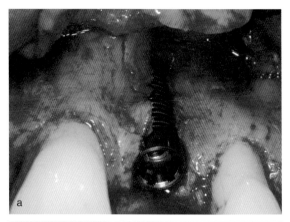
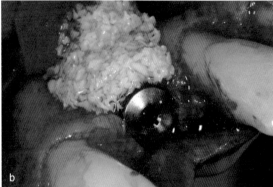
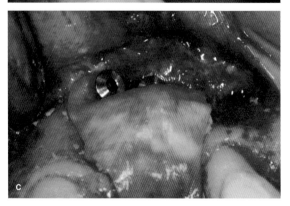

Figure 6.12   (a) Dental implant placed in an inadequate surgical envelope due to bone resorption. (b) Defect corrected with synthetic bone grafting material. The synthetic membrane used to restrain the grafting material is seen at the top of the image. (c) Synthetic membrane in place.

selves), as allografts (where it is obtained from another human of a different genotype) or as xenografts (where material is obtained from another species). Bone grafts may be free or retain a blood supply, although the latter obviously restricts their application.

Autogenous grafts are considered to be the gold standard for bone grafting. They have the advantages of being progressively incorporated into the craniofacial skeleton, able to resist infection, and potentially capable of osteogenesis (Citardi and Friedman, 1994). Bone may be harvested from the implant sites during their preparation using a bone trap, or obtained from either jaw. Where larger quantities of bone are required then the iliac crest is a commonly used donor site. Problems encountered with autogenous grafts include donor site morbidity, site-specific complications (especially if the bone is obtained from a location other than the implantation site), and resorption of the graft with resultant unpredictable contour changes.

Allografts and xenografts are obtained from human and animal sources and are treated to remove material that could cause allergic reactions or infection, leaving the mineral phase largely intact. They may be obtained in the form of blocks or particles depending on their potential application, and provide an inorganic scaffold for bone growth. They thus have similarities to the synthetic graft materials that are available in a range of compositions and formulations. Some patients may be unwilling to be treated with allografts or xenografts for personal or religious reasons and this should be discussed with them when considering treatment options.

There is a range of synthetic bone graft materials available that vary in structure and composition. Most are based on calcium or aluminium. Where these materials are capable of osseoconduction and osseointegration then they are referred to as bioactive. Osseoconduction refers to an ability to support bone growth on its surface and osseointegration refers to the formation and maintenance of a direct bond between the graft and adjacent living bone. This is a favourable situation unlike that in which the tissues form a fibrous capsule around an implant, which is mechanically and biologically unfavourable for a load bearing graft.

Silicate-based alloplasts
Silicate-based alloplastic grafts are based on silicon dioxide, some compounds of which have the ability to bond directly to bone. Two successful biomateri-

als are bioactive glass and glass ionomer in the form of cement or solid implants.

Bioactive glasses

Bioactive glasses are hard, solid, transparent materials composed of varying combinations of sodium oxide, calcium oxide, phosphorus pentoxide and silicon dioxide, with silicate as the primary component. They can be produced in a range of formulations ranging from some which exhibit almost complete solubility in vivo, to others which approach inertness. After implantation of a bioactive glass implant, a silica-rich gel forms on its surface, within which crystals of hydroxyapatite are formed. These provide a mechanism for bonding to bone by reacting with substances such as glycoproteins and collagen on their surfaces. Although there is a strong molecular bond, the glass is not replaced by bone with time. The materials are also rather brittle and tend to be used more for space-filling, although some formulations are strong enough for bone reconstruction; they are not readily shaped at the chair-side and are less suitable for the placing of implants.

Glass-ionomer cements

Glass-ionomer cements represent a hybrid biomaterial containing both organic and inorganic species, and are widely used in dentistry as a restorative material. They set by a two-component reaction producing in effect a bioactive glass with a high aluminium oxide content which has been combined with a polymeric carbon matrix (Wilson et al., 1981; Jonck et al., 1989). The material bonds to bone in a similar manner to the bioactive glasses, although the alumina ions and crystals which are found at the bone–implant interface result in a weaker bond as there is less calcium phosphate crystal formation at the surface. They too are non-resorbable and are used mainly for space filling.

Calcium phosphate-based alloplasts
This group of materials contains some of the best tolerated and most promising alloplastic graft materials, especially the 'apatite' forms of calcium phosphate. All are bioactive, permitting osseoconduction and osseointegration and some forms are resorbable, in both cases varying with the prepara-

tion method and specific composition. They were at one time used principally as ceramics, having been sintered at a high temperature. The two most important apatite preparations are tricalcium phosphate and hydroxyapatite (Costantino *et al.*, 2001).

Tricalcium phosphate

One of the earliest calcium phosphate compounds to be used as an implant was porous beta-tricalcium phosphate, which, unlike ceramic hydroxyapatite slowly dissolves in vivo (Jarcho, 1981). This permits grafting of a bone defect and its subsequent replacement with bone, although usually the new tissue occupies less space than the original graft. An enhanced performance has been reported by combining the tricalcium phosphate with osteogenic proteins.

Hydroxyapatite preparations

Hydroxyapatite is the principal mineral component of bone and has been synthesised for almost 40 years and used clinically for over 25 years. It is typically provided in either ceramic or non-ceramic forms, both of which can permit osseoinduction and osseointegration. The ceramic form is available in both solid and porous preparations, of which the latter are more widely used in reconstruction of the facial skeleton as they permit fibrous ingrowth and are more readily shaped. Granular preparations are more easily contoured at the time of surgery as once in contact with tissue fluids they take on a paste-like consistency, but they tend to migrate until tethered by fibrous tissue (a problem addressed in some preparations by the inclusion of stabilising additives). Porous forms of hydroxyapatite can be either synthetic or produced from coral.

An interesting variant of hydroxyapatite is a non-ceramic or cement form, HA-C. This is composed of tetracalcium phosphate and anhydrous dicalcium phosphate, which react in an aqueous environment to produce hydroxyapatite. HA-C is capable of osseoconduction and osseointegration, but, in contrast to hydroxyapatite is converted to new bone over time without a loss of volume at the recipient site (Costantino *et al.*, 1984). Currently available cements are less suited to load-bearing applications in dentistry.

Calcium carbonate-based materials

These materials are less widely used in dentistry and are fabricated from marine coral; however unlike porous hydroxyapatite implants derived from this material they remain as calcium carbonate and are not converted to calcium phosphate. As a consequence, while the hydroxyapatite-based material is almost non-resorbable when implanted, the calcium carbonate-based material is resorbed and replaced with fibro-osseous tissue when placed in an intra-osseous location. The material is osseoconductive over the internal surfaces of its pores and following initial osseoconduction the calcium carbonate scaffold is removed by osteoclasts and replaced with bone (Papacharalambous and Anastasoff 1993). There is however currently less information on the long-term outcomes of implants of this material.

Bone morphogenetic proteins (BMPs)

Urist first described the osteoinductive properties of demineralised bone matrix (Urist, 1965; Riley *et al.*, 1996) following which several growth factors associated with bone formation have been identified. These are part of a complex process and the BMPs should not be thought of as simple initiators of osseoinduction, which may be placed at an implant site to ensure osseointegration, although they can have beneficial effects in some circumstances.

BMPs are a subdivision of the transforming growth factor (TGF) super-family and eight classes of BMPs have been identified (BMP-2 to BMP-9). There is currently considerable interest in BMP-2 (Stanford *et al.*, 2009). BMP-1 is not part of the TGF family.

Surgical enhancement of implant sites

Grafting techniques

Bone grafts may be used in the form of blocks or particles or powders. The former tend to retain their shape immediately following surgery while the latter need to be restrained mechanically by the adjacent hard and soft tissues, possibly supplemented by an artificial membrane in a technique known as 'guided bone regeneration' (GBR).

Block grafts

This technique basically involves the surgical placement of a solid, as opposed to particulate, graft on the surface of the bone which is to be enhanced, known as the onlay technique, or its insertion into an osteotomy cut in the so-called sandwich technique. There are a number of variations on these basic themes depending on site and desired outcomes. Onlay grafts may be used in either jaw to enhance the alveolar ridge both vertically and horizontally, and are also employed to increase the thickness of the maxillary ridge posteriorly by their insertion below the mucosal lining of the maxillary antrum in the so-called sinus lift procedure. In this situation it is more common to use particulate grafts.

Particulate grafts

These are used to correct localised defects in the bone, often in combination with a restraining membrane with the guided bone regeneration technique.

Bone augmentation – the evidence base

There is some evidence from systematic reviews of the relative efficacy of synthetic bone grafts used for sinus lift procedures (Del Fabbro *et al.*, 2004). This finding was confirmed by the work of Aghaloo and Moy (2007/2008). These authors also considered alveolar ridge augmentation techniques, including guided bone regeneration, onlay or veneer grafting, combinations of onlay, veneer, and interpositional inlay grafting, distraction osteogenesis, ridge-splitting, free and vascularised autografting for discontinuity defects, mandibular interpositional grafting, and socket preservation. They concluded that there was a lack of detailed documentation or long-term follow-up studies on the techniques, with the exception of guided bone regeneration, nevertheless studies meeting the inclusion criteria gave favourable results. It was suggested that procedures for alveolar ridge augmentation may be especially sensitive to operator technique and experience, and that implant survival in these situations may partly reflect the degree of primary (initial) implant stability resulting from its extension into the residual bone at the time of placement.

Esposito *et al.* (2006) have carried out a Cochrane review of bone augmentation procedures related to implant surgery. Their conclusions included the following:

- Major bone grafting procedures of extremely resorbed mandibles may not be justified
- Bone substitutes may replace autogenous bone for sinus lift procedures of extremely atrophic sinuses
- Both guided bone regeneration procedures and distraction osteogenesis can be used to augment bone vertically, but it is unclear which one is more efficient
- It is unclear whether augmentation procedures are needed at immediate single implants placed in fresh extraction sockets, but sites treated with barrier (membrane) plus Bio-Oss™ (natural bone substitute material obtained from the mineral portion of bovine bone) showed a higher position of the gingival margin than sites treated with barriers alone
- More bone was regenerated around fenestrated implants with non-resorbable barriers (i.e. barrier membranes) than without barriers; however, it remains unclear whether such bone is of benefit to the patient
- Bone morphogenetic proteins may enhance bone formation around implants grafted with Bio-Oss™ but there was no reliable evidence supporting the efficacy of other active agents, such as platelet-rich plasma, in conjunction with implant treatment

Their findings also supported those of the workers referred to above in relation to the efficacy of bone substitutes for sinus lift procedures.

Alternative surgical techniques for enhancing implant sites

Guided bone regeneration (GBR)

This technique involves the implantation of biocompatible membranes that allow the passage of tissue fluids but which are intended to act as a cellular barrier. This is thought to prevent the infiltration of fibrous tissue into the graft site and thereby facilitate preferential bone formation. The membranes are also utilised to restrain particulate grafts that otherwise tend to migrate within the tissues. Some grafts incorporate flexible metallic strips to facilitate their placement and contouring, and can be secured with small pins or screws.

Membranes have been made in a variety of materials of which porous polytetrafluoroethylene (PTFE), poly (DL-lactide-epsilon-caprolactone) and collagen, are examples. Non-resorbable membranes are usually removed once their function is complete, thus requiring a second surgical procedure. They are not always easy to manipulate into the desired contour and can become exposed if there is breakdown of an overlying suture line.

Guided bone regeneration is employed in periodontal surgery for defect restoration where it has been shown to be effective in some situations (Murphy and Gunsolley, 2003). Systematic reviews and basic research have however questioned the evidence base for the effectiveness of these techniques in dental implant work (Gielkens *et al.*, 2007; 2008).

Distraction osteogenesis

Distraction osteogenesis is a surgical technique that involves the creation of an osteotomy within an existing bone and the gradual mechanical separation of the cut surfaces using a mechanical distraction device which controls the direction and rate of separation, typically by 1 mm per day (Snyder *et al.*, 1973) (Figure 6.13). During this process new bone is laid down in the defect, resulting ultimately in an altered bone shape and size. The technique is only occasionally used but can be employed, for example, to distract a section of the jaw containing infra-occluded permanent teeth, or

to advance the pre-maxilla. Fixation of the distraction device is via screws, although dental implants have been used for this purpose and then subsequently restored. Since the development of the technique, osseodistraction devices have become more sophisticated, and the feasibility of using trifocal devices has been demonstrated (Sawaki *et al.*, 1997). The benefits of the method include concomitant changes in the associated soft tissues and muscles during the gradual change in the bone's dimensions, the avoidance of the need for bone grafts and the associated potential morbidity from donor sites, and reduced overall operating time.

Key Points: Effects of hypodontia on the oral supporting tissues

Teeth
- Missing units
- Microdontia
- Tapering teeth
- Retained primary teeth
- Delayed eruption
- Infra-occluded teeth
- Tooth wear secondary to reduced numbers of teeth and retention of primary teeth

Bone (effects secondary to missing teeth)
- Reduced amounts of alveolar bone
- Ridge narrowing

Mucosa
- Some evidence for reduced salivary flow in certain patients with an ED
- Resultant problems with mucosal infection and reduced abrasion resistance

---

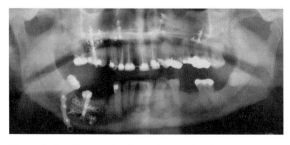

Figure 6.13   Osteogenic distraction used to increase inadequate bulk of alveolar bone in the right mandible. The maxilla has also been repositioned to lower the upper occlusal plane.

References

Aghaloo TL, Moy PK. Which hard tissue augmentation techniques are the most successful in furnishing bony support for implant placement? *Int J Oral Maxillofac Implants* 2007;22(Suppl.):49–70; 2008;23:56 (*erratum*).

Baba K, Tsukiyama Y, Clark GT. Reliability, validity, and utility of various occlusal measurement methods and techniques. *J Prosthet Dent* 2000;83:83–9.

Bergendal B, Norderyd J, Bågesund M, Holst A. Signs and symptoms from ectodermal organs in young Swedish individuals with oligodontia. *Int J Paediatr Dent* 2006; 16:320–326.

Bergendal B. When should we extract deciduous teeth and place implants in young individuals with tooth agenesis? *J Oral Rehabil* 2008;35(Suppl.1):55–63.

Berry DC, Poole DFG. Attrition: possible mechanisms of compensation. *J Oral Rehabil* 1976;3:201–206.

Chung LK, Hobson RS, Nunn JH, Gordon PH, Carter NE. An analysis of the skeletal relationships in a group of young people with hypodontia. *J Orthod* 2000;27: 315–318.

Citardi MJ, Friedman CD. Nonvascularized autogenous bone grafts for craniofacial skeletal augmentation and replacement. *Otolaryngol Clin North Am* 1994;27: 891–910.

Correr GM, Alonso RC, Consani S, Puppin-Rontani RM, Ferracane JL. In vitro wear of primary and permanent enamel. Simultaneous erosion and abrasion. *Am J Dent* 2007;20:394–399.

Costantino PD, Friedman CD, Jones K, *et al.* Hydroxyapatite cement: basic chemistry and histologic properties. *Arch Otolaryngol Head Neck Surg* 1984;240:115–119.

Costantino PD, Hiltzik D, Govindaraj S, Moche J. Bone healing and bone substitutes. *Facial Plast Surg* 2002; 18:13–26.

Costantino PD, Hiltzik DH, Sen C, *et al.* Sphenoethmoid cerebrospinal fluid leak repair with hydroxyapatite cement. *Arch Otolaryngol Head Neck Surg* 2001;127: 588–593.

Del Fabbro M, Testori T, Francetti L, Weinstein R. Systematic review of survival rates for implants placed in the grafted maxillary sinus. *Int J Periodontics Restorative Dent* 2004;24:565–577.

Endo T, Ozoe R, Yoshino S, Shimooka S. Hypodontia patterns and variations in craniofacial morphology in Japanese orthodontic patients. *Angle Orthod* 2006;76:996–1003.

Endo T, Yoshino S, Ozoe R, Kojima K, Shimooka S. Association of advanced hypodontia and craniofacial morphology in Japanese orthodontic patients. *Odontology* 2004;92:48–53.

Eppley BL, Pietrzak WS, Blanton MW. Allograft and alloplastic bone substitutes: a review of science and technology for the craniomaxillofacial surgeon. *J Craniofac Surg* 2005;16:981–989.

Esposito M, Grusovin MG, Coulthard P, Worthington HV. The efficacy of various bone augmentation procedures for dental implants: a Cochrane systematic review of randomized controlled clinical trials. *Int J Oral Maxillofac Implants* 2006;21:696–710.

Friedrich RE, Giese M, Schmelzle R, Mautner VF, Scheuer HA. Jaw malformations plus displacement and numerical aberrations of teeth in neurofibromatosis type 1: a descriptive analysis of 48 patients based on panoramic radiographs and oral findings. *J Craniomaxillofac Surg* 2003;31:1–9.

Gielkens PF, Bos RR, Raghoebar GM, Stegenga B. Is there evidence that barrier membranes prevent bone resorption in autologous bone grafts during the healing period? A systematic review. *Int J Oral Maxillofac Implants* 2007;22:390–398.

Gielkens PF, Schortinghuis J, de Jong JR, *et al.* The influence of barrier membranes on autologous bone grafts. *J Dent Res* 2008;87:1048–1052.

Habal MB, Reddi H. Bone graft and bone induction substitutes. *Clin Plast Surg* 1994;21:525–542.

Hagberg C. Assessment of bite force: A review. *J Craniomandib Disord* 1987;1:162–169.

Haselden K, Hobkirk JA, Goodman JR, Jones SP, Hemmings KW. Root resorption in deciduous canine and molar teeth without permanent successors in patients with severe hypodontia. *Int J Paediatr Dent* 2001;11:171–178.

Hellsing G. On the regulation of interincisor bite force in man. *J Oral Rehabil* 1980;7:403–411.

Hobkirk JA, Goodman JR, Jones SP. Presenting complaints and findings in a group of patients attending a hypodontia clinic. *Br Dent J* 1994;177:337–339.

Hobkirk JA, Nohl F, Bergendal B, Storhaug K, Richter MK. The Management of Ectodermal Dysplasia and Severe Hypodontia. International Conference Statements. *J Oral Rehabil* 2006;33:634–637.

Hobkirk JA, Psarros K. The influence of occlusal surface material on peak masticatory forces using osseointegrated implant-supported prostheses. *Int J Oral Maxillofac Implants* 1992;7:345–352.

Jarcho M. Calcium phosphate ceramics as hard tissue prosthetics. *Clin Orthoped* 1981;157:259–278.

Jonck LM, Grobbelaar CJ, Strating H. Biological evaluation of glass-ionomer cement (ketac-O) as an interface in total joint replacement: a screening test. *Clin Mater* 1989;4:201–224.

Kaercher T. Ocular symptoms and signs in patients with ectodermal dysplasia syndromes. *Graefes Arch Clin Exp Ophthalmol* 2004;242:495–500.

Kao ST, Scott DD. A review of bone substitutes. *Oral Maxillofac Surg Clin North Am* 2007;19:513–521.

Lux CJ, Conradt C, Burden D, Komposch G. Three dimensional analysis of maxillary and mandibular growth increments. *Cleft Palate Craniofac J* 2004;41:304–314.

Lyons MF, Baxendale RH. A preliminary electromyographic study of bite force and jaw-closing muscle fatigue in human subjects with advanced tooth wear. *J Oral Rehabil* 1990;17:311–318.

Murphy KG, Gunsolley JC. Guided tissue regeneration for the treatment of periodontal intrabony and furcation defects. A systematic review. *Ann Periodontol* 2003;8:266–302.

Nowjack-Raymer RE, Sheiham A. Numbers of natural teeth, diet, and nutritional status in US adults. *J Dent Res* 2007;86:1171–1175.

Øgaard B, Krogstad O. Craniofacial structure and soft tissue profile in patients with severe hypodontia. *Am J Orthod Dentofacial Orthop* 1995;108:472–477.

Papacharalambous SK, Anastasoff KI. Natural coral skeleton use as onlay graft for contour augmentation of the face. A preliminary report. *Int J Oral Maxillofac Surg* 1993;22:260–264.

Poyser NJ, Porter RW, Briggs PF, Chana HS, Kelleher MG. The Dahl concept: past, present and future. *Br Dent J* 2005;198:669–676.

Randall RC. Preformed metal crowns for primary and permanent molar teeth: review of the literature. *Pediatr Dent* 2002;24:489–500.

Richter EJ. In vivo vertical forces on implants. *Int J Oral Maxillofac Implants* 1995;10:99–108.

Richter EJ. In vivo horizontal bending moments on implants. *Int J Oral Maxillofac Implants* 1998;13:232–244.

Riley EH, Lane JM, Urist MR, Lyons KM, Lieberman JR. Bone morphogenetic protein-2: biology and applications. *Clin Orthop Relat Res* 1996;324:39–46.

Sawaki Y, Hagino H, Yamamoto H, Ueda M. Trifocal distraction osteogenesis for segmental mandibular defect: a technical innovation. *J Craniomaxillofac Surg* 1997;25:310–315.

Seow WK, Lai PY. Association of taurodontism with hypodontia: a controlled study. *Paediatr Dent* 1989;11:214–219.

Sicher H. *Oral Anatomy*, 3rd edn. CV Mosby Company, St Louis, 1960, pp. 214–244.

Siegel MB, Potsic WP. Ectodermal dysplasia: the otolaryngologic manifestations and management. *Int J Pediatr Otorhinolaryngol* 1990;19:265–271.

Smith BGN, Knight JK. An index for measuring the wear of teeth. *Br Dent J* 1984;156:435–438.

Snyder CC, Levine GA, Swanson HM, Browne EZ Jr. Mandibular lengthening by gradual distraction. Preliminary report. *Plast Reconstr Surg* 1973;51:506–508.

Stanford C, Estafanous E, Ellingsen JE, Oates T, Neppalli K. Thematic abstract review: bone morphogenetic protein-2 (BMP-2): an update. *Int J Oral Maxillofac Implants* 2009;24(Suppl.5):773–775.

Tarjan I, Gabris K, Rozsa N. Early prosthetic treatment of patients with ectodermal dysplasia: a clinical report. *J Prosthet Dent* 2005;93:419–424.

Toolson LB, Smith DE. Clinical measurement and evaluation of vertical dimension. *J Prosthet Dent* 1982;47:236–241.

Urist MR. Bone formation by autoinduction. *Science* 1965;150:893–899.

Walls AW, Steele JG, Sheiham A, Marcenes W, Moynihan PJ. Oral health and nutrition in older people. *J Public Health Dent* 2000;60:304–307.

Walther W. Determinants of a healthy aging dentition: maximum number of bilateral centric stops and optimum vertical dimension of occlusion. *Int J Prosthodont* 2003;16(Suppl.):77–79.

Wilson J, Pigott GH, Schoen F, Hench LL. Toxicology and biocompatibility of bioglasses. *J Biomed Mater Res* 1981;15:805–817.

Yap AK, Klineberg I. Dental implants in patients with ectodermal dysplasia and tooth agenesis: A critical review of the literature. *Int J Prosthodont* 2009;22:268–276.

Yazdanie N, Hobkirk JA. Functional adaptability to changes in lower denture shape. *Eur J Prosthodont Restor Dent* 1997;5:137–143.

Part 3

Age-Related Approaches to Treatment

7 Primary/Early Mixed Dentition

Introduction

As discussed in Chapter 3, the dental care of individuals with developmentally missing teeth is best planned and managed by multidisciplinary teams, the members of which may also provide active treatment where this is in the patient's best interests (Goodman *et al.*, 1994; Hobkirk *et al.*, 1994, 2006; Bergendal *et al.*, 1996; Hobson *et al.*, 2003; Nunn *et al.*, 2003; Bishop *et al.*, 2006, 2007a, 2007b; Worsaae *et al.*, 2007; Nohl *et al.*, 2008; Shafi *et al.*, 2008). All members of the team are essential to its success, although the contribution of their various skills will vary during the care pathway and, in the case of younger patients, the role of the paediatric dentist is likely to predominate (Goodman *et al.*, 1994; Nunn *et al.*, 2003). Young patients present particular challenges in relation to their understanding of their condition and potential treatment options, their ability to cooperate, and the need to establish a long-term relationship with the hypodontia team. Decisions made at this stage and patterns of oral care that are established can have major long-term implications, and treatment planning in the primary and early mixed dentition phase may present more as a behaviour assessment and management challenge than a technical exercise in dental treatment (Nunn *et al.*, 2003). There may also be issues of informed consent or assent, the relationship between the patient and their carers, and their relative aspirations for treatment outcomes.

In general it is important to adopt a flexible approach to allow for active treatment of the patient with hypodontia at an appropriate time for them and their family, which may be several years hence. However, it should be emphasised that regular care with effective prevention is essential to maintain good oral health. Decisions taken at this stage will lay the foundations for what in many cases will be a lifetime of advanced oral care, spreading potentially over six or more decades. There is an opportunity to explain the nature of hypodontia and help with understanding and acceptance of the condition, as well as making the appropriate referrals within the multidisciplinary dental team. There may also be a need for referrals to medical or genetic specialists, who may assist the family (Hobkirk *et al.*, 2006; Gill *et al.*, 2008). The concept of the management of hypodontia by a team of different specialists can be introduced at an early stage, to provide reassurance for the patient and family of coordinated care of the condition for the necessary time period (Gill *et al.*, 2008). In the early stages of diagnosis and treatment it is important to develop and maintain good oral health and establish behaviour management techniques to enable the child and his or her carers to undertake operative procedures (Nunn *et al.*, 2003).

Establishing a relationship

The initial examination of a child is an important opportunity to assess patients from many different aspects. These include their general physical and psychological maturity, the relationship with their parents or carers, the concerns they and their family may have about their dental condition, as well as their medical and dental histories. In addition the child and parents have the opportunity to form a view on the members of the dental team and their philosophy and approach to treatment.

It is very important that the patient feels central to the consultation and not a bystander while their care is discussed. Following the introduction of the dental team and the adults accompanying the child, it is helpful to establish the pathway and reasons for referral, as this helps to clarify the position of everyone involved from the beginning. Every opportunity should be made for patients and carers to express any concerns they may have relating to their appearance, speech or eating, and any resultant impact on their quality of life (Laing *et al.*, 2010). This gives the specialist an insight into the patients' demeanour, communication skills and interpersonal relationships with their carers, and their potential ability to cooperate with dental care. A social history provides a valuable insight into the family structure and support, the schooling experience of the patient, and any potential difficulties with travelling to appointments due to the carers' work or financial commitments. Empathy expressed at this stage regarding the potential significance of key educational events for treatment provision and the potential cost implications of treatment in the longer term may help both the patients and their carers.

Discussions should include any known family history of hypodontia since the inheritance pattern may affect the family's approach to the situation and possible desire for treatment. In some cases a parent may experience feelings of guilt for transmitting the condition and because of its consequences to the child (Gill *et al.*, 2008). At this stage information on patient support groups and the possibility of counselling can be introduced. Where there is no known inheritance pattern, there may be a lack of awareness of the situation and its implications. This requires a careful, staged discussion that allows both children and adults to absorb the information so that ultimately they can begin to discuss among themselves the immediate and longer-term implications of the condition, the potential treatment options and their ramifications, and to seek further clarification of issues. The possibility of referral to paediatric or genetic specialists may be mentioned where appropriate as part of the provision of information (Gill *et al.*, 2008).

A full medical history is important, incorporating not only those matters normally considered relevant to dental care but also issues that may indicate the presence of a syndrome associated with developmentally missing teeth. If this is suspected then further investigation and referral may be indicated. Many such syndromes have implications for the provision of dental care. Patients suffering from one of the ectodermal dysplasias may demonstrate reduced salivary flow, dryness of the eyes and problems with temperature control (Dhanrajani, 2002). They may also have concerns about their appearance, particularly the sparseness of their hair, as well as the associated dental abnormalities (Figure 7.1). A child with Down syndrome may have cardiac defects or behavioural problems that require special consideration. Other syndromes that include hypodontia among their features need to have details clarified, and the implications for treatment considered.

The dental history is important as an indicator of the circumstances of the diagnosis of hypodontia, and the treatment provided generally and specifically, as well as the patient's ability to manage treatment and the techniques used in its provision. In addition a view can be formed as to the level of engagement of the patient and his or her carers with available dental services. It is also essential to enquire in detail about the preventive aspects of the patient's home and surgery care, including diet and oral hygiene habits, and experi-

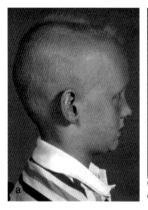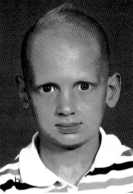

Figure 7.1   Side and front view of child with ectodermal dysplasia.

ence with fluoride supplements and fissure sealants. The importance of good oral health can be emphasised at this time, as it is paramount to the success of any long-term treatment plan. Complex restorative care requires the foundation of healthy periodontal tissues and robust caries prevention, particularly where appliances are to be inserted that have the potential to compromise oral health. Routine prevention and restorative treatment is often most appropriately provided by the general dental practitioner working closely with the specialist team, as part of a shared-care system (Hobson *et al.*, 2003).

Initial examination

Introduction

The initial examination has several functions, all of which are inter-related. The reaction of the child to the clinical environment and their cooperation with the clinical examination gives further insight into behaviour management issues that may be encountered. The initial findings form a baseline from which to monitor the progress of a treatment plan. They also enable the measurement of any deleterious changes to the patient as a result of intervention. In addition, clinical data may be collected for audit or research purposes, and to assist with the development of care pathways for other patients with the condition.

Soft tissues

Oral mucosa

The oral mucosa should be examined for colour and surface abnormalities such as ulcers, swellings or sinuses. In the presence of a removable prosthesis the palatal mucosa may show evidence of denture-related stomatitis (swelling and inflammation) with indications of a fungal infection. Corrective treatment would include education in appropriate oral hygiene and appliance care and wearing habits, together with the prescription of antifungal medication.

The lubrication of the mucosa should be assessed. This is particularly likely to be deficient in patients with hypohidrotic or anhidrotic ectodermal dysplasia. Where this is thought to be inadequate, then salivary flow may be assessed, and indeed this is used as a routine investigation in some clinics. It should be noted that patients with a reduced salivary flow related to an ectodermal dysplasia rarely give a history of a dry mouth since they lack a comparison with a normal situation. However, they will often report that they need frequent drinks, particularly when eating dry foods. Children with xerostomia will be at a higher risk of caries due to lack of salivary buffering capacity and flow-related poor oral clearance of food particles and consequently it is important to know the extent of the xerostomia. An ultrasound image of the salivary glands may be useful when assessing the extent of xerostomia and deciding on appropriate treatment (Heath *et al.*, 2006).

Periodontal tissues

The general status of the periodontal tissues with regard to inflammation and pocketing is an essential initial assessment. A periodontal examination provides an important starting point for determining the oral health of the patient, and for monitoring changes that may occur during treatment. The indices used to measure this depend on clinical choice, but should be relatively rapid and simple, and suitable for assessing both the oral hygiene status and the quality of gingival health (Löe and Silness, 1963; Silness and Löe, 1964; Löe, 1967;

Bollmer *et al.*, 1986; Ciancio, 1986; Chaves *et al.*, 1993; Marks *et al.*, 1993; Vanarsdall, 2007).

The presence and attachment of any fraena should be noted in relation to their potential effects on the periodontal tissues. If the attachment is quite high, it may also complicate the design of a removable prosthesis. An upper midline diastema is frequently associated with an enlarged fraenum, which may extend between the upper central incisors into the palate, as demonstrated by blanching of the palatal tissues when the fraenum is tensed. The fraenum may also appear thickened and fleshy and extend into the lip.

Hard tissues

Bone

A preliminary assessment of the alveolar bone contours is helpful as it will be important initially for the orthodontist in relation to influencing possible tooth movements, and subsequently for the restorative dentist in relation to the provision of replacement teeth. Any reduction in alveolar bone is of particular importance for implant treatment, and may also detract from the aesthetic outcome of treatment with fixed bridgework, as well as reducing the support potentially available for removable prostheses. The width and height of the alveolar bone adjacent to infra-occluded teeth is important in relation to their management and the treatment options subsequent to their removal. In addition there may be bone loss associated with infected primary teeth or periodontal disease around permanent teeth.

Teeth

A full charting of the dentition to identify the teeth present in the mouth is important. Careful examination is necessary to differentiate between the primary and permanent teeth. In patients with severe hypodontia, this may be difficult since some of the permanent teeth may be very microdont and of an abnormal form, and the situation may be further complicated by delayed or ectopic eruption. Several characteristics can be helpful in deciding whether a tooth is primary or permanent, as described below.

- Colour: Primary teeth appear whiter than permanent teeth
- Size: Permanent teeth are usually larger and the occlusal table of primary teeth is narrower
- Wear: A primary tooth may have wear facets if it has been in the mouth beyond its usual lifespan
- Bulbosity: Primary teeth are more bulbous than permanent teeth and have a narrower constriction at the cemento–enamel junction

The identity of a tooth can usually be confirmed radiographically. Primary teeth have short, thin and splayed roots compared to the larger roots of the permanent dentition. There may also be radiographic evidence of root resorption on primary teeth with no permanent successors (Haselden *et al.*, 2001), although this should be considered cautiously as occasionally an ectopic permanent tooth may cause root resorption on an adjacent permanent tooth (Brin *et al.*, 1986).

The mobility of all teeth should be checked. This may give an indication in primary teeth of the extent of root resorption and when exfoliation might be expected (Haselden *et al.*, 2001). Increased mobility in permanent teeth may suggest the possibility of a loss of relative root length within the alveolar bone, either because of periodontal disease or root resorption associated with an adjacent ectopic tooth.

The size and morphology of the teeth, together with radiographic evidence of root anatomy and the extent and structure of supporting bone will indicate the possible future prognosis of a tooth from a functional and aesthetic viewpoint. The health or disease experience of the tooth with regard to caries destruction, extent of any restorations, wear and infractions will also influence its prognosis.

Additional investigations

Radiographs

Radiographs are valuable for the assessment and location of the developing dentition, and to provide an overall picture of the extent of hypodontia for future long-term planning. They are important in assisting with diagnosis, particularly regarding the number of teeth developing, and in treatment planning by assessing pathology. The timing of radiographs is a matter for careful consideration, since it is necessary to balance the exposure to radiation with the quality of the information obtained. In the very young child with delayed eruption or a reduction in the number of primary teeth the taking of radiographs may be difficult due to limited cooperation. In addition the information gained may be of little benefit, because of limited establishment of the dentition, which may lead to an underestimation of the developing permanent dentition. There is evidence to suggest that patients with hypodontia exhibit delayed development of their permanent teeth, such that premature radiography may precede the early signs of late-developing teeth (Ruiz-Mealin et al., 2009).

Nevertheless, it is understandable that parents may be anxious and wish for early confirmation of how many and which teeth are missing. In such circumstances, the advantages and disadvantages of exposing a young child to radiation must be explained to the parents, together with the limitations of the findings at such an early stage. Even though some degree of confirmation may be attained with such radiographs, this will rarely affect treatment planning or treatment at a young age and is probably best delayed until the age of 6 or 7 years, when greater diagnostic and therapeutic benefit can be expected.

Extra-oral radiographs help to scan the entire dentition and assess the number of teeth developing, any obvious ectopic teeth, and other possible pathology. A dental panoramic tomograph can be invaluable in demonstrating which teeth may be missing. Children with known hypodontia of a particular tooth may benefit from having this view taken to screen for further missing teeth elsewhere in the mouth. Cephalometric views may be employed to confirm any altered craniofacial morphology associated with hypodontia (Chung et al., 2000; Bondarets et al., 2002) or to assess skeletal discrepancies that may benefit from early correction with functional or orthopaedic appliances.

The use of supplementary intraoral radiographs can give greater localised clarity than extraoral views when this is considered necessary. Bite-wing radiographs assist in the diagnosis of caries where this is suspected on interstitial surfaces. Periapical radiographs show pathological changes to roots and surrounding supporting tissues, and can also assist in the location of ectopic teeth, using the parallax method. This consists of using two radiographs taken at different horizontal angles with the same vertical angulation, introducing tube shift (Clark, 1909; Jacobs, 1999, 2000; Jones et al., 2000; Mason et al., 2001; Nagpal et al., 2009), whereby the more distant object appears to travel in the same direction of the tube shift, and the closer object appears to move in the opposite direction. This can be described as the SLOB rule (Same Lingual, Opposite Buccal). Combinations of radiographs that can be used in parallax are:

1. Two intraoral periapical views taken at different horizontal angles (horizontal parallax).
2. One periapical and an upper anterior occlusal radiograph (horizontal parallax).
3. An upper anterior occlusal radiograph and a dental panoramic tomograph (vertical parallax).

Vitality testing

Vitality testing of primary teeth has limited validity and can often lead to 'false positive' results (Gopikrishna et al., 2009). However, when there is a question over the status of a permanent tooth that has experienced trauma, this should be investigated as part of the assessment of the dentition. A number of different methods may be used including electrical and thermal stimuli, but it is often very difficult to achieve accurate reporting from young patients (Goho, 1999).

Orthodontic assessment

An orthodontic assessment is essential to enable comprehensive treatment planning to be considered. The skeletal pattern, jaw relationships, soft tissue morphology and patterns of activity, freeway space (FWS), and occlusion should be assessed. This includes the horizontal and vertical relationships between posterior and anterior opposing teeth and involves determination of overjet and overbite. Measurement of spacing within the arches is important and may be accomplished intraorally or on study casts. The positions of teeth within the arch, and their angulations and height within the alveolar bone are important considerations. Ectopic eruption patterns and crossbites may complicate the situation (Carter *et al.*, 2003; Thind *et al.*, 2005).

Freeway space assessment

An assessment of the freeway space can be a useful guide to the vertical dimension of occlusion, which may be judged to be inadequate both on an intraoral basis and also on extraoral examination. Patients with severe hypodontia may exhibit craniofacial growth patterns that produce a markedly reduced lower facial height, increased freeway space and the appearance of over-closure (Sarnäs and Rune, 1983; Øgaard and Krogstad, 1995; Bondarets and McDonald, 2000; Chung *et al.*, 2000). Indeed the impact of a large freeway space may give rise to an unsolicited complaint from patients or carers. Patients with severe hypodontia may have an increased freeway space due to the reduced height of the retained (and probably worn) primary teeth in comparison to the growing jaws and soft tissues (Dermaut *et al.*, 1986; Øgaard and Krogstad, 1995). This will be an important measurement when considering treatment with overdentures to help restore a more normal lower face height.

Infra-occlusion

The extent of infra-occlusion of a tooth may vary from a minor discrepancy to the tooth being only partly visible through (or completely covered by) the oral mucosa. Following eruption, the tooth remains static and is not affected by growth of the neighbouring alveolar bone and vertical changes in the occlusal plane. It can therefore appear clinically as if the tooth has submerged (Sidhu and Ali, 2001). A tooth that is infra-occluded will be immobile, and may frequently be ankylosed, which involves fusion of cementum and dentine to alveolar bone (Kurol and Olson, 1991; Kurol, 2006). The highest incidence of ankylosis has been found to be in primary molars, ranging from 1.5% to 9.9%

(Albers, 1986) with infra-occlusion being slightly higher at 8–14% (Kurol, 1981). It may be tested clinically by tapping the tooth gently and listening for a 'cracked-pot' or metallic tone, which is indicative of the fusion of the cementum or dentine to the alveolar bone. This complication will result in deterioration of the position of the tooth over time, and presages problems in removal resulting from its fusion to the bone. Periapical radiographs may not accurately reflect the histological changes occurring around the roots although partial or total absence of the periodontal ligament may be evident.

Decisions relating to the treatment of such teeth will vary depending on the overall orthodontic assessment along with the degree and rate of infra-occlusion (Ekim and Hatibovic-Kofman, 2001). Brearley and McKibben (1973) have suggested the following classification of infra-occlusion:

- Slight: Occlusal surface located approximately 1 mm below the expected plane of the tooth
- Moderate: Occlusal surface approximately level with the contact point of one or both adjacent teeth (Figure 7.2)
- Severe: Occlusal surface level with or below the interproximal gingival tissue on one or both adjacent teeth (Figure 7.3)

Problems associated with infra-occlusion include mesial tipping of adjacent teeth, particularly the

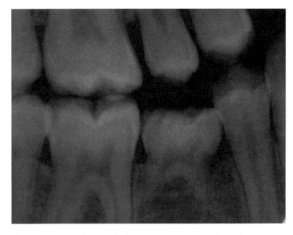

Figure 7.2 Radiograph demonstrating a moderately infra-occluded primary second molar.

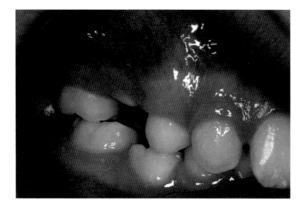

Figure 7.3 Severe infra-occlusion of an upper primary first molar in a 9-year-old patient.

first permanent molar when the second primary molar is infra-occluded, and lack of marginal alveolar bone (which may affect subsequent implant placement). Treatment options consist of either removal of the tooth (usually with moderate to severe infra-occlusion) or building up of the tooth so that the occlusal surface is level with that of the adjacent teeth (slight to moderate infra-occlusion). Decisions as to treatment should be made in conjunction with an orthodontist and, where relevant, restorative assessment.

Treatment

Following a full examination and discussions with the patient and his or her carers it is possible to consider the treatment that would be appropriate for the patient's stage of development. It is important to take into account the patient's and carers' opinions, including their interests in treatment and expectations of its outcomes. These may be influenced by family support groups, published articles and media information. On occasions a compromise may be required, and an initial approach to care agreed so as to be able to assess the realism of their aspirations and ability to accept treatment. It is crucial to avoid causing iatrogenic disease or distressing the patient because of behaviour management issues, as difficulties at this stage can result in long-term problems including disaffection with ongoing dental care.

Treatment planning

Planning involves decision-making in relation to what should be done, and equally as important, its timing. In some situations, a decision may be made to defer any active treatment because of a perceived lack of need by the patient, carers or clinicians, and the status quo accepted at that stage, with an option to review later. Concerns over potential cooperation with oral health maintenance or issues relating to behaviour management may also result in a postponement of active treatment, until the patient is more mature. However, intervention is necessary when there is dental disease, such as caries or periodontal infection, in order to maintain a healthy mouth, which would be essential prior to any later advanced treatment.

Dental care in young patients creates a platform for future treatment. The maintenance of healthy oral tissues is an important basis from which, if it is desirable, more complex treatment can considered, and this can be assessed during these early years. Optimal occlusal development is also important and can be encouraged by appropriate intervention taking advantage of growth patterns and normal tooth movements. These preliminary treatments prepare the patient for more definitive care, later on, when dental development has progressed and a coordinated plan of orthodontic and restorative intervention may be appropriate. They also provide an opportunity to assess the patient's suitability for more complex treatment, which requires greater patient commitment.

Interceptive treatment may be considered in order to facilitate future planning. This includes the removal of primary teeth which can encourage an improved eruption pathway of the successor or adjacent permanent tooth, extraction of infra-occluded teeth whose position is deteriorating and where access may become problematic, or a fraenectomy to facilitate the closure of an upper midline diastema. When a young patient has a concern, for example about the shape of the upper central incisors or the space between these teeth, interceptive treatment can be provided with limited objectives, in the knowledge that the patient will require further definitive management later. This will deal with the patient's immediate concerns and help to develop a relationship with the dental team. Multiple spaces in the primary or early mixed dentition, both anteriorly and posteriorly, may lead to aesthetic and masticatory problems (Laing *et al.*, 2008, 2010) which can usually be resolved with removable prostheses. The possible benefits of interceptive orthodontics should also be considered at this stage.

Consent to treatment

There are several issues relating to consent, since not all young children with hypodontia may want treatment, potentially bringing the patient into conflict with their carers and presenting a challenge for the dentist. Problems sometimes arise where there is a difference of opinion between patients and their carers as to the desirability, necessity and appropriateness of early intervention. Carers may feel strongly that early treatment is desirable for their child, whereas the dental team may have reservations. These issues need to be discussed with all concerned keeping the welfare of the patient foremost. It is also important to ascertain who has parental responsibility for a child under the age of 16 who is undergoing treatment. While these matters are jurisdiction-dependent in the UK, children over the age of 16 years are presumed in law to have capacity to consent to treatment unless there is evidence to the contrary. The Children Act 1989 states who has parental responsibility for a child, thus:

- A mother will always have parental responsibility for her child
- A father will have parental responsibility only if he was married to the mother when the child was born or has gained this responsibility legally by either registering the birth with the mother (only for children born after December 2003) or by way of a parental responsibility agreement made with the mother or in a court
- A child's legally appointed guardian
- A person who has a legally appointed residence order concerning the child
- A local authority designated in a Care Order in respect of the child
- A local authority or person who holds an Emergency Care Order for the child

There remains a degree of inconsistency and ambiguity in the law, and a right to give consent is not balanced with a right to withhold consent (Lowden, 2002). Legally, if a child refuses treatment, their carer can insist that they have the treatment done (Devereux *et al.*, 1993). The issue of Gillick competence (or Fraser competency) is less clear than in the past (Douglas, 1992; Dimond, 2001), although the child is more likely to have a greater influence on whether treatment proceeds when this may be considered to be not life-threatening (Stauch, 1995; Perera, 2008; Cave, 2009). Clinicians must be cautious in proceeding unless the treatment is considered necessary from a health point of view, such as a grossly carious tooth that requires removal. Other treatments, such as the provision of dentures or the restorative building up of teeth, are more aesthetic and best left until requested by the child.

Prevention

It is vital that good oral health is part of the treatment, and that it is maintained both throughout the active treatment phases and thereafter. Achieving good oral health, through the efforts of the patient and their general dental practitioner, may be the only outcome that can be achieved for the patient. The risks of iatrogenic disease as a result of commencing active therapy in an unhealthy mouth should be explained in the initial stages of discussing treatment options. Cooperation with good oral health needs to be discussed with patients and carers as part of the contract established between all the parties regarding treatment. It should be understood that deterioration in oral health will compromise the treatment plan, and may lead to its postponement or cessation. The prevention of dental caries depends on a coordinated approach to four aspects of care, namely diet, oral hygiene, fluoride and fissure sealing (Toumba *et al.*, 2003).

There is well-established guidance on dietary control with regard to refined carbohydrate intake, as well as the need to control acidic drinks associated with erosion. Sticky textured foods should be avoided because of their deleterious effect on fixed orthodontic appliances as well as adhesive restorations. Snacking on sugary foods between meals must be strongly discouraged, making suggestions for alternative, less harmful snacks.

The removal of plaque through efficient oral hygiene measures is acknowledged as important in the prevention of both dental caries and gingival disease. Manual and electric toothbrushes are recommended with the additional use of floss. Single-tuft brushes are particularly appropriate for patients with spaces and irregularly aligned teeth, as well as for cleaning around fixed orthodontic appliances. Patients should be encouraged to brush twice a day for two to 3 minutes and the carers should monitor this.

The caries-protective effect of fluoride has been researched and confirmed over many decades (McDonagh *et al.*, 2000). There are several methods of delivery, with water fluoridation and regular use of fluoride toothpaste being the most effective (Holt and Murray, 1997). Different toothpastes are recommended for different age groups, and pastes with 2800 and 5000 parts per million of available fluoride are produced for use by groups of patients with specific needs. Fluoride mouthwashes are also valuable for the caries-susceptible patient, including those wearing fixed orthodontic appliances. The use of professionally applied fluoride varnishes has also been shown to be useful in preventing dental decay (Marinho, 2009) and should be considered for the hypodontia patient. Care regarding the ingestion of fluoride must always be considered, especially if using higher concentrations than usual. The side effects of ingestion of excessive levels of fluoride include toxicity and fluorosis affecting the permanent dentition.

Fissure sealants are used to form a micromechanically bonded protective layer over the occlusal pits and fissures of caries-susceptible teeth, and their success has been widely reported (Simonsen, 2002). The use of fissure sealants is recommended in several groups of patients, into which patients with hypodontia may fall. Children who have a high caries rate in the primary dentition are recommended to have sealants applied to their permanent molars and premolars on eruption, in order to protect the occlusal surfaces. Children with special needs or those with unusual dental morphology, where the fissure system may be very deep, also benefit from early use of sealants (Nunn *et al.*, 2000). Certainly fissure sealing of the first permanent molars in a child with hypodontia is justifiable and will offer extra protection against dental decay. Patients with hypodontia who have primary teeth that are to be maintained for as long as possible will also benefit from the protection that sealants provide when used in the primary dentition.

Restorative treatment

Initial

As part of the initial phase of preparing the patient for involvement in long-term multidisciplinary care, their early experience with dentistry should be tailored to their dental and psychological needs. Patients with hypodontia will usually have regular contact with the hypodontia team, therefore a key aim of care in the young child is to maintain their enthusiasm and cooperation. Any carious teeth should be restored where possible and restorations and pulp treatment may be routinely used to create a functioning dentition (Yengopal *et al.*, 2009). Techniques such as pulpectomy and the placing of stainless steel crowns may, where necessary, have a large role in maintaining the primary dentition in these patients for as long as possible (Duggal, 2003; Duggal *et al.*, 2003; Attari and Roberts, 2006; Innes *et al.*, 2006, 2009; Rosenblatt, 2008).

Dental treatment can be difficult to carry out in young children and its importance may not be well understood by the patient. This is particularly relevant for children with hypodontia, where there is an increased emphasis on dentistry early on in their lives and care must be taken not to discourage or cause unnecessary distress. This can occur either by excessive focus on dental care or the use of painful procedures that are not strictly necessary. The patient's future care will probably have a relatively large dental component so their early experiences must be as pleasant as possible.

Fayle and Tahmassebi (2003) have suggested that non-pharmacological and pharmacological behaviour management techniques should be employed at an early stage. The benefits of conscious sedation for treatment of children have been well reported, especially if given over the first few visits complex or uncomfortable procedures. It helps to promote a positive psychological response to treatment (Holroyd and Roberts, 2000; Hosey, 2002; Paterson and Tahmassebi, 2003; Hosey and

Fayle, 2006). Consideration should also be given to possible treatment under general anaesthesia, particularly if extensive dentistry due to dental decay is required at an early stage.

Early build-up of primary or microdont teeth

One of the main complaints in the young patient following eruption of the upper and lower incisors is increased spacing due to the size and shape of the teeth, or the absence of teeth. Simple early treatment to improve appearance by using composite resin to enlarge or re-shape the teeth and reduce or close spaces can also bring about increased self-confidence as well as creating a rapport with the dental team. The restorations provided should be conservative in their design so as to minimise damage to the tooth structure. Even if they are only temporary, they will mask the defects until more permanent intervention can begin, typically with orthodontic and restorative treatment. Children with severe hypodontia may only have microdont primary incisors (Figure 7.4)

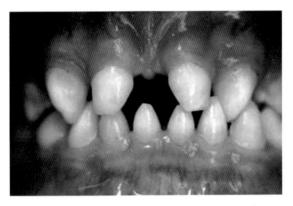

Figure 7.4 Microdont primary incisors associated with severe hypodontia.

with no permanent successors and these teeth may require building up to restore aesthetics and function.

The re-contouring of teeth by the addition of etch-retained composite material, as either facings or a crown addition, can increase the dimensions of the tooth, and modify the contour such that pointed or parallel-sided teeth appear to have more normal morphology. In addition this may result in the closure of some, if not all, of the interdental spaces. Retained but firm primary incisors, particularly those in the lower jaw that may be visible, can also be restored with composite resin, although the extent of the addition may be more limited. The retention of composite restorative materials to the enamel of primary teeth is poor, and the surface area to be etched as well as the crown to root ratio may be limiting features in the size of any modifications. Extension of composite material labially can help increase retention. Newly erupted permanent anterior teeth may be small and require composite resin additions to help with initial aesthetics (Figure 7.5). This can be an easy and pain-free way to provide an 'instant' improvement in the patient's appearance.

Crowns and onlays

The posterior occlusion may require restoration to alter the vertical dimension of occlusion, and thus create adequate space for anterior restorations. There will be a reduction in the freeway space which, if large, may produce an improved overall appearance. This can be achieved with stainless steel crowns on primary molars and first permanent molars, or nickel chromium, gold or porcelain adhesive onlays. Such restorations may also manage carious cavities or enamel defects.

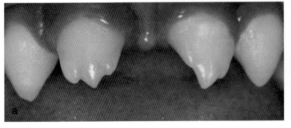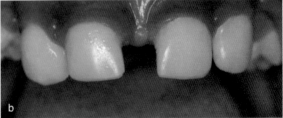

Figure 7.5 (a) Microdont permanent incisors in a patient with hypodontia. (b) Improved aesthetics following composite resin build-ups.

An infra-occluded molar without a successor, which has been identified early, may be restored in an attempt to stimulate the maintenance and regeneration of its periodontal ligament. This will also reduce the risk of tipping of the adjacent teeth, particularly the first permanent molar, leading to space loss. These restorations may be constructed using a variety of materials, although composite resin (prepared either in the laboratory or at the chair-side) and stainless steel crowns are most typically used (Ram and Peretz, 2003; Sabri, 2008). Delay in restoring such a tooth increases the technical difficulty associated with contouring the restoration and shaping its gingival margins.

Removable partial dentures
If there is hypodontia in the primary dentition, carers may ask about early prosthetic replacement. Early provision of prostheses should be patient-led rather than carer-led, and approached with caution due to the associated build up of plaque. Early intervention can also lead to subsequent cooperation difficulties when the permanent dentition requires treatment. Occasionally there may be some benefit in providing a small prosthesis in such cases as a diagnostic appliance to assess the patient's ability to tolerate its use, and having pointed out the potential risks. This often addresses the patient's or carers' concerns. Should there be poor patient compliance with use of the appliance then this will illustrate the problems of early intervention to the carers who then frequently accede to delaying further active intervention.

In the early mixed dentition, if there are concerns about spacing in the posterior quadrants or the need for posterior restorations to gain adequate space for anterior restorations, the construction of removable acrylic prostheses may be considered. These have several advantages – their relative ease of construction, cost, adaptability and reversibility, and the acceptability of the procedure from the patient's viewpoint. For these reasons their use can be valuable as a diagnostic or preliminary treatment. Among the disadvantages – they tend to be bulky, and can be lacking in stability with retention often limited by unhelpful tooth contours, necessitating the use of Adams' clasps and the modification of tooth contours with composite resins to facilitate clasp retention. In addition they are associated with increased levels of caries and periodontal disease unless oral hygiene is meticulous. This is especially a problem for patients with a reduced salivary flow. In addition there is a tendency to denture-related stomatitis if oral and denture hygiene is inadequate or if the denture is worn continually.

In general, partial dentures are rarely used in the early mixed dentition. This is because development of the full adult dentition is necessary prior to orthodontic treatment, which usually precedes the restorative phase of a treatment plan. There are two main exceptions – one is in patients with severe hypodontia in whom overdentures or complete dentures may be used; the other is if the permanent lateral incisors are absent. In the second situation the large diastema in the early mixed dentition may be of significant aesthetic concern to the patient. While awaiting eruption of the permanent canines, approximation of the central incisors can be carried out orthodontically and the child provided with a partial denture to temporarily replace the missing lateral incisors and retain the orthodontic treatment. Close monitoring for the eruption of the permanent canines must be carried out as these teeth may emerge mesial to their normal eruptive positions (Brin *et al.*, 1986).

Overdentures
Overdentures can be provided especially for patients with severe hypodontia (Stephen and Cengiz, 2003). This often involves the use of dentures overlying worn primary teeth with no permanent successors, and using any erupted permanent teeth for added retention (Figure 7.6). Advantages of the procedure include restoration of function and the occlusal vertical dimension (OVD), better retention than with conventional complete dentures, and possible preservation of alveolar bone (Crum and Rooney, 1978). It is important to use the correct size and type of teeth when constructing these dentures so that their appearance is appropriate (Goepferd and Carroll, 1981). The prosthetic teeth should match the teeth that would be present according to the patient's age. Primary prosthetic teeth can be used initially and then changes made as the patient enters the mixed dentition phase. Regular monitoring is essential as the natural primary teeth can be lost or become mobile and therefore adjustments of the dentures may need to be made.

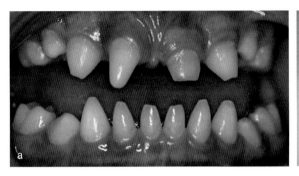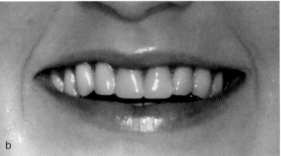

Figure 7.6   (a) Severe hypodontia with associated microdontia of primary teeth. (b) Improved appearance following provision of a maxillary overdenture.

Complete dentures

For children with anodontia, complete dentures, if requested, are the only solution to aesthetic and functional requirements. Carers are usually very keen for their young child to be provided with dentures at an early age. This has been shown to be successful in children even as young as 2 or 3 years and can allow the child to develop normally in terms of speech, chewing, swallowing, facial support and improved self-esteem (Hickey and Vergo, 2001). However, caution must be used with patients who do not want the treatment that is being requested by their carers. Some children are happy to avoid prostheses until they are older, although they may adapt poorly to dentures because they have become used to the absence of a prosthesis for a number of years. A compromise is to provide one denture at a time with a few months in between (Till and Marques, 1992). This allows the child to adapt to having a single prosthesis, usually in the upper arch, before providing them with the corresponding opposing arch prosthesis, an arrangement which is often found to be better tolerated. Complete dentures can offer acceptable aesthetic and functional results, but the underdevelopment of the alveolar ridges may compromise their retention and stability (Pigno *et al.*, 1996).

Although young children often cope very well with partial or complete dentures, sometimes they are not tolerated. In such cases, it may be best to abandon the use of dentures until the child requests such intervention, usually in their early teens. All types of dentures have their disadvantages, and problems such as speech difficulties, dietary limitations and loss of the prosthesis have been reported.

Where considered appropriate, children should be encouraged to persevere as much as possible and adaptation usually occurs.

Orthodontic treatment

It is unusual for extensive orthodontic treatment to be carried out in the primary or early mixed dentitions. There are some situations in which children may benefit from a phase of early orthodontic treatment, and this includes those with hypodontia. When early orthodontic procedures are considered, they should be completed in as short a time as possible so as to avoid reducing patient motivation and compliance with later definitive orthodontic treatment.

Removable appliances are usually simpler than fixed appliances in their technology and the outcome of treatment is more limited than with fixed appliances. They may be considered for simple early treatment if an upper incisor is in crossbite with a lower incisor and simply needs to be tipped 'over the bite'. Treating this early on is more important if there is displacement of the occlusion due to malocclusion- and/or occlusion-induced trauma to the lower incisors.

Fixed appliances enable the operator to move teeth with great accuracy both in position and angulation. A sectional appliance may be used to correct a small abnormality, such as a midline diastema, or a rotation that may be causing occlusal interference. Full-arch appliances are usually used in both arches simultaneously and such treatment is often not started until the permanent dentition has fully erupted. This allows for alignment of all the teeth and the appropriate closure or opening of spaces, as agreed by the multidisciplinary team. By delaying fixed orthodontic treatment until the permanent dentition erupts, treatment may be undertaken in a single phase, rather than in several, which often extends the treatment time and can reduce the patient's motivation and cooperation. In some cases it is necessary to carry out early fixed orthodontic procedures, usually due to the patient's request, low self-esteem or bullying as a result of the patient's appearance. For long-term success, the patient's compliance and understanding that another phase of orthodontic therapy will be required, must be assessed before treatment.

Surgical treatment

Extraction of primary teeth

Primary teeth that are severely affected by caries may be unrestorable because of the extent of tooth destruction or infection. Consequently extraction is the only treatment option. The need for balancing and compensating extractions should be considered, which is when an orthodontic opinion can be helpful. Primary teeth may show root resorption related to ectopic development of permanent teeth. In cases of crowding, the first permanent molars, particularly in the upper arch, may resorb the distal roots of the second primary molars, causing discomfort and ultimately increased mobility. Ectopic maxillary canines, particularly in the absence of lateral incisors, may erupt mesially to their normal positions and affect the primary lateral incisor roots (Brin *et al.*, 1986; Ericson and Kurol, 1986). The loss of primary teeth may encourage the eruption pathway of permanent teeth, thus reducing active orthodontic tooth movement at a later stage (Ericson and Kurol, 1988).

Ankylosed primary teeth that have become infra-occluded may present problems because of their potential to cause food packing thus increasing the risk of caries, or tilting of adjacent teeth resulting in oral hygiene problems and possible gingival disease (Rune and Sarnäs, 1984). If the infra-occlusion is progressive and the tooth loses its occlusal contacts then it is advisable to remove it before access becomes difficult, as at that stage extraction may require a surgical procedure (Jones and Robinson, 2001). When the root fuses to the adjacent bone a careful approach is essential to remove the dental tissue without destroying the surrounding alveolar process and a cautious surgical approach is always advised. Frequently the infra-occlusion causes the bulbosity of the deciduous tooth to become 'locked' below the marginal ridges of the adjacent teeth, which can cause extra difficulty during extraction. In such cases, removal of the mesial and distal portion of the infra-occluded tooth with a straight diamond bur can be undertaken to aid extraction. The first permanent molar may also become tilted mesially due to the lack of a contact point with the primary molar, and orthodontic treatment may be necessary to upright the adult molar in order to aid removal of the primary tooth. If the primary molar is severely infra-occluded then a surgical approach may be necessary, involving the raising of a mucoperiosteal flap and possible alveolar bone removal. Consideration must be given to the position of the mental nerve when carrying out such surgery in the mandible and appropriate precautions must be taken. Similarly, if severely infra-occluded primary molars are to be surgically removed in the maxilla, care must be taken to avoid creating an oral–antral fistula.

Extraction of permanent teeth

Permanent teeth that are affected severely by caries or hypomineralisation may have a poor long-term prognosis despite extensive restorative treatment (Figure 7.7). In these cases a decision may be made in conjunction with the team to accept the loss of

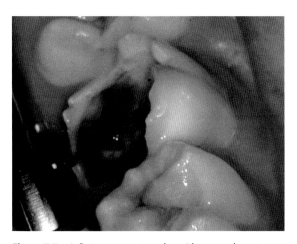

Figure 7.7 A first permanent molar with a poor long-term prognosis.

permanent teeth even though this means a further reduction in their number. The extraction should be carried out as carefully as possible, to preserve the maximum supporting tissues for later treatment options.

Microdont permanent teeth may be deemed to be too small or of a shape that precludes their restoration in a functional or aesthetic manner; their early loss allows full space assessment to be undertaken at treatment planning. The replacement of a unit with a prosthetic tooth of good contour and colour and with a realistic apparent gingival-emergence profile may be preferable to a compromised attempt to retain a tooth.

Ectopic teeth and those exhibiting delayed eruption can be found in both arches in patients with hypodontia. An assessment of these teeth should be made, taking into account such factors as age, general stage of development, root maturity, tooth angulation, and position of the tooth in relation to any erupted teeth (with particular reference to resorption of roots). In order to encourage the eruption of a tooth it may be necessary to expose it surgically, in conjunction with packing of the area or bonding an attachment to the surface of the tooth to enable orthodontic direction of its path of eruption. The most usual attachment is a gold chain, which is bonded to the surface of the unerupted tooth with etch-retained composite resin (Figure 7.8). This is a relatively conservative technique, which depends on good moisture control to allow for effective adhesion (Jones *et al.*, 2000). Some workers have suggested using a magnet bonded to the unerupted tooth (Sandler

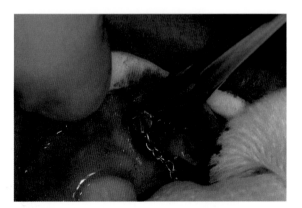

Figure 7.8 Surgical exposure of an unerupted incisor with bonding of a gold chain for orthodontic traction.

et al., 1989; Mancini *et al.*, 1999; Noar and Evans, 1999) as a method of applying a force to guide its eruption.

Soft tissue surgery

In young patients one of the common early treatments is closure of an upper midline diastema to overcome the spacing (a common complaint). The diastema is frequently associated with an enlarged and sometimes fleshy fraenum, which extends between the central incisors and even onto the palatal mucosa. This inhibits the complete closure of the diastema and also encourages its relapse at the end of orthodontic treatment, unless permanent retention is used. The timing of a fraenectomy is subject to debate. The advantage of removing the fraenum before orthodontic treatment is ease of surgical access, especially if it is necessary to extend the incision palatally. On the other hand, it is thought that if surgery is carried out prior to orthodontic treatment then any scar tissue will prevent complete closure of the diastema. Each case is therefore best treated on its individual merits and through discussion with an orthodontist.

Implants in the young patient

Young patients who have severe hypodontia may have difficulties coping with overdentures or complete dentures. This may be due to their age and limited cooperation and perseverance. Small alveolar ridges or decreased salivary volume in patients with ectodermal dysplasia may also contribute to compromised retention. These children may be more content without a prosthesis, not reporting any masticatory difficulties or concerns regarding aesthetics. For some children, though, this is not the case and while it remains controversial there is increasing debate between professionals regarding the provision of implants in young children who have difficulties with a conventional prosthesis so as to improve stability and hence psychosocial and psychological benefits (Kraut, 1996; Pigno *et al.*, 1996).

It has been suggested that implants have a beneficial impact on the preservation of bone in young children with severe hypodontia (von Wowern *et al.*, 1990; Denissen *et al.*, 1993; Murphy, 1995). This is because of the underdevelopment of the alveolar ridges from the lack of teeth and preservation of what bone remains due to loading via the implant. Nevertheless children with hypodontia often have little bone in which to place implants (Smith *et al.*, 1993; Bryant, 1998), which means that bone augmentation may be required prior to placement. The current lack of robust evidence about the effects of such procedures in young children means that such treatment is difficult to justify.

Although reported to be successful in children as young as 5 years old (Smith *et al.*, 1993; Kearns *et al.*, 1999) further surgical revision is invariably required due to these disadvantages. Therefore implants are usually not recommended unless the child is at least over the age of 12 (Bryant, 1998). It has been suggested that developmental factors such as dental and skeletal maturity are more important than chronological age when considering placement of implants in children (Thilander *et al.*, 1994).

If implants are placed in young children with severe hypodontia anterior to the mandibular canine region, where mandibular growth is mostly complete by the age of 11 years, there may be both psychological and functional advantages (Salinas, 2005; Sharma and Vargervik, 2006). Some studies have demonstrated implant success in young patients (Guckes *et al.*, 2002; Imirzalioglu *et al.*, 2002), but there seems to be a consensus that implants should not be routinely recommended for them (Shapiro and Kokich, 1988; Oesterle *et al.*, 1993; Brugnolo *et al.*, 1996; Percinoto *et al.*, 2001; Williams *et al.*, 2004; Brahim, 2005; Sharma and Vargervik, 2006).

At present, the level of evidence for success in young children is weak (Bergendal, 2008; Yap and Klineberg, 2009). While implants have been used in patients aged below 18 years who have severe hypodontia associated with ectodermal dysplasia (Kramer *et al.*, 2007), there is evidence that there is a higher risk of failure (Kearns *et al.*, 1999; Guckes *et al.*, 2002; Bergendal *et al.*, 2008). The main concerns regarding children who have not fully finished growth are that the implants will act similarly to ankylosed teeth, so with vertical development of the jaws, prosthetic infra-occlusion may occur (Cronin *et al.*, 1994; Johansson *et al.*, 1994; Brugnolo *et al.*, 1996; Bryant, 1998; Becktor *et al.*, 2001; Imirzalioglu *et al.*, 2002; Rossi and Andreasen, 2003; Brahim, 2005).

Key Points: Treatment in the primary/early mixed dentition

- Children can often be challenging to treat and this can be complicated by carer concerns
- Every effort must be made to ensure that both child and carer are informed of all possible treatment options
- Where possible the child should be made to feel part of the decision-making process
- It is important not to pressurise children with hypodontia to have treatment in the early mixed dentition and their views must be considered
- Children with hypodontia may require extensive treatment later in life so it is important not to lose their compliance
- Prevention and maintaining good oral health are fundamental to treating children with hypodontia
- Management during early mixed dentition can vary from no active treatment to 'interim' restorative procedures (e.g. dentures, build-ups and bridges)
- Young patients and their carers must be informed that due to growth any treatment given at this age may be an intermediate phase which can be built on when the patient is older

Dental implants in the primary/early mixed dentition
- Dental implant treatment can be valuable in the skeletally mature child. Its use in young children is at present controversial due to a lack of clinical data
- At present the level of evidence for implant success in young children is weak
- A high rate of implant loss before loading has been reported in young patients
- Osseointegrated implants are effectively ankylosed and subsequent jaw growth can cause them to become 'infra-occluded' and unsuitably aligned for prosthodontic reconstruction
- It is now generally considered that implants should not be used until after skeletal maturity

Other potentially unfavourable consequences include:

- Implant 'infra-occlusion' due to bone growth whereby the length and height of the mandible continues to develop into early adulthood (Salinas, 2005; Ersoy *et al.*, 2006; Heij *et al.*, 2006; Fudalej *et al.*, 2007)

- Implant exposure due to bone resorption associated with jaw growth
- Limitation of jaw growth if implants are connected by a rigid prosthesis crossing the midline (Oesterle *et al.*, 1993; Cronin and Oesterle, 1998; Nohl *et al.*, 2008)
- A high rate of implant loss before loading (one retrospective analysis of outcomes showed a rate of loss of 64.3% in patients aged 5–2 years) (Bergendal *et al.*, 2008)

References

Albers DD. Ankylosis of teeth in the developing dentition. *Quintessence Int* 1986;17:303–308.

Attari N, Roberts JF. Restoration of primary teeth with crowns: A systematic review of the literature. *Eur Arch Paediatr Dent* 2006;7:58–62.

Becktor KB, Becktor JP, Keller EE. Growth analysis of a patient with ectodermal dysplasia treated with endosseous implants: A case report. *Int J Oral Maxillofac Implants* 2001;16:864–874.

Bergendal B. When should we extract deciduous teeth and place implants in young individuals with tooth agenesis? *J Oral Rehabil* 2008;35(Suppl.1):55–63.

Bergendal B, Bergendal T, Hallonsten AL, *et al.* A multidisciplinary approach to oral rehabilitation with osseointegrated implants in children and adolescents with multiple aplasia. *Eur J Orthod* 1996;18:119–129.

Bergendal B, Ekman A, Nilsson P. Implant failure in young children with ectodermal dysplasia: A retrospective evaluation of use and outcome of dental implant treatment in children in Sweden. *Int J Oral Maxillofac Implants* 2008;23:520–524.

Bishop K, Addy L, Knox J. Modern restorative management of patients with congenitally missing teeth: 1. Introduction, terminology and epidemiology. *Dent Update* 2006;33:531–537.

Bishop K, Addy L, Knox J. Modern restorative management of patients with congenitally missing teeth: 3. Conventional restorative options and considerations. *Dent Update* 2007a;34:30–38.

Bishop K, Addy L, Knox J. Modern restorative management of patients with congenitally missing teeth: 4. The role of implants. *Dent Update* 2007b;34:79–84.

Bollmer BW, Sturzenberger OP, Lehnhoff RW, *et al.* A comparison of 3 clinical indices for measuring gingivitis. *J Clin Periodontol* 1986;13:392–395.

Bondarets N, McDonald F. Analysis of the vertical facial form in patients with severe hypodontia. *Am J Phys Anthropol* 2000;111:177–184.

Bondarets N, Jones RM, McDonald F. Analysis of facial growth in subjects with syndromic ectodermal dysplasia: a longitudinal analysis. *Orthod Craniofac Res* 2002;5:71–84.

Brahim JS. Dental implants in children. *Oral Maxillofac Surg Clin North Am* 2005;17:375–381.

Brearley LJ, McKibben DH Jr. Ankylosis of primary molar teeth. I. Prevalence and characteristics. *ASDC J Dent Child* 1973;40:54–63.

Brin I, Becker A, Shalhav M. Position of the maxillary permanent canine in relation to anomalous or missing lateral incisors: a population study. *Eur J Orthod* 1986;8:12–16.

Brugnolo E, Mazzocco C, Cordioli G, Majzoub Z. Clinical and radiographic findings following placement of single-tooth implants in young patients–Case reports. *Int J Periodontics Restorative Dent* 1996;16:421–433.

Bryant SR. The effects of age, jaw site, and bone condition on oral implant outcomes. *Int J Prosthodont* 1998;11:470–490.

Carter NE, Gillgrass TJ, Hobson RS, *et al.* The interdisciplinary management of hypodontia: orthodontics. *Br Dent J* 2003;194:361–366.

Cave E. Adolescent consent and confidentiality in the UK. *Eur J Health Law* 2009;16:309–331.

Chaves ES, Wood RC, Jones AA, *et al.* Relationship of 'bleeding on probing' and 'gingival index bleeding' as clinical parameters of gingival inflammation. *J Clin Periodontol* 1993;20:139–143.

Chung LK, Hobson RS, Nunn JH, Gordon PH, Carter NE. An analysis of the skeletal relationships in a group of young people with hypodontia. *J Orthod* 2000;27:315–318.

Ciancio SG. Current status of indices of gingivitis. *J Clin Periodontol* 1986;13:375–382.

Clark C. A method of ascertaining the position of unerupted teeth by means of film radiographs. *Proc R Soc Med* 1909;3:87–90.

Cronin RJ Jr, Oesterle LJ. Implant use in growing patients. Treatment planning concerns. *Dent Clin North Am* 1998;42:1–34.

Cronin RJ Jr, Oesterle LJ, Ranly DM. Mandibular implants and the growing patient. *Int J Oral Maxillofac Implants* 1994;9:55–62.

Crum RJ, Rooney GE Jr. Alveolar bone loss in overdentures: A 5-year study. *J Prosthet Dent* 1978;40:610–613.

Denissen HW, Kalk W, Veldhuis HA, van Waas MA. Anatomic consideration for preventive implantation. *Int J Oral Maxillofac Implants* 1993;8:191–196.

Dermaut LR, Goeffers KR, De Smit AA. Prevalence of tooth agenesis correlated with jaw relationship and dental crowding. *Am J Orthod Dentofacial Orthop* 1986;90:204–210.

Devereux JA, Jones DP, Dickenson DL. Can children withhold consent to treatment? *BMJ* 1993;306:1459–1461.

Dhanrajani PJ. Hypodontia: Etiology, clinical features, and management. *Quintessence Int* 2002;33:294–302.

Dimond B. Legal aspects of consent 8: Children under the age of 16 years. *Br J Nurs* 2001;10:797–799.

Douglas G. The retreat from Gillick. *Mod Law Rev* 1992; 55:569–576.

Duggal MS. Paediatric dentistry in the new millennium: 1. Quality care for children. *Dent Update* 2003;30: 230–234.

Duggal MS, Gautam SK, Nichol R, Robertson AJ. Paediatric dentistry in the new millennium: 4. Cost-effective restorative techniques for primary molars. *Dent Update* 2003;30:410–415.

Ekim SL, Hatibovic-Kofman S. A treatment decision-making model for infra-occluded primary molars. *Int J Paediatr Dent* 2001;11:340–346.

Ericson S, Kurol J. Radiographic assessment of maxillary canine eruption in children with clinical signs of eruption disturbance. *Eur J Orthod* 1986;8:133–140.

Ericson S, Kurol J. Early treatment of palatally erupting canines by extraction of the primary canines. *Eur J Orthod* 1988;10:283–295.

Ersoy AE, Ellialti DB, Dogan N. Implant-supported prosthetic applications on development of children and adolescents: A pilot study in pigs. *Implant Dent* 2006;15: 412–419.

Fayle SA, Tahmassebi JF. Paediatric dentistry in the new millennium: 2. Behaviour management–helping children to accept dentistry. *Dent Update* 2003;30: 294–298.

Fudalej P, Kokich VG, Leroux B. Determining the cessation of vertical growth of the craniofacial structures to facilitate placement of single-tooth implants. *Am J Orthod Dentofacial Orthop* 2007;131(Suppl.4): S59–67.

Gill DS, Jones S, Hobkirk J, *et al.* Counselling patients with hypodontia. *Dent Update* 2008;35:344–352.

Goepferd SJ, Carroll CE. Hypohidrotic ectodermal dysplasia: A unique approach to esthetic and prosthetic management. *J Am Dent Assoc* 1981;102:867–869.

Goho C. Pulse oximetry evaluation of vitality in primary and immature permanent teeth. *Pediatr Dent* 1999;21: 125–127.

Goodman JR, Jones SP, Hobkirk JA, King PA. Hypodontia: 1. Clinical features and the management of mild to moderate hypodontia. *Dent Update* 1994;21:381–384.

Gopikrishna V, Pradeep G, Venkateshbabu N. Assessment of pulp vitality: a review. *Int J Paediatr Dent* 2009;19: 3–15.

Guckes AD, Scurria MS, King TS, McCarthy GR, Brahim JS. Prospective clinical trial of dental implants in persons with ectodermal dysplasia. *J Prosthet Dent* 2002;88: 21–25.

Haselden K, Hobkirk JA, Goodman JR, Jones SP, and Hemmings KW. Root resorption in deciduous canine and molar teeth without permanent successors in patients with severe hypodontia. *Int J Paediatr Dent* 2001;11:171–178.

Heath N, Macleod I, Pearce R. Major salivary gland agenesis in a young child: consequences for oral health. *Int J Paediatr Dent* 2006;16:431–448.

Heij DG, Opdebeeck H, van Steenberghe D, *et al.* Facial development, continuous tooth eruption, and mesial drift as compromising factors for implant placement. *Int J Oral Maxillofac Implants* 2006;21:867–878.

Hickey AJ, Vergo TJ Jr. Prosthetic treatments for patients with ectodermal dysplasia. *J Prosthet Dent* 2001;86: 364–368.

Hobkirk JA, Goodman JR, Jones SP. Presenting complaints and findings in a group of patients attending a hypodontia clinic. *Br Dent J* 1994;177:337–339.

Hobkirk JA, Nohl F, Bergendal B, Storhaug K, Richter MK. The management of ectodermal dysplasia and severe hypodontia. International conference statements. *J Oral Rehabil* 2006;33:634–637.

Hobson RS, Carter NE, Gillgrass TJ, *et al.* The interdisciplinary management of hypodontia: the relationship between an interdisciplinary team and the general dental practitioner. *Br Dent J* 2003;194:479–482.

Holroyd I, Roberts GJ. Inhalation sedation with nitrous oxide: A review. *Dent Update* 2000;27:141–146.

Holt RD, Murray JJ. Developments in fluoride toothpastes – An overview. *Community Dent Health* 1997;14:4–10.

Hosey MT. UK National Clinical Guidelines in Paediatric Dentistry. Managing anxious children: The use of conscious sedation in paediatric dentistry. *Int J Paediatr Dent* 2002;12:359–372.

Hosey MT, Fayle S. Pharmaceutical prescribing for children. Part 5. Conscious sedation for dentistry in children. *Prim Dent Care* 2006;13:93–96.

Imirzalioglu P, Uckan S, Haydar SG. Surgical and prosthodontic treatment alternatives for children and adolescents with ectodermal dysplasia: A clinical report. *J Prosthet Dent* 2002;88:569–572.

Innes NP, Stirrups DR, Evans DJ, Hall N, Leggate M. A novel technique using preformed metal crowns for managing carious primary molars in general practice – A retrospective analysis. *Br Dent J* 2006;200:451–454.

Innes N, Evans D, Hall N. The Hall Technique for managing carious primary molars. *Dent Update* 2009;36: 472–478.

Jacobs SG. Localization of the unerupted maxillary canine: How to and when to. *Am J Orthod Dentofacial Orthop* 1999;115:314–322.

Jacobs SG. Radiographic localization of unerupted teeth: Further findings about the vertical tube shift method and other localization techniques. *Am J Orthod Dentofacial Orthop* 2000;118:439–447.

Johansson G, Palmqvist S, Svenson B. Effects of early placement of a single tooth implant. A case report. *Clin Oral Implants Res* 1994;5:48–51.

Jones J, Robinson PD. Submerging deciduous molars – An extraction in time! *Dent Update* 2001;28:309–311.

Jones SP, Hodges SJ, Bloom KL. Orthodontic Practice Now – The management of ectopic maxillary canines. *Dentalpractice* 2000;38(Suppl.12):9–13.

Kearns G, Sharma A, Perrott D, *et al.* Placement of endosseous implants in children and adolescents with hereditary ectodermal dysplasia. *Oral Surg Oral Med Oral Pathol Oral Radiol Endod* 1999;88:5–10.

Kramer FJ, Baethge C, Tschernitschek H. Implants in children with ectodermal dysplasia: A case report and literature review. *Clin Oral Implants Res* 2007;18:140–146.

Kraut RA. Dental implants for children: Creating smiles for children without teeth. *Pract Periodontics Aesthet Dent* 1996;8:909–1013.

Kurol J. Infra-occlusion of primary molars: An epidemiologic and familial study. *Community Dent Oral Epidemiol* 1981;9:94–102.

Kurol J. Impacted and ankylosed teeth: why, when, and how to intervene. *Am J Orthod Dentofacial Orthop* 2006;129(Suppl.4):S86–90.

Kurol J, Olson L. Ankylosis of primary molars–a future periodontal threat to the first permanent molars? *Eur J Orthod* 1991;13:404–409.

Laing ER, Cunningham SJ, Jones SP, Moles D, Gill DS. The psychosocial impact of hypodontia in children. *J Orthod* 2008;35:225.

Laing E, Cunningham SJ, Jones S, Moles D, Gill D. Psychosocial impact of hypodontia in children. *Am J Orthod Dentofacial Orthop* 2010;137:35–41.

Löe H. The Gingival Index, the Plaque Index and the Retention Index systems. *J Periodontol* 1967;38:610–616.

Löe H, Silness J. Periodontal disease in pregnancy: I Prevalence and severity. *Acta Odontol Scand* 1963;21:533–551.

Lowden J. Children's rights: A decade of dispute. *J Adv Nurs* 2002;37:100–107.

Mancini GP, Noar JH, Evans RD. The physical characteristics of neodymium iron boron magnets for tooth extrusion. *Eur J Orthod* 1999;21:541–550.

Marinho VC. Cochrane reviews of randomized trials of fluoride therapies for preventing dental caries. *Eur Arch Paediatr Dent* 2009;10:183–191.

Marks RG, Magnusson I, Taylor M, *et al.* Evaluation of reliability and reproducibility of dental indices. *J Clin Periodontol* 1993;20:54–58.

Mason C, Papadakou P, Roberts GJ. The radiographic localization of impacted maxillary canines: a comparison of methods. *Eur J Orthod* 2001;23:25–34.

McDonagh MS, Whiting PF, Wilson PM, *et al.* Systematic review of water fluoridation. *BMJ* 2000;321:855–859.

Murphy WM. Clinical and experimental bone changes after intraosseous implantation. *J Prosthet Dent* 1995;73: 31–35.

Nagpal A, Pai KM, Setty S, Sharma G. Localization of impacted maxillary canines using panoramic radiography. *J Oral Sci* 2009;51:37–45.

Noar JH, Evans RD. Rare earth magnets in orthodontics: An overview. *Br J Orthod* 1999;26:29–37.

Nohl F, Cole B, Hobson R, *et al.* The management of hypodontia: present and future. *Dent Update* 2008;35: 79–88.

Nunn JH, Murray JJ, Smallridge J. British Society of Paediatric Dentistry: A policy document on fissure sealants in paediatric dentistry. *Int J Paediatr Dent* 2000;10:174–177.

Nunn JH, Carter NE, Gillgrass TJ, *et al.* The interdisciplinary management of hypodontia: background and role of paediatric dentistry. *Br Dent J* 2003;194:245–251.

Oesterle LJ, Cronin RJ Jr, Ranly DM. Maxillary implants in the growing patient. *Int J Oral Maxillofac Implants* 1993;8:377–387.

Øgaard B, Krogstad O. Craniofacial structure and soft tissue profile in patients with severe hypodontia. *Am J Orthod Dentofacial Orthop* 1995;108:472–477.

Paterson SA, Tahmassebi JF. Paediatric dentistry in the new millennium: 3. Use of inhalation sedation in paediatric dentistry. *Dent Update* 2003;30:350–358.

Percinoto C, Vieira AE, Barbieri CM, Melhado FL, Moreira KS. Use of dental implants in children: A literature review. *Quintessence Int* 2001;32:381–383.

Perera A. Can I decide please? The state of children's consent in the UK. *Eur J Health Law* 2008;15:411–420.

Pigno MA, Blackman RB, Cronin RJ Jr, Cavazos E. Prosthodontic management of ectodermal dysplasia: A review of the literature. *J Prosthet Dent* 1996;76:541–545.

Ram D, Peretz B. Restoring coronal contours of retained infra-occluded primary second molars using bonded resin-based composite. *Pediatr Dent* 2003;25:71–73.

Rosenblatt A. The Hall technique is an effective treatment option for carious primary molar teeth. *Evid Based Dent* 2008;9:44–45.

Rossi E, Andreasen JO. Maxillary bone growth and implant positioning in a young patient: A Case report. *Int J Periodontics Restorative Dent* 2003;23:113–119.

Ruiz-Mealin EV, Gill DS, Parekh S, Jones SP, Moles DR. A radiographic study of tooth development in hypodontia. *J Orthod* 2009;36:291.

Rune B, Sarnäs KV. Root resorption and submergence in retained deciduous second molars. A mixed-longitudinal study of 77 children with developmental absence of second premolars. *Eur J Orthod* 1984;6: 123–131.

Sabri R. Management of over-retained mandibular deciduous second molars with and without permanent successors. *World J Orthod* 2008;9:209–220.

Salinas T. Implant placement in developing patients. *Pract Proced Aesthet Dent* 2005;17:14.

Sandler PJ, Meghji S, Murray AM, *et al.* Magnets and orthodontics. *Br J Orthod* 1989;16:243–249.

Sarnäs KV, Rune B. The facial profile in advanced hypodontia: A mixed longitudinal study of 141 children. *Eur J Orthod* 1983;5:133–143.

Shafi I, Phillips JM, Dawson MP, Broad RD, Hosey MT. A study of patients attending a multidisciplinary hypodontia clinic over a five year period. *Br Dent J* 2008; 205:649–652.

Shapiro PA, Kokich VG. Uses of implants in orthodontics. *Dent Clin North Am* 1988;32:539–550.

Sharma AB, Vargervik K. Using implants for the growing child. *J Calif Dent Assoc* 2006;34:719–724.

Sidhu HK, Ali A. Hypodontia, ankylosis and infraocclusion: Report of a case restored with a fibre-reinforced ceromeric bridge. *Br Dent J* 2001;191: 613–616.

Silness J, Löe H. Periodontal disease in pregnancy: II Correlation between oral hygiene and periodontal condition. *Acta Odontol Scand* 1964;22:121–135.

Simonsen RJ. Pit and fissure sealant: Review of the literature. *Pediatr Dent* 2002;24:393–414.

Smith RA, Vargervik K, Kearns G, Bosch C, Koumjian J. Placement of an endosseous implant in a growing child with ectodermal dysplasia. *Oral Surg Oral Med Oral Pathol* 1993;75:669–673.

Stauch M. Rationality and the refusal of medical treatment: A critique of the recent approach of the English courts. *J Med Ethics* 1995;21:162–165.

Stephen A, Cengiz SB. The use of overdentures in the management of severe hypodontia associated with

microdontia: A case report. *J Clin Pediatr Dent* 2003;27: 219–222.

Thilander B, Odman J, Gröndahl K, Friberg B. Osseointegrated implants in adolescents. An alternative in replacing missing teeth? *Eur J Orthod* 1994;16: 84–95.

Thind BS, Stirrups DR, Forgie AH, Larmour CJ, Mossey PA. Management of hypodontia: orthodontic considerations(II). *Quintessence Int* 2005;36:345–353.

Till MJ, Marques AP. Ectodermal dysplasia: Treatment considerations and case reports. *Northwest Dent* 1992; 71:25–28.

Toumba KJ, Tahmassebi JF, Balmer R. Paediatric dentistry in the new millennium: 5. Clinical prevention: The role of the general dental practitioner. *Dent Update* 2003;30:503–510.

Vanarsdall DC. *Concise Encyclopedia of Periodontology.* Munksgaard, Blackwell, 2007.

von Wowern N, Harder F, Hjørting-Hansen E, Gotfredsen K. ITI implants with overdentures: A prevention of bone loss in edentulous mandibles? *Int J Oral Maxillofac Implants* 1990;5:135–139.

Williams P, Travess H, Sandy J. The use of osseointegrated implants in orthodontic patients: I. Implants and their use in children. *Dent Update* 2004;31:287–290.

Worsaae N, Jensen BN, Holm B, Holsko J. Treatment of severe hypodontia-oligodontia–an interdisciplinary concept. *Int J Oral Maxillofac Surg* 2007;36:473–480.

Yap AK, Klineberg I. Dental implants in patients with ectodermal dysplasia and tooth agenesis: A critical review of the literature. *Int J Prosthodont* 2009;22:268–276.

Yengopal V, Harneker SY, Patel N, Siegfried N. Dental fillings for the treatment of caries in the primary dentition. *Cochrane Database Syst Rev* 2009, Apr 15, CD004483.

8 Late Mixed and Early Permanent Dentition

Introduction

The late mixed and early permanent dentition stage is a period when the permanent dentition is beginning to become established. As well as dental changes, pronounced general changes are also taking place, such as puberty, rapid facial growth and psychological development. It is a period when the consequences of hypodontia may start to become apparent to patients and their families. Consequently they may begin to feel concerned about spacing between the incisor teeth or the presence of small misshapen teeth. Children may also be bullied at school about their dental appearance.

Orthodontic treatment can often be considered in the late mixed and early permanent dentition stage. It may involve the use of fixed or removable appliances (e.g. functional appliances) once the majority of permanent teeth have erupted. The relative roles of the orthodontist and restorative dentist in providing care will vary depending on the severity of the hypodontia. At one extreme, where there are only a few missing units, ortho-

dontic space closure may be the treatment of choice and may be the only procedure required. At the other extreme, as represented by a dentition with large numbers of missing permanent teeth, restorative treatment may be the principal approach with orthodontics producing only small changes.

The aim of this chapter is to present an overview of the main orthodontic and restorative considerations when providing care during the late mixed and early permanent dentition stage. Box 8.1 summarises important principles of treatment planning and Table 8.1 summarises the most common forms of treatment according to the stage of development.

Late mixed and early permanent dentition stage

The last primary teeth to exfoliate are usually the second molars. These are replaced by the second premolars at the age of 11–12 years. In hypodontia there is often a generalised delay in dental development, on average approximately 1.5 years (Ruiz-

Hypodontia: A Team Approach to Management, First Edition
© J.A. Hobkirk, D.S. Gill, S.P. Jones, K.W. Hemmings, G.S. Bassi, A.L. O'Donnell and J.R. Goodman
Published 2011 by Blackwell Publishing Ltd

Mealin *et al.*, 2009). This delay appears to increase as the severity of hypodontia increases. For example, Ruiz-Mealin *et al.* (2009) showed that for each developmentally absent tooth the delay in dental development increased by a mean of 0.13 years. It is worth noting that this delay does not occur in all individuals.

A delay in a patient's dental development can mean postponing the preparation of a comprehensive treatment plan. It is not possible to assess whether a space for a missing maxillary lateral incisor should be opened or closed until the maxillary canine has erupted and a decision can be made as to whether this tooth could provide a reasonable substitute for the missing lateral incisor. It is often not sensible to commence with fixed appliance treatment until all the permanent teeth mesial to the first molars have erupted since ideally all teeth that require movement should be incorporated into the appliance during one episode. The delay in onset of orthodontic treatment can be frustrating for the family if the child's school peers may have already commenced such therapy. Sometimes the family may pressurise clinicians to begin orthodontic treatment even though the dentition has not been established. Pressure to comply with the family's wishes in these circumstances should be resisted because it may result in prolonged orthodontic treatment because at some point the newly erupted teeth will need to be incorporated into the appliance. If the remaining permanent teeth are close to eruption, one method of accelerating their emergence is to remove their primary predecessors (Kerr, 1980). This does, however, subject the patient to an unpleasant dental experience and the benefits

of the procedure must be discussed carefully with them and their family. Evidence suggests that earlier extraction of primary teeth may accelerate eruption of their successors (Kerr, 1980), although the risk of space loss must be considered carefully (as this will ultimately delay eruption).

Once in the late mixed or early permanent dentition stage, patients will ideally undergo a comprehensive assessment by a multidisciplinary team. Treatment at this stage will often involve input from an orthodontist and restorative and paediatric dentists. Generally speaking, patients with severe hypodontia require more restorative than orthodontic input, while milder situations can sometimes be managed by orthodontics alone. A patient with hypodontia may also have superimposed the general features of a malocclusion (e.g. a Class II or Class III incisor relationship) and it is important that this is also managed within the overall treatment plan.

In Chapter 4, the principles of treatment planning were outlined. The purpose of this chapter is to consider the orthodontic and restorative management of patients during the late mixed and early permanent dentition stage. Preventative dental care is important at all stages of dental development and the reader is referred to Chapter 5 for further information on this subject.

Orthodontic treatment

Orthodontic treatment is often commenced in the late mixed dentition or early permanent dentition stage. Treatment is directed at correcting general features of the malocclusion as well as those specific to hypodontia. There are a number of benefits in undertaking orthodontic treatment at this early stage:

1. Patients, as well as family members, are often beginning to develop concerns about how their teeth appear.
2. Fixed orthodontic appliances are usually more acceptable to patients in this age group as their peers are often also undergoing treatment.
3. Rapid facial growth during this period can facilitate overbite reduction and space closure as the dentition is in a continual state of passive eruption.

Table 8.1   Common forms of treatment according to developmental stage.

Age/dentition	Treatment	Comments
Under 6 years/ preschool (primary dentition)	Removable dentures for psychological and functional reasons	Will require regular adjustments during growth Retention and stability may be problematic in children with poorly developed alveolar ridges
7–12 years (mixed dentition)	Composite resin build-ups to improve the appearance of microdont permanent teeth or worn primary teeth	
	Removable dentures	
	Possibly interceptive extractions to guide eruption	Problems may include palatal maxillary canines and infraocclusion
	Simple orthodontic treatment for space redistribution (e.g. a diastema that cannot be closed restoratively)	Long-term retention required
Over 12 years (permanent dentition)	Orthodontic treatment Resin-bonded bridges following orthodontic treatment for tooth replacement	Pontics can be placed on the fixed appliance and retainer following orthodontics as a temporary measure Other methods of tooth replacement include: – maintaining the primary predecessor – dentures – fixed bridges – transplantation
	Composite resin build-up of microdont or hypoplastic teeth	Disguising intense hypoplastic patches can be difficult
	Overdentures (severe hypodontia)	Abutments help maintain alveolar bone, improve retention and stability and provide proprioception
16–20 years (established dentition)	Single tooth implants or implant fixed bridges or implant-retained overdentures	Placed when the majority of facial growth is complete (tends to be earlier in females (17 years) than males (21 years)) Bone augmentation procedures may be required before implant placement
	Orthodontics in combination with orthognathic surgery	For patients with severe skeletal discrepancies at the completion of facial growth

The benefits of orthodontic treatment

Orthodontic treatment can facilitate the restorative management of hypodontia in many cases. In others, where full space closure is possible, it may help to avoid the need for restorative treatment altogether. There are many potential benefits of orthodontic treatment in patients with hypodontia, as described below.

Idealisation of spaces for prosthodontic tooth replacement
The distribution of space is often asymmetrical and not ideal for the placement of optimally sized

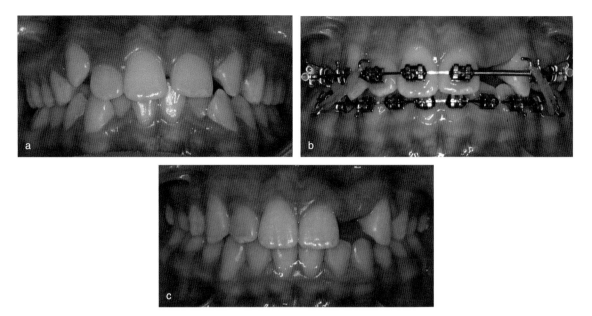

Figure 8.1   Orthodontic treatment to idealise the size of space for prosthodontic replacement of UL2. It is essential to ensure that the correct spacing is produced both between the crowns and roots of standing teeth (a) before, (b) during, and (c) after orthodontic treatment.

pontics. As well as improving aesthetic outcomes, space idealisation allows for the placement of correctly sized pontics that are more biomechanically sound for long-term success (Figure 8.1). Space was discussed in more detail in Chapter 4 and it is important that it is considered in three dimensions.

Root separation and paralleling
Space idealisation is not only important between the crowns of adjacent teeth but also between their roots. Correct root positioning facilitates the placement of implant-retained restorations; even if tooth-retained bridgework is the intended restorative solution, correctly angulated abutment teeth offer better resistance to functional loading.

Space closure to minimise the need for prosthodontic intervention
Space within the dental arch is often required for the correction of certain features of a malocclusion (e.g. crowding, overjet correction). Extraction of retained primary teeth, with no permanent successors, may provide the necessary space required for correcting malocclusion. This can in some cir-

cumstances preclude the need for prosthodontic treatment.

Ideal positioning of microdont teeth for restorative build up
Microdont teeth (e.g. peg-shaped lateral incisors), particularly when in the aesthetic zone, may benefit from restorative build up in order to create ideal balance and symmetry. The correct positioning of these teeth (mesiodistally, anteroposteriorly and vertically) can facilitate the placement of aesthetic restorations with good emergence profiles (Figure 8.2).

Uprighting of tilted molars that may be potential abutments
Molar teeth may become excessively tilted, particularly when the adjacent primary molars are severely infra-occluded. Such teeth benefit from uprighting to make them favourable bridge abutments.

Correction of a deep overbite
A deep incisor overbite can place undesirable forces on restored anterior teeth, and can also be

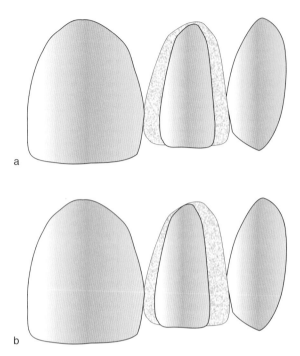

a

b

Figure 8.2   The ideal positioning of a microdont lateral incisor for restorative enlargement. (a) The tooth can be placed in the middle of the space to allow equal build-up on the mesial and distal aspects. (b) Alternatively the tooth can be positioned slightly more mesially in order to reduce the mesial emergence profile of the restoration and enhance the aesthetic result.

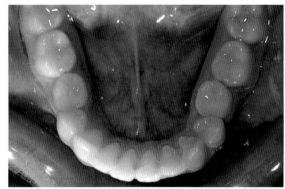

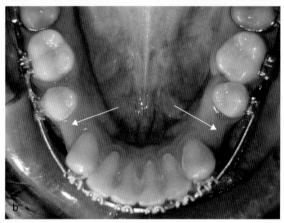

b

Figure 8.3   Implant site development. (a) The aim is to move the first premolars distally into the sites of the missing second premolars, following extraction of the infra-occluded primary second molars. (b) The well-developed ridge (arrow)* for the placement of first premolar implants not only provides valuable bone volume but also lessens the risk of damage to the mental nerve during implant placement. The rotational positions of the lower canines will be idealised towards the end of orthodontic treatment.

traumatic and prevent upper incisor retraction during overjet correction. Both fixed and removable orthodontic appliances can help in overbite correction.

Intrusion of overerupted teeth

Teeth opposing edentulous ridges or worn primary teeth often undergo overeruption. Such overerupted teeth can impinge on the vertical space required for prosthodontic tooth replacement, and orthodontic intrusion may help to facilitate restorative treatment in such cases.

Implant site development

Orthodontic tooth movement is associated with the generation of alveolar bone. When a tooth erupts, or is moved into an edentulous space, alveolar bone is developed at the site of tooth movement. If the tooth is later orthodontically moved away from the site, a thick ridge of alveolar bone

will remain in the area previously occupied by the tooth (Figure 8.3).

Studies suggest that this bone is very stable over time, undergoing very little resorption (Spear *et al.*, 1997) and it can provide a suitable surgical envelope for implant placement. Intentional movement of teeth to stimulate ridge development is known as 'implant site development'. This may be used:

- To allow maxillary canines to erupt into missing lateral incisor sites followed by later retraction, leaving sufficient bone volume for implant replacement of lateral incisors

- To move the first premolar into the second premolar site leaving a thick ridge of bone in the first premolar site for implant replacement (implant placement in the first premolar site also carries less risk of mental nerve damage compared to that in the second premolar region)

Orthodontic appliances

There are a number of orthodontic approaches available to achieve the goals outlined above. Depending on the specific aims and objectives of orthodontic treatment, a range of appliances may be used including:

- Fixed appliances
- Functional appliances
- Bite planes
- Headgear and temporary anchorage devices (TADs)

Fixed appliances are most commonly used as they allow extremely controlled tooth movement. Removable appliances can be incorporated into fixed-appliance treatment if necessary. For example, an anterior bite plane may be used to help reduce a deep overbite, or a functional appliance may be used to help correct an anteroposterior and vertical inter-arch discrepancy.

Problems encountered during orthodontic treatment

Orthodontic treatment in people with hypodontia can be difficult for a number of reasons, including the following:

- Deep overbite management
- Anchorage management
- Long edentulous spans and atrophic ridges
- Bonding abnormally shaped (sometimes hypomineralised) teeth
- Rotated teeth
- Retention of primary teeth
- Microdontia and arch coordination
- Late developing teeth
- Root paralleling
- Appliance breakages
- Retention

Deep overbite

The incisor overbite is the vertical overlap of the lower incisors by the uppers when the molar teeth are in contact. Ideally the overbite should measure 2–4 mm or the upper incisors should overlap the lower incisors by a quarter to a third of their crown height. There are several reasons for treating a deep overbite, including those listed here.

- As part of comprehensive orthodontic treatment, the upper incisors cannot be fully retracted from a Class II position if the overbite has not been fully reduced
- The overbite may be traumatic to the hard and/ or soft tissues
- A deep overbite may place unfavourable forces on restorations in the incisor region, predisposing to restorative failures

Patients with hypodontia may have a deep overbite, particularly when the incisors in the lower arch are missing (which allows the opposing incisors to overerupt). Such an overbite may be challenging to treat, particularly in severe hypodontia, as the premolars and second molars may be absent, thus jeopardising the success of conventional orthodontic treatment mechanics for overbite control. However, there are several orthodontic approaches available for reducing deep overbites within the growing patient:

- Incisor intrusion
- Molar extrusion
- Incisor proclination

In a typical orthodontic case, all three mechanisms may be used when a fixed appliance technique has been adopted for overbite control. Frequently an orthodontist will place a reverse curve of Spee into the lower archwire to encourage extrusion of the premolars and first molars (if the second molars are incorporated into the appliance) and intrusion of the incisors (Clifford *et al.*, 1999). In moderate or severe cases of hypodontia, where a number of lower incisors, premolars and molars are missing, these mechanics may not be as effective, particularly if growth is unfavourable, for example in a patient with a counter-clockwise (forward) mandibular growth rotation (Figure 4.14).

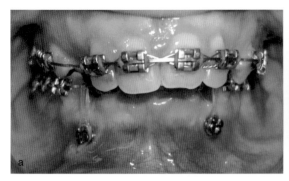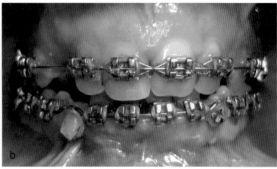

Figure 8.4   The use of temporary anchorage devices (TADs) to reduce a deep incisor overbite in an adult patient. (a) TADs were inserted into the edentulous sites where LR3 and LL3 were missing, applying a gentle intrusive force via an elastic chain to the lower archwire in the incisor region. (b) Reduced overbite after 6 months of gentle intrusion. Note the now clearly visible lower incisor brackets and the displacement of the archwire towards the TAD. The head of the TAD on the patients' right was covered with composite resin to help reduce soft tissue irritation.

In such cases, overbite reduction can be problematic and the use of an upper removable appliance with an anterior bite plane should be considered from an early stage, to encourage lower molar eruption. Alternatively, temporary anchorage devices may be used to apply intrusive forces to the lower incisors (Figure 8.4). These are essentially a type of endosseous implant, placed temporarily to provide anchorage for orthodontic tooth movement. Treatment with a functional appliance can also be an effective means of reducing a deep overbite when there is a superimposed Class II malocclusion. Likewise, cervical-pull headgear can assist overbite control by causing molar extrusion where distalisation of the upper molars or anchorage control is required to correct a Class II molar relationship.

If all measures fail because growth is unfavourable, then the only options remaining for the orthodontist are either to accept the deep overbite, together with the limitations that this may pose for malocclusion correction and restorative treatment, or to consider orthognathic surgery to achieve full correction. A careful risk–benefit analysis should be undertaken with respect to the latter approach and surgical correction should occur only once the majority of facial growth is complete.

Anchorage management

Anchorage control is the resistance to the three-dimensional unwanted forces generated in reaction to the active forces of an appliance. These will be equal in magnitude and opposite in direction to the active forces. The previous discussion on overbite reduction dealt with vertical anchorage issues. Anchorage in the anteroposterior dimension can also be compromised in patients with developmentally missing teeth. A common example is when molars and premolars are missing so there is inadequate posterior anchorage to retract the maxillary incisors or canines into a Class I position. The reverse situation is sometimes encountered when anterior teeth are missing, producing inadequate anchorage to protract the posterior teeth and thus close spaces by mesial molar movement. In this latter situation, loss of anchorage control can lead to over retraction of the upper incisors with a resultant Class III incisor relationship.

There are numerous mechanisms for anchorage reinforcement depending on whether this needs to be achieved in the upper or lower arch, in the anterior or posterior region, and the degree of reinforcement which is required (Table 8.2).

Temporary anchorage devices are a useful adjunct in the management of hypodontia. Edentulous sites can provide a convenient location for placing these devices without risking damage to adjacent roots (Figure 8.5). Several problems exist with the use of headgear, including safety concerns, because of the potential risk of eye injury (Blum-Hareuveni et al., 2004), and problems with patient compliance. Temporary anchorage devices are not without problems; these relate to poor primary stability if the cortical bone is thin (in chil-

Table 8.2   Methods of orthodontic anchorage management.

	MAXILLARY		MANDIBULAR	
	Posterior	Anterior	Posterior	Anterior
Low/medium anchorage	Nance palatal arch	Class III elastics	Lingual arch	Class II elastics
	Class II elastics	–	Class III elastics	–
High anchorage	Headgear	Protraction headgear	TADs	TADs
	TADs	TADs	–	–

TAD, temporary anchorage device.

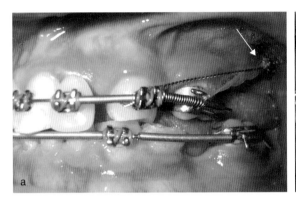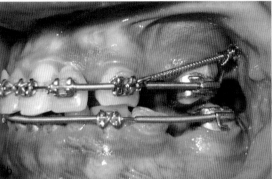

Figure 8.5   Temporary anchorage devices (TAD) are useful adjuncts to orthodontic space redistribution. (a) This patient has a TAD in the upper left tuberosity region (arrow) to stabilise the canine position (because the first molar was moved distally, using a compressed coil spring). (b) Space is created for one missing premolar (there was no mesial movement of the canine and the first molar moved closer to the TAD).

dren) and soft tissue irritation if they are placed into mobile mucosa when there is a limited width of attached gingivae. Biomechanically, it may also be challenging to deliver the ideal force vectors for the required tooth movements because of the limitations placed on positioning the temporary anchorage device, particularly in the vertical dimension.

Bonding abnormally shaped teeth
Conventional orthodontic brackets are mass-produced and therefore the bracket base, which is bonded onto the labial tooth surface, conforms to the shape of an average-shaped and average-sized tooth. When hypodontia is associated with microdontia, the bracket base does not match the tooth surface accurately. This can result in a number of problems including the incorrect delivery of the prescription within the bracket slot and bond failure. This is a nuisance during orthodontic treat-

ment as it prolongs treatment and requires the patient to attend for additional visits, which are inconvenient and frustrating. If bond failures are a recurrent problem the use of orthodontic bands with pre-soldered brackets may be considered or the labial tooth surface can be modified with composite resin to produce a more normal anatomical form that better accommodates the bracket base. It is important, as part of informed consent, to warn patients about the risks of bond failure and the added inconvenience associated with these during treatment.

Rotated teeth
Tooth rotation tends to be more prevalent in those with hypodontia, suggesting common linking genetic mechanisms for these dental anomalies (Baccetti, 1998). Severe rotation of the premolar teeth can occasionally be encountered in patients

affected by hypodontia. Such rotations can be challenging for the orthodontist to correct for a number of reasons. Often the orthodontic bracket cannot be placed in the ideal labial position at the start of treatment because of the rotation and has to be repositioned several times before the tooth position is fully corrected. This can add considerable time (3–6 months) to the initial alignment stages of treatment.

A second problem encountered with rotations is that the corrected tooth position is highly prone to relapse once orthodontic appliances are removed. This is because the transeptal periodontal fibres take considerable time to remodel to the corrected tooth position (Reitan, 1967). The potential energy stored in the stretched elastic fibres of de-rotated teeth provides the driving force for relapse. Achieving good intercuspation of premolar rotational corrections can help in retaining the corrected tooth positions. Pericision, which involves surgically severing the transeptal fibres, may also help to improve the stability of the rotation correction (Edwards, 1988) but is performed infrequently.

Long edentulous spans, atrophic ridges and pontics

The presence of long edentulous spans or several retained primary molar teeth can complicate orthodontic management for several reasons:

1. Long spans of unprotected archwire can be uncomfortable for the patient, causing trauma to the lips or cheeks. It is therefore important to cover such spans with metal or plastic sleeving to minimise this risk. The covering also helps protect the archwire from occlusal forces and may reduce the risk of archwire fracture. The ends of the archwire must be turned down tightly to minimise the risk of disengaging from the molar teeth.

Edentulous areas can also be troublesome if there is alveolar atrophy. This may limit tooth movement into the area due to a lack of alveolar bone, making space closure for missing units unfeasible.

Anteriorly positioned edentulous areas often impair dental aesthetics. During orthodontic treatment a bracket can be bonded to a shade-matched acrylic pontic tooth and secured to the archwire to improve the appearance (Figure 8.6). Such pontics also act as useful space-maintaining devices during the space closure phase of orthodontic therapy, although they have a tendency to rotate during the early phases of treatment because of the small

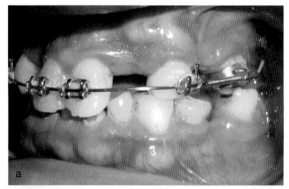
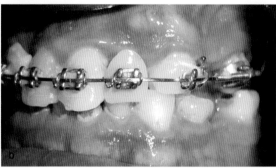

Figure 8.6 An acrylic pontic secured onto an archwire during orthodontic treatment improve appearances. (a) Patient before pontic placement and (b) after placement. A bracket attached to the pontic was secured onto the archwire.

archwire dimensions employed, which can be problematic. Additionally the patient must take care not to incise with the pontic as there is a risk of bond failure. Alternatively therefore the pontic may be attached temporarily to an adjacent tooth during the early phases of treatment using composite resin so as to limit these complications.

Retention of primary teeth

There are a number of advantages in retaining healthy primary teeth in patients with hypodontia. These teeth can often survive for many years and help to maintain aesthetics and function in any given area (Laing *et al.*, 2010). An additional benefit of retaining primary teeth is that their presence tends to maintain alveolar bone at a site that may be crucial for future prosthodontic treatment. Following extraction of the lower second primary molar the ridge may reduce in width by 25% over 4 years (Ostler and Kokich, 1994). The use of primary teeth as abutments for bridges has been rarely reported in the literature and the outcome of the procedure remains uncertain (Einwag, 1984).

Although the retention of primary teeth can have advantages, it can also pose some problems particularly during orthodontic management. The two principal difficulties associated with the retention of these teeth are an obstruction to the correct positioning of the permanent teeth and the introduction of a tooth size discrepancy that does not allow the achievement of an ideal occlusion. For example, retention of the second primary molars can lead to Class II half-unit molar relationship because the lowers tend to be larger than the uppers. If this is not acceptable, either the mesiodistal width of the lower second primary molar should be reduced to allow the lower molar to move forwards into a Class I relationship, or the lower primary molar should be extracted to permit this outcome. Mesiodistal tooth reduction is preferable as retention of the roots helps to prevent alveolar ridge atrophy. The presence of divergent primary molar roots has previously been cited as a contraindication for mesiodistal tooth reduction. However, more recently it has been stated that this may not be as problematic as previously thought because the roots of the divergent primary teeth are more likely to undergo resorption than those of the adjacent permanent tooth (Kokich, 2002). Tooth reduction will almost certainly lead to dentine exposure and it is important that the dentine tubules are sealed with a flowable composite material to reduce sensitivity and protect the pulp–dentine complex from bacterial ingress.

Root paralleling

Root paralleling is important if all prosthodontic options are to remain viable following orthodontic treatment. It is particularly crucial when implant-retained restorations are to be considered. Achieving correct root paralleling is an area that was previously of less significance in orthodontic treatment and consequently more likely to be overlooked. It is disappointing for a patient if fixed appliances have to be reinserted at a later date to achieve this goal and there may be consequent medicolegal implications.

It is important that all patients are reviewed by a prosthodontist before fixed appliances are removed in order to determine any final root repositioning that may be required. A periapical radiograph using the paralleling technique should be taken perpendicular to the edentulous space to be restored, in order to determine root position and separation. If the space available is inadequate, for example in the lateral incisor area, a number of strategies exist to increase the space:

- Distal movement of the canine into space already present, or space created by interproximal enamel reduction or distal molar movement
- Further correction of the angulation (tip) of the canine and central incisor crowns
- Inclination (torque) adjustment of the canine and central incisor

The angulation of teeth can be altered by the introduction of second order (tip) bends into the orthodontic archwire, or by repositioning the brackets of central incisors and/or canines. In the anterior region, not only angulation but incorrect inclination (torque) can affect the proximity of the root apices between teeth. This is due to the wagon-wheel effect described by Andrews (1972), whereby the anterior teeth follow an arc and over proclination can lead to approximation of their root apices. It is important during the treatment planning stages to recognise these potential difficulties, selecting appropriate bracket prescriptions and ensuring correct bracket positioning. Other factors that can complicate correct root positioning are:

- Abnormal crown morphology leading to incorrect bracket placement
- Long edentulous spans introducing flexibility into the orthodontic archwire and reducing its efficacy for tooth alignment
- Long spans of wire are also more prone to distortion which may compromise tooth positioning
- The presence of tooth-size discrepancies may lead to inadequate space when the correct occlusal relationship has been achieved

Microdontia and arch coordination

The presence of microdontia, particularly when the buccolingual tooth dimension is affected, can complicate arch coordination. Because a fixed appliance will align the labial tooth surfaces, the palatal aspect of a microdont tooth will tend to move into a scissor-bite relationship. Subsequently the lack of an occlusal stop means the teeth can overerupt and introduce occlusal interferences as well as reduce vertical space for restoring the opposing arch. Fortunately this problem is relatively rare, but when it does occur it can be difficult to manage. The range of orthodontic techniques for scissor-bite correction include upper arch contraction, lower arch expansion and inclination adjustments. When these fail, building up the tooth to correct the microdontia may be considered.

Late developing teeth

There is large variability in the timing of tooth development and there is good evidence that in hypodontia it tends to be delayed (Ruiz-Mealin *et al.*, 2009). Occasionally, one tooth (commonly the second premolar) can be very delayed in development compared to the others, a problem which appears to be more common in the maxilla (Ravin and Nielsen, 1977). If the delay is substantial, it may not be practical to await eruption of the relevant tooth before commencing orthodontic treatment, and it is advisable that this be initiated and the space maintained to allow later eruption of the delayed tooth. Sometimes it may not be for many years following orthodontic treatment and long-term space maintenance is therefore important. The patient should also be warned that the tooth may erupt into a poorly aligned position which can either be accepted or corrected with a removable or shortened sectional fixed appliance.

Retention

Retention is an essential stage following orthodontic treatment designed to maintain the corrections that have been achieved during treatment. Numerous factors may be involved in orthodontic relapse including the natural tendency that teeth have to revert to their original positions (physiological recovery), late mandibular growth that can lead to late lower incisor crowding and occlusal changes, and relapse because the teeth have been placed into an inherently unstable position (e.g. lower incisor proclination) (Richardson, 1994). Procedures that may be prone to relapse in hypodontia include:

- Space closure
- Idealisation of spaces
- Correction of rotations

- Correction of root positions adjacent to edentulous spaces (Olsen and Kokich, 2010)
- Alignment of impacted maxillary canines

A number of different retainers are available for the maintenance of corrections achieved during orthodontic treatment. The choice of retainer depends on several factors including individual patient preference, the orthodontist's choice, patient motivation and durability of the device.

The Hawley retainer is the most durable device available (Figure 8.7a). It consists of an acrylic base

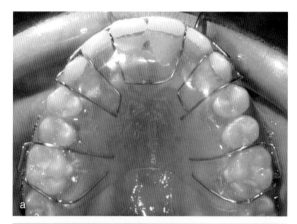

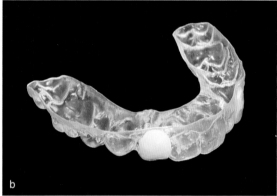

Figure 8.7 (a) A Hawley retainer in situ with pontics replacing the lateral incisors. Metal stops have been placed mesial and distal to the upper lateral incisor spaces to help maintain the space even if the acrylic pontic wears interproximally during repeated insertion and removal (or if it fractures off the appliance). (b) An Essix style vacuum-formed retainer with acrylic pontics replacing the missing lateral incisors. There must be an adequate number of standing teeth of normal form (non-microdont) to provide good retention for the appliance.

plate with Adams clasps to provide retention, and a labial bow that may be acrylated or fitted (used in order to maintain incisor alignment). Pontics can be placed in the positions where teeth are missing to help restore the patient's appearance and to maintain spaces. The mesial and distal surfaces of pontics can wear during repeated insertion and removal of the appliance, and it is possible for them to break off, therefore mesial and distal metal stops should also be placed across edentulous spaces for extra security in space maintenance. Some feel that unsupported pontics can place additional pressure on the edentulous ridge, which may exacerbate bone resorption and complicate future restorative treatment. Small rests can therefore be placed onto the cingulum plateau of teeth adjacent to the edentulous ridge to improve support of the pontic and overcome this potential problem.

The vacuum-formed Essix retainer is another popular device. Again pontics can be placed into the edentulous spaces to help restore appearance (Figure 8.7b). Particular advantages of this form of retainer are its ease of manufacture and its aesthetic appearance. However it is not as durable as the Hawley retainer and should be removed for eating – which may not be desirable for a patient with missing anterior teeth. Also, this type of retainer depends on the presence of teeth for retention, so it may not be suitable for patients with several missing units or generalised microdontia. Poor retainer retention is a recipe for orthodontic relapse.

Fixed retainers can provide a useful form of retention with the advantage of not being dependent on patient compliance for insertion (Figure 8.8). They also provide better retention than removable retainers and lessen the risk of root re-approximation following space opening (Olsen and Kokich, 2010). Their disadvantages include difficulties with oral hygiene and the risk of partial de-bonds with the subsequent hazard of relapse and secondary caries. The palatal surface of laboratory constructed restorations can be modified in order to facilitate retainer placement. Additionally, it may be possible to incorporate a retention element into the design of resin-bonded bridge work to replace missing lateral incisors. In the latter example, splinted retainers can be placed on the central incisors.

Appliances breakages

Patients with hypodontia may be more prone to breakages of fixed appliance than the average orthodontic patient. There are a few reasons for this:

- Large spans of unsupported archwire, which can place excess forces on the brackets mesial and distal to the span due to distortion from occlusal forces
- Poor adaptation of bracket bases to microdont tooth surfaces
- Hypomineralisation, which may affect bond strengths

Restorative management of patients

The standard restorative treatment-planning principles apply to every patient. In addition to normal clinical and radiographic examinations, a number of diagnostic procedures will invariably be helpful. These include a Kesling set-up (Kesling, 1956), a wax try-in and a diagnostic wax-up (Figure 8.9). Changes to the contour of teeth can often be quickly simulated in the mouth by direct placement of composite resin with a 'free-hand' technique. For more extensive changes a matrix based on a diagnostic wax-up can facilitate this. In more difficult cases it is often helpful to consider a period of provisional restorations before definitive treatment is carried out.

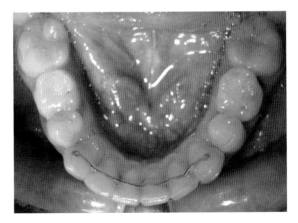

Figure 8.8   A fixed orthodontic retainer made from 0.0175-inch diameter spiral wire (Twistflex) bonded with composite resin to maintain lower incisor alignment.

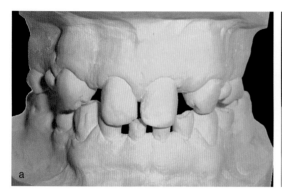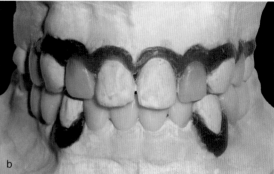

Figure 8.9   (a) Pre-operative study cast showing irregular tooth spacing. (b) Post-operative Kesling set-up and diagnostic wax-up showing improved appearance and occlusion.

Table 8.3   Advantages and disadvantages of re-contouring at different times during orthodontic treatment.

	Advantages	Disadvantages
Before orthodontics	The restoration can act as a space maintainer during orthodontics Correction of the labial contour may facilitate orthodontic bonding	Adequate space must be present –
During orthodontics	Excess space can be created, and later closed, to allow interproximal finishing	Gingival inflammation may prevent good moisture control Orthodontic re-bracketing may necessitate dropping down in the archwire sequence
After orthodontics	Resolution of gingival inflammation allows good moisture control	Space maintenance is required during orthodontic treatment

Re-contouring

Composite resin build-ups of microdont teeth can be undertaken before, during or after orthodontic treatment. Table 8.3 summarises the advantages and disadvantages of each approach. Advances in composite resin technology have allowed this treatment to be used in a wide range of clinical situations. Its minimally invasive nature is particularly attractive for patients affected by hypodontia, who often present at a relatively young age. Composite resin is particularly useful during growth periods because it is easily modified as the gingival margins mature. Porcelain veneers or bonded crowns offer superior aesthetics but should only be considered once the gingival margins are fully mature at the completion of facial growth. Patients and their carers or parents should be made aware of the requirement for the lifelong maintenance and replacement of all restorative procedures.

Re-contouring of teeth is commonly carried out in the following situations:

- For conversion of canine teeth to simulate lateral incisors
- For closure of a median diastema
- For reshaping of microdont teeth
- For occlusal enhancement of infra-occluded teeth

Re-contouring teeth with composite resin is the treatment of choice in the developing dentition. Good appearance can be achieved with modern materials – incremental build-up using opaque, dentine and enamel layers can provide excellent appearance. These build-ups can be time consuming, but in simpler situations only an enamel build-up is required. Moisture control is usually best achieved using a rubber dam, but there are instances when the use of retraction cord, local anaesthetic and astringent salts provides more satisfactory management of the soft tissues. Most recontouring techniques can be provided directly at the chair-side, although as the number of teeth to be treated or the severity of the microdontia increases so an indirect technique using laboratory-made restorations becomes advantageous. It is important to use sufficient bulk of material as fractures often occur when composite materials are placed in thin sections.

Canines simulating lateral incisors

If a canine tooth is large and its shade has a strong or deep chroma it will be very difficult to re-contour or modify it to resemble a lateral incisor. Similarly, the gingival contour may not be similar to that of a lateral incisor, especially if the tooth is wide in a mesiodistal dimension. Whether such a tooth can be satisfactorily re-contoured can only be made once it has erupted. The positioning of the canine tooth next to the central incisor is sometimes an orthodontic convenience and it can avoid a protracted course of orthodontic treatment. The position of the root apex or bodily position of the tooth often influences the ease of orthodontic treatment. The available evidence suggests that orthodontic space closure produces results that are well accepted by patients and encourages periodontal health in comparison with prosthetic replacements in selected cases (Robertsson and Mohlin, 2000). However, many consider that the best aesthetics can only be achieved if the appropriate teeth are placed or restored in the correct positions.

Correct orthodontic positioning of a canine can facilitate restorative treatment where the aim is for the tooth to mimic the lateral incisor. If the canine is extruded during orthodontic treatment, it will help to improve the relationship between the gingival heights of the canine and central incisor. Ideally, the lateral incisor's gingival level (or the canine if it is mimicking the lateral incisor) should lie approximately 1 mm coronal to that of the central incisor. Creating this relationship is only important if the smile-line is high and the gingival margins are exposed during smiling. It should also be born in mind that extrusion of the canine will necessitate greater enamel reduction of its tip as the incisal edge of the lateral incisor should lie 0.5–1 mm more apical to that of the central incisor for ideal aesthetics (Bukhary et al., 2007). Placing

the canine slightly upright (rather than the usual mesial angulation) will also enhance its mimicry of the lateral incisor, and it will appear narrower mesiodistally if it is not excessively angulated. The inclination of the maxillary canine should be adjusted to reduce root prominence and minimise root bulge.

Bleaching the canine tooth with an external technique, using 10–15% carbamide peroxide gel, is viewed as the treatment of choice for improving the shade of the tooth. Reduction of the tooth could occur at the cusp tip, mesial and distal proximal surfaces, buccal or labial contour bulge and occasionally the palatal surface. Palatal reduction may be important to allow the tooth to be fully retracted during orthodontic treatment. Clinicians should be mindful of the limitations of enamel dimensions in these areas, particularly at the cervical margins where there may be less than 1 mm of residual enamel. Commonly, the incisal edge requires addition of composite resin to the mesial and distal surface (Figure 8.10). Occasionally, a full composite labial veneer may provide the best result if colour-matching is important. The final result may depend on the smile-line – if it is high then gingival aesthetics may be particularly important. (Jepson et al., 2003, Millar and Taylor, 1995).

When closing the maxillary lateral incisor space it is necessary to pay attention to the position of the first premolar which has taken on the role of the maxillary canine. This can be achieved through a number of orthodontic modifications (Rosa and Zachrisson, 2007):

- Slight mesio-palatal rotation: To help hide the palatal cusp from exposure during smiling
- Intrusion: To help match the level of the gingival margin to that of the central incisor if the smile-line is high and the patient is concerned about it (the requires restorative build-up of the height of the first premolar to match that of the central incisor)
- Buccal movement of the root: To produce a canine eminence

Median diastema

Patients commonly express concerns about the appearance of a midline maxillary diastema. If the size of the maxillary incisors is within acceptable limits, then this is usually best managed by closing

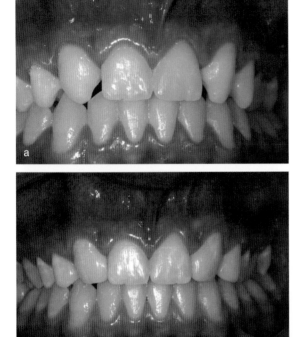

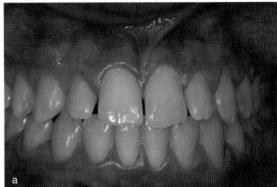

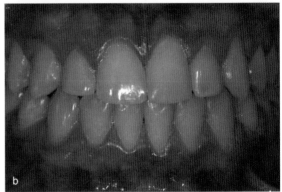

Figure 8.10   (a) Maxillary canines placed adjacent to central incisors in the lateral incisor positions. (b) Re-contoured canines with reduced cusp tips and composite additions to improve their appearance as a diagnostic procedure.

Figure 8.11   (a) Residual median diastema and microdont lateral incisors at the end of orthodontic treatment. (b) Median diastema closed and lateral incisors re-contoured with composite resin.

the space orthodontically, although long-term retention with a fixed retainer is often required to maintain the new tooth positions. Diagnostically, it is important to establish whether the maxillary midline fraenum is involved with diastema formation; then it may be necessary to perform a fraenectomy to improve the stability of orthodontic space closure.

It is not always appropriate to close a diastema orthodontically because of microdontia or a tooth size discrepancy, or because the patient is unwilling to undertake orthodontic appliance therapy. When spacing is considered to be unsightly, composite resin additions are usually the treatment of choice (Sabri, 1999) (Figure 8.11). On occasions it may be acceptable to only partly reduce the diastema to maintain the proportions of the teeth. Current aesthetic principles would suggest that the

ideal width to length ratio of the central incisor should be 0.75–0.85 (Wolfart *et al.*, 2005).

Microdont teeth

Microdontia may be localised or generalised, with the upper lateral incisors commonly affected in patients with hypodontia. If the tooth is microdont it may be peg-shaped or have a normal shape but be reduced in size. Such teeth can often be enlarged using either conventional or adhesive restorations. Goodacre *et al.* (2001) set out minimal dimensions for the success of the former and considered that there should be a minimum of 3 mm axial wall preparation for anterior teeth and 4 mm for molar teeth, assuming that preparations had a 10–20-degree taper. The use of adhesive restorations in these situations may prove advantageous, requiring less tooth preparation (Figure 8.12), and is

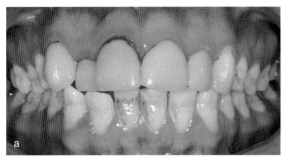

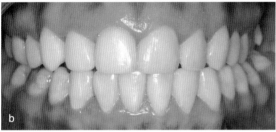

Figure 8.12 (a) Generalised microdontia and hypoplasia. Previous treatment had been restricted to the upper anterior teeth. (b) Multiple composite restorations used to restore normal contour to the teeth following orthodontic treatment.

often preferable. However, when the clinical crowns are very small then the service life of such restorations tends to be reduced. If the microdontia is extensive it may be preferable to consider treatment with partial or complete overdentures, although most patients prefer management with fixed restorations in the form of composite resin build-ups if possible.

While treatment of the anterior teeth is often all that is indicated during the early teenage years, on occasions full-mouth treatment is required, including management of the posterior teeth. When planning such procedures in younger patients it should be borne in mind that their tolerance of dental treatment may be reduced.

It is essential for the orthodontist to consult with the restorative dentist about the positioning of microdont teeth to facilitate restorative measures, considering the three dimensions addressed by Kokich and Spear (1997) in relation to the positioning of a peg-shaped lateral incisor:

- Dimension 1: Mesiodistally – the peg-shaped tooth can be placed slightly mesially in the space to minimise the mesial emergence profile

of the restoration (Figure 8.2). The lateral incisor commonly has a greater distal emergence profile
- Dimension 2: Vertically – the tooth should be positioned in such a way that the gingival margin lies 1 mm below that of the central incisor, and level to the lateral incisor on the contralateral side if the smile-line is high.
- Dimension 3: Anteroposteriorly – positioning depends on the final restoration planned. If it will be composite or porcelain veneer then the lateral incisor should be positioned with minimal overjet in order to maximise the labial build-up, but for a full-coverage crown an overjet of 0.5–1 mm should be left to minimise the amount of palatal reduction required.

It is also important to ensure that the correct mesiodistal space is created to allow the lateral incisor to be built up to natural looking width. If the contralateral tooth is of normal dimensions, it can be used as a guide; if the tooth is missing or is also peg-shaped, then the decision about how much space to create should be based on aesthetic and occlusal principles.

Occlusally, if the teeth are aligned and a normal overjet and overbite is created then the correct amount of space should be available for the lateral incisor (assuming that there is no tooth size discrepancy). A Kesling set-up can be employed before treatment to determine this space, or a tooth size analysis can be undertaken to calculate the ideal mesiodistal width of the lateral incisor.

Aesthetically, the golden proportion has been suggested as a guide to the space needed for the lateral incisor, with the width of the lateral incisor being approximately 62% that of the central incisor when viewed from the front (Levin, 1978). More recently it has been questioned whether one proportion can be the ideal standard for all, as perceptions of appearance have a large subjective component (Bukhary et al., 2007). In the Bukhary study, slightly greater dimensions were found to be the most aesthetically pleasing.

Infra-occluded teeth

Infra-occluded primary molars are commonly encountered in people with hypodontia. Rarely, the patient may complain about poor appearance or functional problems associated with the presence of these teeth. If he or she has a high level of plaque control, restoration of these teeth may be considered if there is a risk of mesiodistal or vertical space loss (see Chapter 4). Direct composite restorations or indirect composite onlays made in the laboratory can be used, providing the best appearance (Evans and Briggs, 1996; Robinson and Chan, 2009). Gold onlays have a less-appealing appearance but have been shown to be more effective in the long-term (Chana *et al.*, 2000).

In Chapter 4 it was noted that the progression of infra-occlusion depends on the degree of remaining vertical facial growth, and this is largely dependent on the age and gender of the patient at the time of assessment. It has been argued that if considerable progression of infra-occlusion is anticipated then early extraction of these teeth may be beneficial by helping to retain the height of the associated alveolar bone (Ostler and Kokich, 1994). If the ankylosed tooth is retained then the vertical alveolar discrepancy may undergo progression. However, there is some evidence, albeit not conclusive, that if the infra-occluded tooth is extracted early then the alveolus in the single-unit edentulous site will continue to develop vertically under the influence of the eruption of the adjacent non-ankylosed teeth (Ostler and Kokich, 1994).

Replacement of teeth

At the end of orthodontic treatment the patient is generally keen to have any missing teeth replaced to improve appearance and function. There may be indications to replace these teeth on the grounds of maintaining oral health, and it is certainly helpful to replace them for preventing orthodontic relapse. Planning of tooth replacement should follow standard prosthodontic and orthodontic protocols (Hemmings and Harrington, 2004; Shillingburg *et al.*, 1997; Wise, 1995), and the options are as follows:

- Accept the space and do not restore
- Use a removable partial denture
- Use a resin-bonded bridge
- Use a conventional bridge
- Use an implant-supported crown
- Perform autotransplantation

It is rare for patients to accept spaces in the anterior part of their mouths although they may be prepared to accept missing molars and function with a shortened dental arch (Kayser, 1981). It should be stressed that this is only appropriate if there is an absence of dental pathology. The presence of toothwear, dysfunction of the temperomandibular joint, or periodontal drifting of teeth would suggest that this approach is inappropriate.

Dentures

Dentures are relatively simple and quick to provide for patients and are often well tolerated by young people. The use of partial dentures is quite common. Complete dentures are rarely required as anodontia is a very uncommon condition. Similarly, a partial or complete overdenture is often indicated when there are multiple missing teeth, or discrepancies with the occlusion and retention of some primary teeth. Many partial dentures conform to the existing dentition and are more aesthetically pleasing than removable orthodontic retainers with pontics. They can therefore be worn during the day, providing the best appearance. The orthodontic retainer is used at night for reasonable orthodontic stability. If designed to cover less of the gingival tissues, they are less injurious to the periodontium. The provision of partial dentures should follow standard design principles (Figure 8.13).

Overdentures

Overdentures can provide a useful treatment option in patients with few erupted teeth. They permit changes to the occlusal vertical dimension (OVD) in patients with an increased freeway space (FWS) and provide additional lip support, with the teeth helping to improve stability and retention of the appliance. Retained roots may also encourage the maintenance of alveolar bone, however if roots are retained it is essential that patients have good dietary and plaque control. They must remove dentures during sleep because of the high risk of caries developing in the abutment teeth.

Overdentures may be partial or complete and their exact design will evolve during the planning procedure, particularly during the wax try-in stage. The main factors taken into account with the design are:

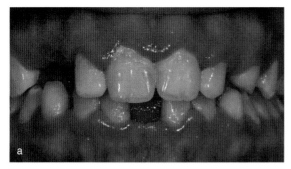

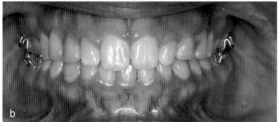

Figure 8.13   (a) Patient in mixed dentition stage with recent loss of primary teeth and poor oral hygiene. (b) Oral hygiene has been improved. Interim replacement with acrylic upper and lower partial dentures.

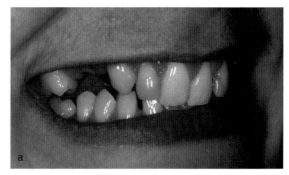

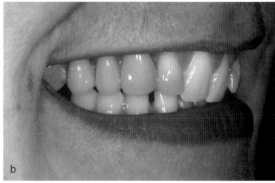

Figure 8.14   (a) Hypodontia with missing UR4, UR5 and infra-occlusion of UR3. (b) Appearance and occlusion improved with a partial overlay denture.

- Missing hard or soft tissues to be replaced prosthetically
- Additional lip support, if any, to be provided
- Prosthetic changes to be made in the OVD
- The level and orientation of the occlusal plane to be created
- Any skeletal discrepancies requiring prosthetic correction
- Occlusal stability (anterior guidance and posterior stability)

As simple a design as possible should be used, allowing for anticipated growth in the facial skeleton. One that uses an acrylic base is usually best suited because of the ease with which it can be modified, most commonly by adjustments to the fitting surface or re-lining. If the patient can be successfully treated with a single denture in one jaw only, then this is better tolerated than dentures in both jaws. For young patients it is important to use a shade and a mould similar to those of primary teeth; typically they are smaller and paler than those used in adult patients. Often quite dramatic improvements to the appearance and function can

be obtained with these appliances, using relatively simple procedures (Hobkirk and Brook, 1980), but concerns have been raised about the long-term use of removable prostheses and periodontal health (Yeung et al., 2000). If excellent oral hygiene and maintenance care are carried then satisfactory long-term performance can be expected (Bergman, 1995).

Figure 8.14 shows restoration of the maxillary occlusal plane with a partial overdenture in a patient with severe hypodontia. A complete overdenture, by contrast, covers all the teeth in one jaw and can be used to improve the OVD and incisal relationship. It also provides lip support, which can further enhance facial aesthetics (Figure 8.15).

Dentures with metal frameworks are more durable than those with acrylic bases. They also have reduced bulk and are better tolerated by patients. However, their additional cost is not often justified until growth has stopped (Sundram and Walmsley, 2003). Consequently, partial dentures

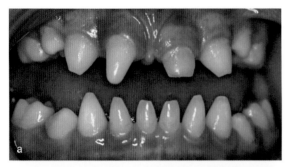

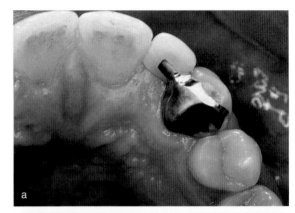

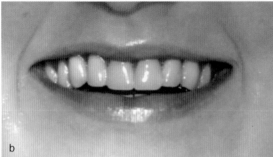

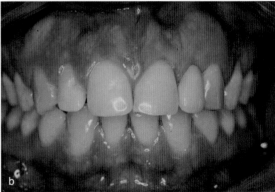

Figure 8.15 (a) Microdont teeth and retained primary teeth in a patient with severe hypodontia. (b) Complete overdenture used to improve appearance and occlusion (the patient did not want a lower denture).

Figure 8.16 (a) Palatal view of a resin-bonded cantilever bridge replacing a lateral incisor. (b) Labial view.

with acrylic bases that promote good maintenance during the teenage years have much to commend them (Winstanley, 1984; Hemmings *et al.*, 1995).

Resin-bonded bridges

Resin-bonded bridges have been used successfully since 1977 (Howe and Denehy, 1977). The technique has been developed over many years and good success rates are expected (St George *et al.*, 2002a, St George *et al.*, 2002b). Reported survival rates suggest an 80% success rate over a period of 6 years or longer (Creugers *et al.*, 1992; Rammelsberg *et al.*, 1993, Probster *et al.*, 1997; Behr *et al.*, 1998; Djemal *et al.*, 1999; Pjetursson *et al.*, 2008), but the success rates in patients under 20 years of age have been shown to be reduced (Dunne and Millar, 1993). This might be due to a smaller bonding area on potential abutment teeth. There is some evidence that tooth preparation with interproximal groves, boxes and occlusal rests may increase survival of the bridges (Barrack and Bretz, 1993; Nohl *et al.*, 2008), although many experts consider that minimal tooth preparation is required to obtain

similarly good survival in younger patients (Djemal *et al.*, 1999).

It has been shown in a number of studies that cantilever bridge designs have a higher success rate than fixed–fixed designs (Hussey and Linden, 1996). They potentially produce a better appearance because there is less metal coverage of the abutment tooth (Figure 8.16). The path of insertion of the bridge often allows better closure of interdental spaces with cantilever bridges. One further advantage is that when replacing a lateral incisor tooth with a cantilever bridge bonded to the canine tooth, metal coverage of the central incisor tooth may be avoided, and this can improve appearance particularly if the incisal edge is translucent or thin.

Orthodontic retention is another consideration in the design of a resin-bonded bridge. It is often possible to incorporate a groove within the framework that allows the subsequent placement of a 'twistflex' wire retainer. Alternatively, a fixed–

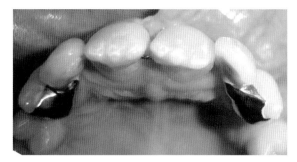

Figure 8.17   Relapse of resin-bonded cantilever bridges.

fixed adhesive bridge design may prevent orthodontic relapse. Careful follow-up will be required
to ensure that one of the bridge retainers is not de-
bonded – if this goes unnoticed, there is a risk of
caries developing in the affected abutment and of
drifting of the de-bonded tooth.

One disadvantage of cantilever designs is that
orthodontic stability is not obtained. This can be
particularly troublesome if rotational movements
have been corrected as part of the orthodontic
treatment (Figure 8.17). Orthodontic stability will
be enhanced to a greater or less extent when:

- a tooth pontic fills the space and provides tight
  contact points
- a wide contact point or 'wrap around' the interproximal area is provided by the pontic
- a splinted or fixed–fixed framework design is
  employed
- a removable retainer is used in conjunction
  with a resin-bonded bridge.

Certainly the most effective splinting is obtained
with a splinted or fixed–fixed framework (Figure
8.18). If a median diastema has been closed orthodontically and lateral incisors are missing, a double
cantilever design can be appropriate (Figure 8.19).
Using grooves or tubes in combination with a
twistflex wire retainer increases the bulk of the
restorations and complexity of the treatment.
Splinted designs incur a slight increase in failure
(Garnett *et al.*, 2006 and Djemal *et al.*, 1999).

If opaque resin cements are used it is unusual to
have a poor appearance with 'greying' of the incisal
edge of the abutment teeth due to the colour of the
metal framework altering the apparent colour of
the abutment tooth. However, care should be taken

with the design if the incisal edges of potential
abutment teeth are thin or particularly translucent.
It is preferable to try and cover as much of the
enamel surface as possible, including an extension
up to the incisal edge of most teeth, sometimes
incorporating an overlap of the incisal edge as
well. However, if appearance is particularly important, there may have to be some compromise with
a reduction of the extent of the bonding area or the
use of a retaining wing that finishes short of the
incisal edge.

Posterior bridges are subject to higher occlusal
loading. In order to counteract this, the framework
has to be robust and provide maximum coverage
of the abutment teeth. This may be acceptable in
the upper arch, but there is often significant aesthetic compromise in the lower arch when the
occlusal surface of a tooth is covered to enhance
the retention and stability of a bridge (Figure 8.20).

Careful technique is important for ensuring the
success of resin-bonded bridges. Consider the
following:

- Maintaining a dry field (e.g. using a rubber
  dam)
- Carrying out metal preparation immediately
  before cementation (this requires the use of an
  intraoral sand-blaster using 50-micron aluminium oxide grit)
- Using an opaque resin cement (manipulated
  according to the manufacturer's instructions)
- Managing the occlusion with a bridge designed
  to avoid stress on the cement lute (often requires
  sharing occlusal loads across bridge abutments;
  in cantilever designs occlusal loads on the
  pontic should be minimised) (see Chapter 5)
- Ensuring components are thick enough to be
  durable (this reduces the flexure of frameworks
  and minimises the risk of cementation failure;
  if the connector height is minimal it may be
  sensible to consider crown-lengthening surgery
  or an alternative treatment)

If orthodontic treatment has been carried out it
is usually wise to avoid restorative treatment
involving tooth replacement with fixed bridges
for 3–6 months (Jepson *et al.*, 2003). Small tooth
movements do occur as part of a 'settling in' of the
occlusion, however if partial dentures or retainers
are worn for a long period of time there can be

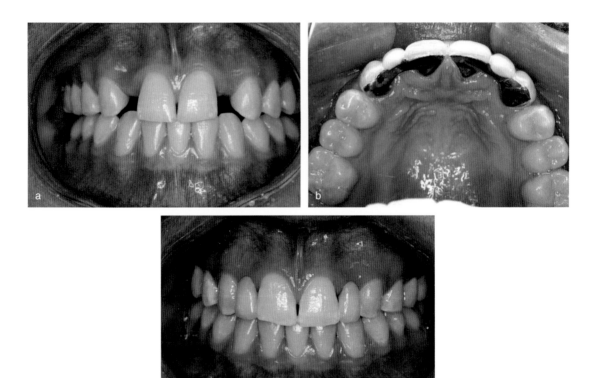

Figure 8.18 (a) Completed orthodontic treatment with symmetrical spacing provided for lateral incisor replacement. (b) Palatal view and (c) labial view of fixed–fixed splinted resin-bonded bridges replacing the lateral incisors. The metal retaining wings have been extended up to the incisal edges for maximum coverage.

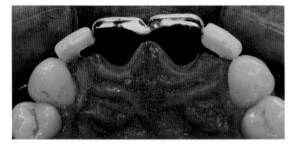

Figure 8.19 Double cantilever splinted resin-bonded bridge replacing lateral incisors.

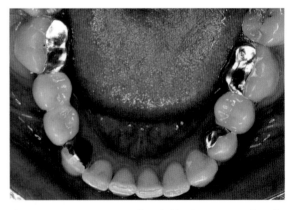

Figure 8.20 Posterior resin-bonded bridges. Maximal tooth coverage is required in this situation, which may compromise the aesthetics.

problems with periodontal inflammation and soft tissue control during restorative procedures.

Conventional bridges
The use of conventional bridges, typically in the form of porcelain fused to metal, should normally be confined to older patients, because in younger patients there is a significant risk of pulp exposure, leading to periapical pathology at an early age. It has been noted that failure rates of conventional bridges are higher in younger patients (Roberts, 1970), although survival is better than with resin-

bonded bridges (Reuter and Brose, 1984; Scurria *et al.*, 1998). The main concern is that when a conventional bridge fails it may lead to the loss of the abutment tooth. While survival of conventional bridges is in the order of 10–15 years, this is relatively short in terms of a patient's lifetime. Nevertheless there are circumstances when individual teeth have been heavily restored or endodontically treated and a conventional bridge is appropriate. In general, it is better to use the natural tooth as an abutment for as long as possible and certainly this is preferable to considering a dental implant in a growing patient. It is acknowledged that success rates for conventional bridges in younger patients are lower than those in more mature patients.

Dental implants
Dental implants should only be placed when the majority of skeletal growth has completed because earlier insertion will lead to infra-occlusion, significantly compromise aesthetics and create an angular bony defect around adjacent teeth (Thilander *et al.*, 1994, 1999, 2001). Although growth studies indicate that facial growth continues well into adulthood (Behrents, 1985), recent research suggests that clinically insignificant growth will occur after the second decade (Fudalej *et al.*, 2007). The only precise method of determining whether progression of facial growth is minimal is to record two serial lateral cephalometric radiographs 6–12 months apart (Heij *et al.*, 2006). They should be superimposed on cranial base structures and the vertical difference in the mandibular outline measured. If there is a minimal difference it can be assumed that the majority of facial growth is complete and implants can be safely placed.

With the success of resin-bonded bridges being in excess of 7–8 years on average, many patients maintain satisfactory appearance and function into their third or fourth decades before detailed discussions about treatment with dental implants become necessary. It is recognised that dental implants may be extremely helpful in maintaining implant-retained overdentures in the growing patient (Kearns *et al.*, 1999, Durstberger *et al.*, 1999), but some crestal bone loss occurs around all dental implants. An acceptable rate of loss is less than 0.2 mm per year (Albretsson *et al.*, 1986) with typical rates varying between 0.02 and 0.1 mm per year (Bryant 1998). Of course these may be acceptable for implant treatment in middle-aged or older patients, but the implications for young patients are more significant. Only a small amount of growth occurs in the facial bones during adult life (Cronin and Oesterle, 1998; Oesterle and Cronin, 2000). This is clearly not the situation in children, which is why reported results of treatment with dental implants in children and adolescents have been variable (Bergendahl *et al.*, 1996, Koch *et al.*, 1996, Gukes *et al.*, 2002, Heij *et al.*, 2006). Ethical issues and concerns about potential failure rates exist as there are limited published controlled clinical trials in this area.

Autotransplantation of teeth
Autotransplantation is the surgical repositioning of a tooth within the same person. This form of tooth replacement has become a popular strategy within some centres particularly for the replacement of central incisors lost in traumatic injuries. In hypodontia, it is possible to transplant an upper third molar into a second primary molar site when the second premolar is developmentally absent or remove a premolar from a crowded arch and transplant it into an opposing arch with spacing and missing premolars.

Studies suggest that autotransplantation can have a long-term success rate of over 90% (Andreasen *et al.*, 1990a). Some of the advantages and disadvantages are outlined in Table 8.4. One major advantage, when used in a growing child, is that a successful transplant will continue to erupt to compensate for vertical skeletal facial growth (unlike a dental implant). Such eruption is particularly beneficial as it helps to develop the height of the alveolar ridge which can facilitate future implant treatment should the transplant fail. Similarly, the transplanted tooth may be moved orthodontically (Lagerstrom and Kristerson, 1986).

Autotransplantation is an extremely technique sensitive procedure which may be why it is performed in only a few centres. A number of principles need to be adhered to when considering transplantation including:

- Minimal damage should be caused to the periodontal ligament and root cementum during surgical removal and transplantation, by using a strict surgical protocol and ensuring the root morphology favours extraction. Damage to the root surface will almost certainly lead to

Table 8.4   The relative advantages and disadvantages of autotransplantation.

Advantages	Unlike an implant, a non-ankylosed transplant will undergo continual eruption
	Alveolar bone volume is maintained due to the presence of a functional tooth
	An intact periodontal ligament allows orthodontic tooth movement
	Revascularisation of the pulp chamber may occur
	No need for restorative treatment that may involve preparation of adjacent teeth
	Good reported long-term outcomes
Disadvantages	Risk of ankylosis
	Requires strict surgical protocols
	Need for endodontic treatment
	Probable need for re-contouring of the transplanted tooth
	Patient must be highly motivated

ankylosis and subsequent replacement resorption (Andreasen *et al.*, 1990c)

- The root length should be three-quarters developed with an open apex to allow pulpal revascularisation (a transplant with an open apex is likely to undergo revascularisation and will not require root canal treatment) (Andreasen *et al.*, 1990b)
- There should be adequate bone at the recipient site
- Root canal treatment should be carried out at the correct time in teeth transplanted with a closed apex
- The patient should be well motivated

In patients with hypodontia the edentulous alveolus is often thin or hypoplastic. This makes autotransplantation difficult, and it is difficult to justify pre-operative bone grafting or bone augmentation in a growing patient to permit autotransplantation.

Key Points: Treatment of patients with hypodontia in the late mixed and early permanent dentition

- Dental development can be delayed in patients with hypodontia, lengthening courses of treatment
- Orthodontics aims to create ideal tooth spacing and occlusal relationships
- Root paralleling should be checked with periapical radiographs prior to orthodontic de-bonding
- Restorative treatment at this stage aims to improve the contour of teeth and replace missing teeth during important school years. Composite resin is best for re-contouring and resin-bonded bridges for fixed tooth replacement
- Dentures or overdentures may be necessary for optimal treatment of severe hypodontia
- Prosthodontic treatment should have low maintenance and should not compromise future care (particularly the use of implants) when growth has been completed. Orthodontic retention with fixed or removable retainers is vital in this respect

Conclusion

The management of hypodontia during the late mixed and early permanent dentition stage is pivotal in the long-term management of patients. Decisions made at this stage can have lasting implications so it is essential that careful treatment planning is carried out within a multidisciplinary context. Treatment will often involve a combination of orthodontics and restorative dentistry. The broad aims of orthodontic treatment are either space redistribution or closure and correction of a superimposed malocclusion if present. It is impor-

tant for the restorative dentist to examine patients before de-bonding orthodontic appliances to ensure that the restorative treatment objectives can be satisfied.

Restorative treatment aims to restore appearance and function using fixed restorations if at all possible. This is important for the patient's development in adolescence. Any treatment provided at this stage should not compromise future treatment when the patient has completed growth. Long-term retention is important and splinting of teeth should be considered.

References

Andreasen JO, Paulsen HU, Ahlquist R, Bayer T, Schwartz O. A long-term study of 370 autotransplanted premolars. Part I. Surgical procedures and standardised techniques for monitoring healing. *Eur J Orthod* 1990a;12:3–13.

Andreasen JO, Paulsen HU, Yu Z, Bayer T, Schwartz O. A long-term study of 370 autotransplanted premolars. Part II. Tooth survival and pulp healing subsequent to transplantation. *Eur J Orthod* 1990b;12:14–24.

Andreasen JO, Paulsen HU, Ahlquist R, Bayer T, Schwartz O. A long-term study of 370 autotransplanted premolars. Part III. Periodontal healing subsequent to transplantation. *Eur J Orthod* 1990c;12:25–37.

Albretsson T, Zarb GA, Worthington P, Eriksson AR. The long-term efficacy of currently used dental implants: A review and proposed criteria of success. *Int J Oral Maxillofac Implants* 1986;1:11–25.

Andrews LF. The six keys to normal occlusion. *Am J Orthod* 1972;62:296–309.

Baccetti T. Tooth rotation associated with aplasia of non-adjacent teeth. *Angle Orthod* 1998;68:471–474.

Barrack GM, Bretz WA. A long-term prospective study of etched-cast restorations. *Int J Prosthodont* 1993;6:428–434.

Behr M, Liebrock A, Stich W, *et al.* Adhesive-fixed partial dentures in anterior and posterior areas. *Clin Oral Investig* 1998;2:31–35.

Behrents RG. *Atlas of Growth in the Aging Craniofacial Skeleton. Craniofacial Growth Series*. Centre for Human Growth and Development, University of Michigan, 1985.

Bergendahl B, Bergendahl T, Hallonsten A-L, *et al.* A multidisciplinary approach to rehabilitation with osseointegrated implants in children and adolescents with multiple aplasia. *Eur J Orthod* 1996;18:119–129.

Bergman B. A 25 year longitudinal study of patients treated with removable partial dentures. *J Oral Rehabil* 1995;22:595–599.

Blum-Hareuveni T, Rehany U, Rumelt S. Blinding endophthalmitis from orthodontic headgear. *N Engl J Med* 2004;351(26):2774–2775.

Bryant S R. The effects of age, jaw site and bone condition on oral implant outcomes. *Int J Prosthodont* 1998;11:470–490.

Bukhary SM, Gill DS, Tredwin CJ, Moles DR. The influence of varying maxillary incisor dimensions on perceived smile aesthetics. *Br Dent J* 2007;203(12):687–693.

Chana H, Kelleher M, Briggs P, Hopper R. Clinical evaluation of resin-bonded gold alloy veneers. *J Prosthet Dent* 2000;83:294–300.

Creugers, NH, Kayser AF. An analysis of multiple failures of resin-bonded bridges. *J Dent* 1992;20:348–351.

Cronin RJ, Oesterle LJ. Implant use in growing patients, treatment planning concerns. *Dent Clin North Am* 1998;42:1–34.

Clifford PM, Orr JF, Burden DJ. The effects of increasing the reverse curve of Spee in a lower archwire examined using a dynamic photo-elastic gelatine model. *Eur J Orthod* 1999;21:213–222.

Djemal S, Setchell D, King P, Wickens J. Long-term survival characteristics of 832 resin-retained bridges and splints provided in a post-graduate teaching hospital between 1978 and 1993. *J Oral Rehabil* 1999;26:302–320.

Dunne S M, Millar B J. A longitudinal study of the clinical performance of resin-bonded bridges and splints. *Br Dent J* 1993;174:405–412.

Durstberger G, Celar A, Watzek G. Implant-surgical and prosthetic rehabilitation of patients with multiple dental aplasia. A clinical report. *Int J Oral Maxillofac Implants* 1999;14:417–423.

Edwards JG. A long-term prospective evaluation of the circumferential supracrestal fiberotomy in alleviating orthodontic relapse. *Am J Orthod Dentofacial Orthop* 1988;93:380–387.

Evans RD, Briggs PF. Restoration of an infra-occluded primary molar with indirect composite onlay: A case report and literature review. *Dent Update* 1996;23:52–54.

Einwag JA. Ground devitalized deciduous molar as an abutment for a fixed bridge – An example. *Quintessence Int* 1984;35:1481–1483.

Fudalej P, Kokich VG, Leroux B. Determining the cessation of vertical growth of the craniofacial structures to facilitate placement of single-tooth implants. *Am J Orthod Dentofacial Orthop* 2007;131(Suppl.4):S59–67.

Garnett MG, Wassell RW, Jepson NJ, Nohl FS. Survival of resin-bonded bridgework in hypodontia patients. *Br Dent J* 2006;201:527–534.

Goodacre Ch, Campagni WV, Aquilino SA. Tooth preparations for complete crowns: an art form based on scientific principles. *J Prosthet Dent* 2001;85:363–376.

Gukes AD, Scurria MS, King TS, McCarthy GR, Brahim JS. Prospective clinical trial of dental implants in persons with ectodermal dysplasia. *J Prosthet Dent* 2002;88:21–25.

Heij DO, Opdebeeck H, Steenberghe D, *et al.* Facial Development, Continuous Tooth Eruption, and Mesial Drift as Compromising Factors for Implant Placement. *Int J Oral Maxillofac Implants* 2006;21:867–878.

Hemmings K, Harrington Z. Replacement of Missing teeth with fixed Prosthesis. *Dent Update* 2004;31:137–141.

Hemmings KW, Howlett JA, Woodley NJ, Griffiths BM. Partial dentures for patients with advanced tooth wear. *Dent Update* 1995 22:2 52–59.

Hobkirk JA, Brook AH. The management of patients with severe hypodontia. *J Oral Rehabil* 1980;7:289–298.

Howe DF, Denehy GE. Anterior partial fixed dentures utilising the acid-etch technique and a cast metal framework. *J Prosthet Dent* 1977;37:28–31.

Hussey DL, Linden GJ. The clinical performance of cantilevered resin-bonded bridgework. *J Dent* 1996;24: 251–256.

Jepson NJ, Nohl FS, Carter NE, *et al.* The interdisciplinary management of hypodontia: restorative dentistry. *Br Dent J* 2003 Mar 22;194(6):299–304 *(review)*.

Kayser AF. Shortened dental arches and oral function. *J Oral Rehabil* 1981;8:457–462.

Kearns G, Sharma A, Perrott D, *et al.* Placement of endosseous implants in children and adolescents with hereditary ectodermal dysplasia. *Oral Surg Oral Med Oral Pathol* 1999;88:5–10.

Kerr WJ. The effect of the premature loss of deciduous canines and molars on the eruption of their successors. *Eur J Orthod* 1980;2:123–128.

Kesling HD. The diagnostic set-up with considerations of the third dimension. *Am J Orthod* 1956;42:740–748.

Koch G, Bergendahl T, Kvint S, Johansson UB. *Consensus Conference on Oral Implants in Young Patients.* Göteborg, Graphic systems, 1996.

Kokich VG, Spear FM. Guidelines for managing the orthodontic-restorative patient. *Semin Orthod* 1997; 3:3–20.

Kokich VO Jr. Congenitally missing teeth: orthodontic management in the adolescent patient. *Am J Orthod Dentofacial Orthop* 2002;121:594–595.

Lagerstrom L, Kristerson L. Influence of orthodontic treatment on root development of autotransplanted premolars. *Am J Orthodont* 1986;89:146–150.

Laing E, Cunningham SC, Jones SP, Moles D, Gill DS. The psychosocial impact of hypodontia in children. *Am J Orthod Dentofacial Orthop* 2010;137:35–41.

Levin EI. Dental esthetics and the golden proportion. *J Prosthet Dent* 1978;40:244–252.

Millar BJ, Taylor NG. Lateral thinking: The management of upper lateral incisors. *Br Dent J* 1995;179:99–106.

Nohl F, Cole B, Hobson R, *et al.* The management of hypodontia: Present and Future. *Dent Update* 2008;35: 79–90.

Oesterle LJ, Cronin RJ Jr. Adult growth, ageing and the single tooth implant. *Int J Oral Maxillofac Implants* 2000;15:252–260.

Olsen TM, Kokich VG Sr. Postorthodontic root approximation after opening space for maxillary lateral incisor implants. *Am J Orthod Dentofacial Orthop* 2010;137: 158.e1–158.

Ostler MS, Kokich VG Sr. Alveolar ridge changes in patients congenitally missing mandibular second premolars. *J Prosthet Dent* 1994;71:144–149.

Probster B, Henrich GM, Gutenberg J. 11-year follow up study of resin bonded fixed partial dentures. *Int J Prosthodont* 1997;10:259–268.

Pjetursson BE, Tan WC, Tan K, *et al.* A systematic review of the survival and complications rates of resin-bonded bridges after an observation period of at least 5 years. *Clin Oral Implants Res* 2008;19:131–141.

Rammelsberg P, Pospiech P, Gernet W. Clinical factors affecting adhesive fixed partial dentures. A six year study. *J Prosthet Dent* 1993;70:300–307.

Ravin JJ, Nielsen HG. A longitudinal radiographic study of the mineralization of 2nd premolars. *Scand J Dent Res* 1977;85:232–236.

Reitan K. Clinical and histologic observations on tooth movement during and after orthodontic treatment. *Am J Orthod* 1967;53:721–745.

Reuter JE, Brose MO. Failures in full crown retained dental bridges. *Br Dent J* 1984;157:61–63.

Roberts DH. The relationship between age and the failure of bridge prosthesis. *Br Dent J* 1970;128:175–177.

Robertsson S, Mohlin B. The congenitally missing upper lateral incisor. A retrospective study of orthodontic space closure versus restorative treatment. *Eur J Orthod* 2000;22:697–710.

Robinson S, Chan M. New teeth from old: treatment options for retained primary teeth. *Br Dent J* 2009;207: 315–320.

Rosa M, Zachrisson BU. Integrating space closure and esthetic dentistry in patients with missing lateral incisors. *J Clin Orthod* 2007;41:563–573.

Richardson ME. The etiology of late lower arch crowding alternative to mesially directed forces: a review. *Am J Orthod Dentofacial Orthop* 1994;105:592–597.

Ruiz-Mealin EV, Gill DS, Parekh S, Jones SP, Moles DR. A radiographic study of tooth development in hypodontia. *J Orthod* 2009;36:291.

Sabri R. Management of missing maxillary lateral incisors. *J Am Dent Assoc* 1999;130:80–84.

Scurria MS, Bader, Shugars DA. Meta-analysis of fixed partial denture survival; prostheses and abutments. *J Prosthet Dent* 1998;79:459–464.

Shillingburg HT Jr, Hobo S, Whitsett LD, Jacobi R, Brackett SE. *Fundamentals of Fixed Prosthodontics*, 3rd edn. 1997, Quintessence Publishing, Carol Stream, IL.

Spear F, Mathews D, Kokich V. Interdisciplinary management of single-tooth implants. *Semin Orthod* 1997;3:45.

St George G, Hemmings KW and Patel K. Resin-retained bridges re-visited. Part 1. History and Indications. *Prim Dent Care* 2002a;9(3):87–91.

St George G, Hemmings KW and Patel K. Resin-retained Bridges revisited. Part 2. Clinical considerations. *Prim Dent Care* 2002b;9(4):139–144.

Sundram F, Walmsley A. The management of severe hypodontia in a young adult patient: A case report. *Dent Update* 2003;30(6):326–330.

Thilander B, Odman J, Grondahl, Friberg B. Osseointegrated implants in adolescents. An alternative in replacing missing teeth? *Eur J Orthod* 1994;16:84–95.

Thilander B, Odman J, Jemt T. Single implants in the upper incisor region and their relationship to the adjacent teeth. An 8-year follow-up study. *Clin Oral Implants Res* 1999;10:346–355.

Thilander B, Odman J, Lekholm U. Orthodontic aspects of the use of oral implants in adolescents: A ten year follow-up study. *Eur J Orthod* 2001;23:715–731.

Winstanley RB. Prosthodontic treatment of patients with hypodontia. *J Prosthet Dent* 1984;52:687–691.

Wise MD. *Failure in the Restored Dentition: Management and Treatment*. Quintessence Publishing, Chicago, 1995.

Wolfart S, Thormann H, Freitag S, Kern M. Assessment of dental appearance following changes in incisor proportions. *Eur J Oral Sci* 2005;113:159–165.

Yeung AL, Lo EC, Chow TW, Clark RK. Oral health status of patients 5–6 years after placement of cobalt-chromium removable partial dentures. *J Oral Rehabil* 2000;27:183–189.

9 The Established Dentition with Hypodontia

Introduction

The management of patients with hypodontia in the mixed dentition stage was discussed in Chapter 8. A seamless transition of treatment into the *established* stage of dental development is crucial in delivering a coordinated care pathway for these patients and avoiding unnecessary delays in their treatment. In patients with severe hypodontia, the limited permanent dentition may be developed by the age of 8 or 9 years, whereas in milder forms the dentition may not fully establish until 13–15 years of age. For the purposes of this book, the established dentition is considered to be the stage at which definitive or long-term restorative work is to be undertaken.

Factors that may influence the treatment of hypodontia in this patient group can broadly be divided into *systemic* issues and *local* issues.

Key systemic issues that may influence treatment planning

Identifying the patient's treatment objectives

A critical factor that should be determined at the beginning of treatment is the patient's motivation for what is often an extensive period of dental care (Dhanrajani, 2002; Bishop *et al.*, 2006; Naini and Gill, 2008a, 2008b). As discussed in Chapter 3, it is imperative to take a multidisciplinary approach in the management of patients with hypodontia and to ascertain the patient's concerns and treatment objectives (Hobkirk *et al.*, 1994; Dhanrajani, 2002; Francischone *et al.*, 2003; Hobson *et al.*, 2003; Hobkirk *et al.*, 2006). It is also important to recognise that these may change over time either because it has not technically been possible to achieve the original goals, or because there has been an altera-

Hypodontia: A Team Approach to Management, First Edition
© J.A. Hobkirk, D.S. Gill, S.P. Jones, K.W. Hemmings, G.S. Bassi, A.L. O'Donnell and J.R. Goodman
Published 2011 by Blackwell Publishing Ltd

tion in the patient's perception of what is important in his or her dental treatment (Nohl *et al.*, 2008; Shafi *et al.*, 2008). An example of this might be a patient in whom a second premolar space existed in the mandible at the end of orthodontic treatment, where the original plan had been to restore it using an implant. However, after the completion of orthodontic treatment the patient might be sufficiently satisfied with the improvement that the premolar space is no longer an issue, and might prefer it to be left unrestored (Morgan and Howe, 2003). This may particularly be the case when the restorative phase is complex and bony augmentation procedures are required prior to implant placement (Nohl *et al.*, 2008).

Identifying patient expectations

Once the objectives of treatment have been established, the patient's expectations of the potential procedures and their outcomes need to be explored, and if necessary clarified (Bishop *et al.*, 2006; Naini and Gill, 2008a, 2008b). Patients with hypodontia may have already undergone several years of interceptive or definitive treatment in their childhood and adolescent years. It is important that they maintain realistic expectations of the likely timescale of any remaining treatment and what it will involve, including its long-term prognosis and any anticipated maintenance requirements. Any limitations of treatment should be thoroughly explained as part of gaining informed consent. The vast majority of patients who seek treatment for hypodontia do so at an early stage in their lives and therefore any restorative treatment is likely to have future maintenance implications (Hobkirk *et al.*, 1995). The expectations of treatment can sometimes be unrealistic, which is often understandable if small teeth and gaps in the arches have been present for most of a patient's life. In these situations it is not unusual for a patient to request 'large white teeth', but the degree to which this can be achieved should be carefully discussed.

Social issues

When patients have reached the established dentition phase and completed other dental treatment

(such as initial restorative care involving resin-retained bridges or orthodontics), they are often undertaking higher education at a college or university or are in full-time employment. Thus various social factors can significantly influence their availability for treatment, particularly if it extends over many months. The ability of a patient to attend and undergo this kind of care, for example complicated implant treatment, needs to be ascertained. Consider whether simpler treatment could be provided as an interim measure, postponing the more time-intensive procedures until the patient can commit to them (Goodman *et al.*, 1994; Hobkirk *et al.*, 1995; Morgan and Howe, 2003; Nohl *et al.*, 2008).

Health-related issues

Although the majority of patients with hypodontia have an unremarkable medical history, some do have an associated syndrome and can have a number of related health problems that may impact on potential treatment (Shroff *et al.*, 1996). Collagen defects sometimes occur and may complicate the provision of tissue-borne prostheses, even if they are being used as an interim measure. Furthermore, collagen defects may result in friable gingival tissues that inhibit the moisture control needed for conservative adhesive dentistry techniques to be successful. As described in Chapter 1, patients with hypodontia as part of a syndrome such as hypohidrotic ectodermal dysplasia with immune deficiency (HED-ID) have an associated deficiency in the immune system, which may have a particular impact on treatment options such as dental implants (Açikgöz *et al.*, 2007). See the OMIM database (Online Mendelian Inheritance in Man) available at www.ncbi.nlm.nih.gov/Omim/.

Key local issues that may influence treatment planning

Evidence of commitment to oral care

As with all patients requiring restorative care, the health of the periodontium is fundamental to a successful treatment outcome (Swartz *et al.*, 1996). Chapter 3 describes the benefits of using a pro

Table 9.1   A summary of basic periodontal examination (BPE) scores.

Score	Description
0	No bleeding No pocketing detected
1	Bleeding on probing No pocketing greater than 3.5 mm
2	Plaque-retentive factors present No pocketing greater than 3.5 mm
3	Pockets greater than 3.5 mm but less than 5.5 mm in depth
4	Pockets greater than 5.5 mm in depth
*	Total attachment loss 7 mm or greater, or furcation involvement

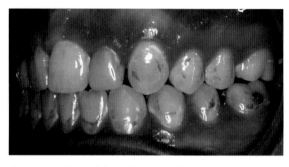

Figure 9.1   Enamel decalcification following removal of a fixed orthodontic appliance in a patient who had suboptimal oral hygiene.

forma sheet to collect data within a multidisciplinary team environment and to ensure that essential information is noted at the initial appointment. The example of a pro forma in Chapter 3 (Figure 3.2) includes a basic periodontal examination (BPE), which provides an indication of the condition of the periodontium and the effectiveness of the patient's oral hygiene. The basic periodontal examination (BPE) scores are summarised in Table 9.1. A patient must be able to demonstrate a commitment to oral care, with a stable periodontal condition and the absence of active dental disease, before embarking on complex treatment. Where disease is present this must be treated as an initial phase of care, following which a period of monitoring may be required to assess the patient's ability to maintain a stable and healthy oral environment. If a healthy dental condition cannot be maintained, the appropriateness of undertaking complex treatment must be questioned, and the treatment plan may need to be modified accordingly.

Initial treatment to achieve a stable and healthy dental state may include oral hygiene instruction, supra- and subgingival scaling, topical fluoride application, treatment of carious teeth including restorative or endodontic therapy, and the extraction of teeth with a poor prognosis (Goodman et al., 1994; Bishop et al., 2006). However, careful consideration needs to be given before extracting teeth, particularly if implant treatment is planned, so that the tooth is removed at the most appro-

priate time. If there is a long interval between extraction and implant placement, excessive bone resorption may complicate implant therapy. Following this initial treatment the patient should be reviewed, after an appropriate time period, to ensure that his or her dental condition is stable before commencing more advanced procedures. However, even though there may be an improvement in oral care at this stage, careful re-evaluation is required throughout treatment to avoid any unnecessary complications. These may arise, for example, if the patient's oral hygiene and diet control are sub-optimal during fixed orthodontic appliance therapy, resulting in decalcification of the enamel after appliance removal (Figure 9.1).

Tissue responses to previous treatment

When a patient presents for definitive care in the established dentition, there is an ideal opportunity to evaluate the tissue responses to previous treatment. An example of this is an assessment of the gingival biotype, which may be an important factor when considering tooth replacement options (Figure 9.2). If previous surgery (such as that for the removal of impacted or ectopic teeth) has resulted in gingival recession around the remaining teeth in that area, it is possible that further recession will occur when other surgical procedures (such as implant treatment) are performed. Similarly, if previous attempts to extrude teeth with orthodontic appliances have been unsuccessful, and it is considered desirable to increase the occlusal vertical dimension (OVD) during later

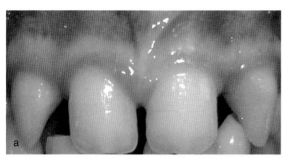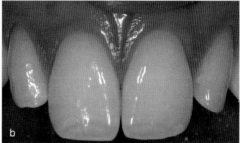

Figure 9.2   (a) Thick gingival biotype with broad interdental papillae. (b) Thin gingival biotype showing scalloped contour. A thin gingival biotype may be more prone to recession, particularly if a mucoperiosteal flap is raised for surgical interventions such as implant placement.

treatment by discluding the posterior teeth using an anterior bite plane, it is unlikely that the molar teeth will erupt passively in order to re-establish occlusal contact. This may necessitate additional restorative treatment in the form of cast occlusal restorations on the molars to provide the increase in OVD. These will also carry an added burden of maintenance care.

Dental aesthetics

One of the primary reasons for which a patient with hypodontia may seek treatment is to correct a perceived problem with the appearance of his or her teeth. Issues may include spacing resulting from missing or microdont teeth, malformations of the teeth or their malalignment (Peck *et al.*, 1996, 2002; McKeown *et al.*, 2002). The effect the appearance of the teeth can have on a patient's self-confidence should not be underestimated, and this may be a key factor that motivates them to undergo extensive courses of treatment (Gill *et al.*, 2007; Naini and Gill, 2008a, 2008b). However, there is much variation in what is perceived to be an acceptable dental appearance, and the desires of the individual patient should always be borne in mind. For example some patients may feel that a small diastema between the maxillary central incisor teeth gives character to a smile, whereas others wish for all spacing to be closed. In situations where it is not possible to do this with orthodontic treatment, a similar effect may be achieved by enlarging the teeth with either composite resin or with veneers. This may significantly increase the

patient's maintenance requirements in the medium- to long-term, which needs to be balanced against the improvement in aesthetics achieved (Bishop *et al.*, 2006).

Function

It is surprising that many patients with even severe hypodontia do not complain of problems relating to oral function (Hobkirk *et al.*, 1994). This is particularly the case when the primary teeth remain in situ in place of the missing secondary teeth (Laing *et al.*, 2008). However, when multiple secondary teeth are absent and the primary teeth have exfoliated, function often becomes more of an issue, especially if the missing teeth are grouped together in one posterior sextant. In this situation the missing teeth should be replaced in a manner that restores normal oral function as much as possible, for which implant treatment is frequently the first option to be considered.

Tooth size and form

The features associated with hypodontia have been considered in Chapter 2. Malformations in the size and form of the teeth frequently occur in patients with the condition and can affect any tooth series (Goodman *et al.*, 1994; Bishop *et al.*, 2006; Addy *et al.*, 2006). However, the most commonly affected teeth are the maxillary lateral incisors, even in mild cases of hypodontia. Frequently, the absence of a maxillary lateral incisor is associated with the presence of a microdont lateral incisor tooth on the contralateral side. In such circumstances a decision often needs to be made between extracting the microdont tooth and closing the lateral incisor spacing bilaterally, or building up the microdont incisor and opening the spacing on the contralateral side to allow for prosthetic replacement of the missing tooth with a bridge or implant (Goodman *et al.*, 1994; Millar and Taylor, 1995; Francischone *et al.*, 2003; Jepson *et al.*, 2003; Forgie *et al.*, 2005; Kokich and Kinzer, 2005; Thind *et al.*, 2005; Addy *et al.*, 2006). Several factors may need to be taken into account when deciding which option to pursue, as follows.

Prognosis of the microdont tooth

Where a microdont lateral incisor has a poor prognosis due to a short root or additional morphological deformation such as a *dens invaginatus* (Figure 9.3) with pulpal disease, it may be preferable to extract the tooth and close the spacing.

Gingival margins of the canines

The scope for disguising a canine as a lateral incisor is a significant factor when deciding whether to open or close a lateral incisor space. The definitive levels of the gingival margins do not stabilise until adult life. Since patients often present for ortho-

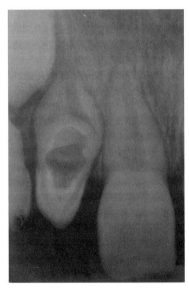

Figure 9.3 Radiograph of an upper lateral incisor presenting as a dens invaginatus (dens-in-dente).

dontic treatment before the gingival margin levels have fully matured, a decision is required as to whether to open or close the lateral incisor space at this stage – a judgement that is partly influenced by the anticipated level at which the gingival margin is likely to stabilise. When assessing whether the maxillary canine teeth can be disguised as lateral incisors, a satisfactory aesthetic result can normally be achieved as long as the gingival margins of the canine teeth are not apical to those of the central incisors (Figure 9.4). This assumes the gingival margins of the teeth are visible when smiling, and in patients with a low smile-line the gingival level may be less important (Gill *et al.*, 2007). It may be possible to alter the gingival margin by moving the canine tooth in a vertical direction orthodontically (Kokich and Kinzer, 2005). If the gingival margin is considered to be too apical, orthodontic extrusion will allow the gingival complex to be at a more coronal level. However, both the palatal cingulum and cusp tip of the canine will need to be reduced, and the extent to which this can be performed is often the limiting factor on how much extrusion is feasible.

Size of the canines

According to the golden proportion philosophy of aesthetics the maxillary lateral incisor teeth should be approximately two-thirds the size of the upper central incisors (Ricketts, 1982; Gill *et al.*, 2007; Naini and Gill, 2008a). It can therefore be helpful to assess the height and width of the canines and central incisors to determine how close their relative dimensions conform to this guide. Sometimes it is possible to reduce the size of the canine teeth, but any such re-contouring should ideally be confined to within the enamel. The adjusted area should be polished and a concentrated fluoride paste applied. If the canine teeth are of a substantial size, it may not be possible to achieve an aesthetically pleasing result by moving them next to the central incisor teeth and closing the lateral incisor space (Figure 9.5). If appearance is a high priority for the patient in this situation, enlarging the lateral incisor space to permit its prosthetic replacement is likely to be preferable.

Contour of the canines

The labial contour of the canines is often bulbous whereas that of the maxillary incisors is less so.

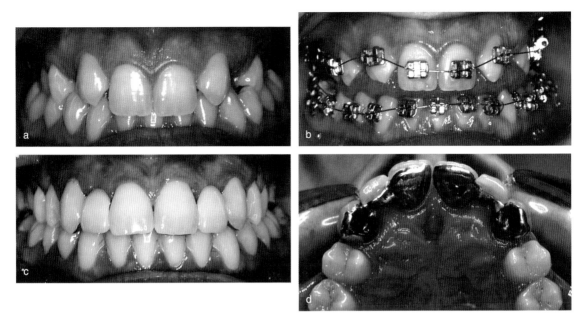

Figure 9.4   (a)–(d) The gingival margins of the upper canine teeth are significantly more apical than those of the maxillary central incisors. For this reason, this patient's maxillary lateral incisor spaces were re-created for prosthetic replacement. Note the incisal overlap of the resin-bonded bridge retainers to ensure all excursive contacts remain on the metal framework and do not pass across the junction between the retainer and the abutment tooth. The aesthetics were not compromised.

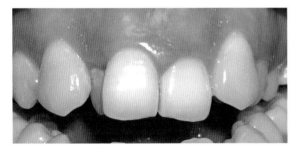

Figure 9.5   Large canine teeth that would be difficult to disguise as lateral incisors.

Therefore when attempting to disguise upper canine teeth as lateral incisors, the labial surface may need to be re-contoured. This should be confined to the enamel so as to avoid the need for restorations such as veneers or crowns. However, as the enamel is reduced in thickness so the colour of the darker dentine will become more visible, thus exacerbating any colour differences between the canine and central incisor teeth. If this difference in colour is significant, it may be preferable to enlarge the lateral incisor space to permit the use of a prosthetic replacement and allow a gradation in colour from the central incisor tooth to the prosthetic lateral incisor and finally to the canine.

Colour of the canines

The maxillary canines are naturally darker in colour than the incisors. The difference between the two teeth can vary considerably but, as mentioned above, if it is significant a more aesthetically pleasing result may be achieved by placing a prosthetic replacement in a suitably expanded lateral incisor space. However if other factors suggest the canine should be moved into the lateral incisor space, it may be possible to improve the colour of the canine tooth by vital bleaching or the use of composite resin or porcelain veneers. Matching the colour of the central incisor and canine teeth is more difficult if the central incisor has several obviously different shades or translucencies. In this situation bleaching the central incisors in addition to the canine teeth may produce a more harmonious appearance, or it may be a factor that favours enlarging the lateral incisor space and matching the prosthetic replacement with the shade of the central incisor tooth.

Shape of the canines

There can be a wide variation in the shape of the maxillary canine tooth but often it has a noticeable cusp tip. In some circumstances the shape and position of the tip of the maxillary canine may be such that 3–4 mm would need to be removed to achieve the desirable incisal level and shape. Such an extensive amount of tooth reduction may require the addition of a restorative material such as composite resin to protect the exposed dentine and give the desired aesthetic result. However such restorations can be prone to chipping or fracture, and therefore it may be preferable in these circumstances to use a prosthetic lateral incisor. Alternatively orthodontic intrusion of the canine could be considered although the effect that this would have on the gingival margin of the tooth would need to be assessed and a judgement made as to whether this would produce a satisfactory result.

Symmetry

Although a canine tooth may be acceptably disguised as an absent lateral incisor following space closure, the appearance may be compromised if it is carried out unilaterally. This may result in an asymmetric labial segment which is particularly obvious when there is a large canine on one side of the midline and a microdont lateral incisor on the contralateral side. In such circumstances, a more aesthetically pleasing and symmetrical outcome may be obtained by either re-opening the lateral incisor space for prosthetic replacement or by extracting the lateral incisor on the contralateral side and closing both spaces.

Space requirements

Where the maxillary dentition demonstrates generalised spacing it is often appropriate to localise this space into the lateral incisor site, thus allowing for its prosthetic replacement (Figure 9.6). A crowded dentition on the other hand is more conducive to closing the space.

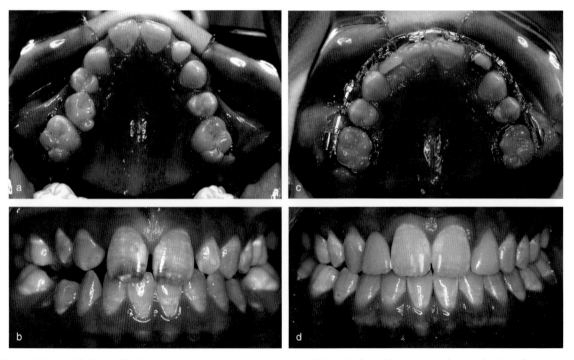

Figure 9.6   (a)–(d) Generalised anterior spacing that was concentrated into the lateral incisor sites for prosthetic replacement of the UR2 and restorative build-up of the microdont UL2.

Anteroposterior incisor relationship

This may influence the decision to close or re-open maxillary lateral incisor spaces. Where the incisor relationship is Class III, any attempt to close anterior spacing risks worsening the relationship through retraction of the upper labial segment. In such circumstances it is often better to consider re-opening the spaces for prosthetic replacement of lateral incisors, thus maintaining the labial segment in a more forward position. In patients with Class II malocclusions, the upper incisor spacing can be utilised for overjet reduction in a Class II division 1 incisor relationship, or to provide space for torquing of the upper central incisors in a Class II division 2 incisor relationship. In such circumstances, closure of the lateral incisor space may be preferable.

Relationship between the arches

Where the posterior teeth interdigitate well with their opposing teeth and the canine teeth are in a Class I relationship, it is often better to open the lateral incisor space.

Orthodontic tooth movements required

Moving teeth in older patients is inherently more difficult and often takes longer than in their younger counterparts. The position of the root apex often provides a useful guide as to where the crown can relatively easily be moved, through mainly tilting movements. If the root apex of the canine is in the lateral incisor position and the tooth needs to be bodily moved through the bone, it can significantly increase the treatment time for a patient. Therefore, on balance, it may be desirable to leave the canine in its incorrect position and disguise it as a lateral incisor if possible (Kokich and Kinzer, 2005).

Buccal bony contour

The alveolar bone develops in the presence of teeth and a failure of tooth development almost invariably results in deficiencies of bone volume at that site. In the clinical scenario of a missing maxillary lateral incisor, the canine often erupts into an ectopic position such that there is spacing mesially and distally to the crown. If the canine has erupted significantly mesially with its root apex above the crown, there can be a marked buccal bony concav-ity at the site where the canine tooth should have erupted. Thus if implant treatment was being considered, a bony augmentation procedure may become necessary to house an implant fixture of the appropriate diameter in the canine position. In this situation it may be beneficial to open the lateral incisor space by moving the canine into its correct position, thereby 'bringing' the alveolar complex with the tooth and obviating the need for a bone-grafting procedure. Furthermore, the bone in the lateral incisor region, into which site the canine had erupted, maintains its volume and an implant can often be placed at this site without requiring bone augmentation (Kinzer and Kokich, 2005).

Where the canine has erupted into its correct position and a deficiency in bone volume exists in the missing lateral incisor region, it may be possible to orthodontically move the canine into the lateral incisor site to allow the alveolar bone to develop there, before retracting the canine back into its correct position again. Although this potentially allows for implant replacement of the lateral incisor without the need for a bone graft, it can significantly increase the orthodontic treatment time and increase the risk of causing root resorption of the canine tooth.

Long-term maintenance

Most restorative dental treatment requires a certain degree of maintenance, the burden of which can vary widely. Generally speaking, if the lateral incisor space is closed then the restorative maintenance requirements are reduced compared with opening the space for prosthetic replacement (Kokich and Kinzer, 2005). As will be discussed later in this chapter, maintenance issues can significantly increase the future costs for a patient both in terms of time needed to attend for treatment and the financial commitment.

Missing teeth

The number of missing teeth does not always directly relate to the complexity of care required to treat a particular patient. Relatively straightforward removable prosthetic appliances can sometimes be used to help patients with severe hypodontia or anodontia (Figure 9.7) (Esposito and Cowper, 1991; Stephen and Cengiz, 2003), whereas

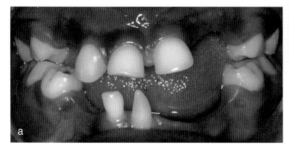
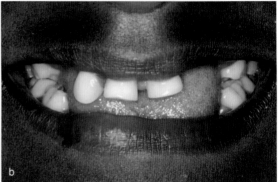
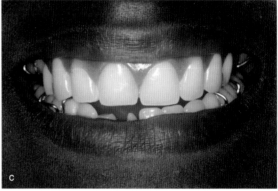

Figure 9.7   (a)–(c) Patient with severe hypodontia treated using removable prostheses.

a patient with milder hypodontia may require complex orthodontic treatment, surgical bone augmentation and dental implants (Hobkirk and Brook, 1980; Nohl *et al.*, 2008).

However, with increasing numbers of missing teeth, there tends to be a reduction in the quantity of dental hard and soft tissues and this can provide significant challenges in the provision of care for these patients (Figure 9.8). A key factor for successful orthodontic treatment is the management of anchorage, which is often difficult where there are multiple missing teeth (Nohl *et al.*, 2008). In these circumstances it may be possible to enhance anchorage with the use of extraoral headgear or with temporary anchorage devices (also known as TADs, bone anchorage devices, orthodontic mini-screws or orthodontic mini-implants).

The need for a high level of patient motivation and cooperation with orthodontic headgear has led to increasing use of temporary anchorage devices for hypodontia patients. Temporary anchorage devices are placed into the buccal or palatal/lingual cortical plate of bone within the alveolus under local or topical anaesthesia. They do not osseointegrate but simply rely on a self-tapping screw thread engaging into the cortical bone. They remain in place during orthodontic treatment to provide absolute anchorage that resists unwanted reciprocal tooth movements but can be simply removed once tooth movement is completed (Costa *et al.*, 1998; Yao *et al.*, 2005; Lee *et al.*, 2007). They have the potential to facilitate treatment in difficult hypodontia cases so as to create the optimal spacing for prosthodontic restoration (Nohl *et al.*, 2008).

Space

In the established dentition, there are unlikely to be any further changes in the alignment of the dentition associated with erupting teeth, since at this

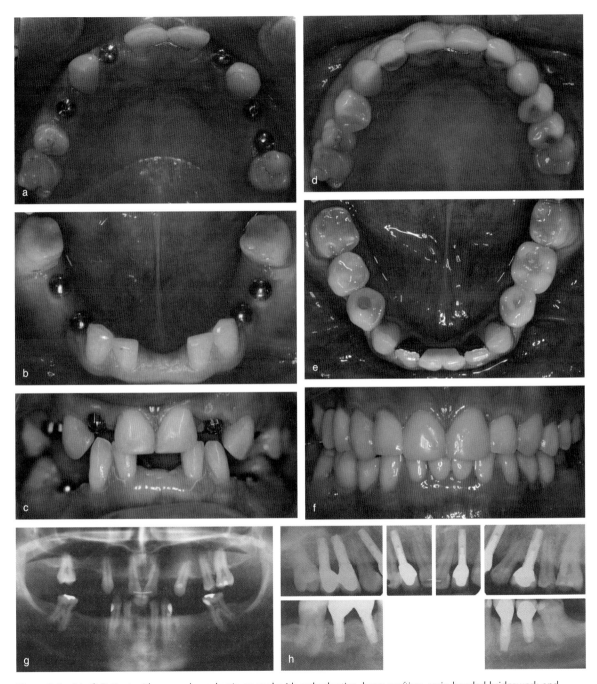

Figure 9.8   (a)–(f) Patient with severe hypodontia treated with orthodontics, bone grafting, resin-bonded bridgework and dental implants. (g) and (h) Radiographs of the same patient.

stage of the dentition any teeth that had the potential to erupt would have done so. A treatment plan can be devised based on the existing spaces, although it needs to be borne in mind that some minor changes in anterior alignment may result from late mandibular growth. Such changes are common to patients with or without hypodontia. Where space exists in the established dentition in

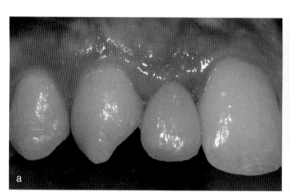
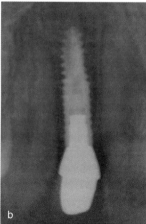

Figure 9.9   (a) Missing lateral incisor (UR2) replaced with an implant crown. (b) A narrow implant was used due to the reduced inter-radicular space between the adjacent teeth. Adequate biological width has allowed satisfactory interdental papilla formation.

a patient with hypodontia it should be assessed in all dimensions, namely the:

● Mesiodistal dimension
● Buccolingual space
● Vertical space

Mesiodistal dimension
The mesiodistal space between teeth should be assessed at both the crown and root level. Implants are increasingly being used to replace missing teeth, and require sufficient space to house the implant fixture and allow for an appropriate biological space surrounding it. Most regular-sized implants are approximately 4 mm in diameter, and allowing for 1.5 mm of biological space either side of the implant, a useful guide to the space required is 7 mm. In certain situations, such as for the replacement of maxillary lateral incisors or mandibular incisor teeth, it is possible to use narrower diameter implants such that only 6–6.5 mm of mesiodistal space is necessary (Figure 9.9). If implant treatment is being considered, either as part of the devised treatment plan or for future use, careful planning with the orthodontist is necessary to ensure the appropriate space is created between the crowns and roots of adjacent teeth (Richardson and Russell, 2001; Kinzer and Kokich, 2005; Bishop *et al.*, 2007b; Simeone *et al.*, 2007). Measurements

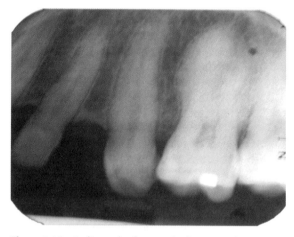

Figure 9.10   Radiograph of roots of adjacent teeth converging into a potential implant site.

at the crown level should be performed at both the cervical and incisal/occlusal aspects of the teeth so that a judgement can be made on the orthodontic movement required. This may involve simple tipping movements of the crown or more mechanically demanding axial correction with uprighting of roots or bodily tooth movement.

At the root level, radiographs are needed to assess the angulation of the roots in relation to the crown (Figure 9.10). Careful root control will need to be achieved by the orthodontist during treatment. The roots of teeth adjacent to a potential implant zone must be parallel or – better still – divergent at the completion of orthodontic treatment to facilitate implant placement without risk of root damage. If there is a degree of dilaceration of the root of an adjacent tooth into a potential implant zone, there may be insufficient inter-radicular distance for an implant, even though the measurements at crown level are adequate.

In some circumstances it may be possible to correct the position of the root orthodontically by over-correcting the tooth inclination but this may adversely affect the long axis of the crown, which can then require correction with restorative treatment such as re-contouring and composite resin additions. In severe cases, dilacerations may impede the use of implants, necessitating either the elective extraction of the dilacerated tooth or the use of an alternative restorative strategy.

A particular problem exists in patients who present with hypodontia with associated micro-dontia. Here, a balance often needs to be achieved between providing the optimal mesiodistal space to allow for implant treatment, or achieving a smaller space so that the replacement tooth is pro-portionally harmonious with the adjacent natural teeth. In these circumstances, alternative tooth replacement options such as resin-bonded bridge-work may need to be considered, with the pontic being of a similar size to the adjacent teeth. Alternatively, if resin-bonded bridges are not deemed to be appropriate, perhaps because of a lack of bonding surface area on potential abutment teeth, spacing of the neighbouring teeth could be incorporated into the orthodontic treatment plan to allow these teeth to be restoratively increased in size. This would result in the implant crown and the restored adjacent teeth being in the correct proportions.

A further consideration when assessing the mesiodistal space in a dentition occurs when the primary molar teeth are retained but the premolars are absent. The primary molars, particularly the second molars, are wider mesiodistally than the premolar teeth, and sometimes this extra space can be utilised when aligning the arch. However, in many instances the roots of the second primary molar are sufficiently intact for the tooth to remain in situ into adulthood. Replacement will ultimately

be required and at that stage the prosthetic tooth would be of a similar size to the primary molar. If this would not produce an acceptable occlusal result then consideration may need to be given to extraction of the primary molar earlier in the treatment planning process. This may also be the case if a resin-bonded bridge is going to be used to replace the missing premolar when the primary molar tooth has exfoliated. In this situation it may be desirable to extract the primary molar, partially close the resultant space as part of the overall orthodontic treatment plan, and thereby produce a more favourable size ratio between abutment and pontic. Reducing the size of a primary molar tooth during orthodontic treatment, by disking the mesial and distal surfaces could also be considered to achieve the correct width for premolar replacement at a later stage. However, this is often more complicated in the second premolar region because the divergent roots of the corresponding primary molar tooth may prevent the adjacent teeth being moved into this area.

Buccolingual space

An assessment of the buccolingual dimensions of the site of a missing tooth is increasingly important as the use of implants becomes more common. The position of the replacement tooth crown should be determined and the implant placement planned according to this. These initial investigations may reveal an inadequate buccolingual width to insert an implant in the desired position, in which case bone augmentation procedures may need to be considered. Where a primary tooth remains in situ a cursory examination may suggest an adequate buccolingual bone volume. However, careful pal-pation of the region often reveals a marked concav-ity of the bone beyond the roots of the primary tooth (Figure 9.11) that may require augmentation for implant restoration at the site (Figure 9.12).

Vertical space

Where a tooth is absent, there is the potential for the opposing tooth to overerupt and encroach on the prosthetic space. An overerupted tooth may be intruded orthodontically using active appliances, or by the use of a bite plane to utilise the Dahl effect, since localised overeruption can complicate the restorative replacement of a tooth. While it may be possible to control the occlusal contacts of the prosthetic tooth in the static intercuspal or retruded positions, it is more difficult to control contacts during excursive mandibular movements. The replacement tooth may consequently need to be

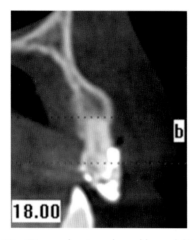

Figure 9.11 CT scan showing a buccal bony deficiency beyond the roots of a retained primary tooth.

reduced in length to avoid deleterious dynamic occlusal contacts (although this may compromise its appearance).

When a permanent tooth does not develop, the alveolar and surrounding tissues also often fail to fully form. This can lead to buccolingual deficiencies in the bone, and sometimes, more significantly, to a lack of vertical alveolar development. This is usually seen in the posterior region of the jaws and can result in infra-occlusion of a retained primary tooth. Where multiple teeth are absent in the same part of the mouth, the lack of alveolar development can result in a significant alteration of the occlusal plane (Figure 9.13). Re-establishing the correct level of the alveolus in these circumstances can be challenging because bone augmentation procedures tend to be less successful when a gain in height is attempted.

Distraction osteogenesis is an alternative method of re-establishing the correct alveolar height but it has not gained widespread use due to difficulties in wearing the appliance and the high degree of

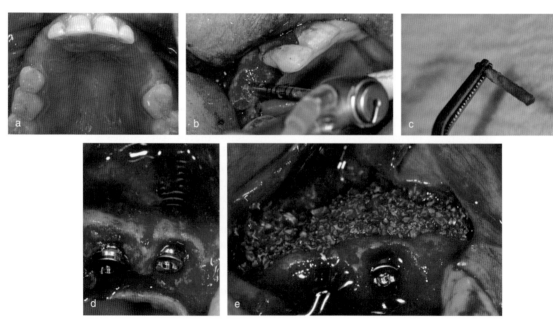

Figure 9.12 Pre-operative view of the maxilla (a) suggesting adequate ridge width for implant treatment following recent removal of the retained primary teeth. However, a buccal bony concavity existed beyond the crest of the ridge and therefore a core of bone was harvested (b) and (c) using a trephine bur at one of the implant sites. (d) Dental implants inserted into the available bone. Note buccal fenestration of the implants apically despite adequate crestal bone width. (e) Buccal bone augmentation completed after milling the core of bone and combining this with xenograft bone particles (Bio-Oss™). A double layer of xenograft membrane (BioGide™) was then placed.

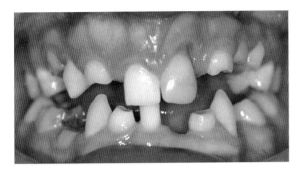

Figure 9.13   Retained primary teeth with disruption of the maxillary and mandibular occlusal planes.

patient compliance needed (Gaggl *et al.*, 1999a, 1999b; Arvystas, 2003). Furthermore in cases where hypodontia is present in the posterior maxilla, there may be insufficient bone beneath the maxillary sinus to allow the distraction process to occur.

Bone

Bone is a crucial tissue when considering the management of patients with hypodontia. Deficiencies in bone volume and quality can affect orthodontic and restorative treatment and significantly increase the overall treatment time.

Implant replacement of missing teeth has become the treatment of choice in many cases (Richardson and Russell, 2001; Francischone *et al.*, 2003; Kinzer and Kokich, 2005; Bishop *et al.*, 2007b), and unlike alternative replacement therapies (such as bridgework or removable dentures) it is critically dependent on the volume and quality of bone in potential implant sites. Bone volume can readily be established both clinically and radiographically, but its quality is more difficult to ascertain. Radiographs provide very limited information on the quality of the bone, and while computed tomography (CT) scans give much more detailed data, there is still no strong evidence that this correlates well with bone quality. CT scans however do give a good indication of the bone density at potential implant sites (Arai *et al.*, 1999; Fortin *et al.*, 2002; Nohl *et al.*, 2008).

Fortunately, modern implant surfaces are sufficiently characterised to allow osseointegration to occur even where the bone quality is suboptimal.

Where there are deficiencies of volume, the bone can be augmented with a variety of procedures, although this will increase the time taken for treatment to be completed. Many patients would have already attended numerous dental appointments and this additional treatment time may not therefore be acceptable to them. Therefore alternative treatment options such as bridges or dentures may need to be considered.

Where mandibular teeth are developmentally absent, there may be a distinct lack of cancellous bone such that the cortical plates are almost fused together (Ostler and Kokich, 1994; Santos, 2002). This can pose a significant challenge for orthodontic tooth movements into this area as the cortical plates inhibit such movements. It may be tempting in these circumstances to open the space to allow for prosthetic replacement of the missing tooth, but this decision should be carefully evaluated, as the restorative options available may be limited. Implant therapy in these cases is likely to involve significant bone grafting and therefore it would be prudent to assess the adjacent teeth for their suitability as abutment teeth for bridgework (Bishop *et al.*, 2007a).

Soft tissues

The oral soft tissues of primary concern in the management of hypodontia are the gingivae, which are often lacking in volume where teeth have not formed, a feature frequently combined with a thin gingival biotype. Both of these factors can make predictable correction of a gingival discrepancy difficult. This is particularly the case where vertical soft-tissue grafting is necessary, when there is poor formation of the interdental papilla. Various soft tissue surgical procedures have been described to augment the lack of gingival tissues, such as free gingival grafts, subepithelial connective tissue grafts and localised pedicle flaps. Although these procedures are more commonly employed during implant treatment, they can be used where other options, such as bridges, are to be used to replace the missing teeth. In the aesthetic zone, a marked buccal concavity may be unacceptable to a patient and augmentation of the gingival tissue prior to fitting a bridge can be performed to improve the soft tissue appearance at the site.

In the older patient with an established dentition, there may be a history of periodontal disease resulting in gingival recession. Where this involves teeth that need to be orthodontically moved this can be critical if the direction of tooth movement is towards the area of gingival recession. Thus, if a tooth with a labial recession defect needs to be moved labially, there is an increased risk of the recession worsening. Gingival augmentation procedures may be necessary prior to orthodontic treatment to minimise the chances of this occurring. Similarly where the roots of teeth that are to be torqued labially with orthodontic treatment are already palpable, gingival augmentation may be advisable to reduce the risk of gingival recession or dehiscence defects developing during orthodontic tooth movement.

Where hypodontia is associated with the ectodermal dysplasias, the oral soft tissues can be thick and inelastic thereby hindering access when performing treatment. Also varying degrees of macroglossia may be encountered, which can further restrict access to treatment and complicate moisture control for adhesive techniques.

Treatment

Establishing treatment objectives

Treatment for patients with hypodontia can be extensive and requires a significant investment by the patient in terms of time and possible financial costs. A patient in the established dentition stage with hypodontia may have already attended a hypodontia clinic many times but it is still important to establish and re-evaluate their treatment objectives. These may alter as a patient proceeds through their care pathway as described above. For example, if it has not been possible to accomplish the desired orthodontic movements to allow for implant replacement of a tooth, a patient may decide to pursue the bridge option rather than further orthodontic treatment to idealise the space for an implant (Dhanrajani, 2002; Bishop *et al.*, 2007a, 2007b; Nohl *et al.*, 2008).

As with any good care pathway, a significant amount of time should be devoted to determining how the treatment objectives are to be achieved. Such planning is often a key factor in a successful outcome. A variety of methods is available to help

a patient visualise what would be achievable with treatment. An orthodontic Kesling set-up can be invaluable for demonstrating the tooth movements that are possible, and when coupled with a restorative diagnostic wax-up the patient can very quickly conceptualise the predicted endpoint of treatment (Kesling, 1956). However, it can sometimes be difficult for a patient to translate a Kesling set-up or diagnostic wax-up into the intraoral situation, a problem addressed by a number of computer software programs which can aid the patient in visualising the proposed treatment outcome. Often such programs involve capturing a digital image of the dental arches and using a variety of on-screen menus to simulate the proposed treatment. The patient can, for example, see the appearance of fixed orthodontic appliances when placed on the teeth and how space may increase in one area of the mouth as it is consolidated in another.

When using these programs it is important to ensure that the treatment being described to the patient is actually achievable, as it is very easy to produce a highly desirable end result that in fact cannot be clinically achieved. For example, when there is a significant vertical discrepancy in the hard and soft tissues where the permanent teeth have failed to develop, it is unlikely it will be possible to predictably harmonise the gingival levels of the replacement teeth with the adjacent natural teeth. Similarly where microdont teeth are present with spacing between them, there is a limit on the degree to which composite resin build-ups or veneers can close the spacing. This is often dictated by the emergence profile that can be achieved with the restorations without producing a plaque trap. In such a situation the patient should be informed as to whether orthodontic treatment is likely to be required to at least partially close the spacing or they may assume the wax-up or image shown to them can be achieved without the use of orthodontic appliances.

Developing a treatment plan

Once the aims of treatment have been established a plan can be developed to achieve these objectives. This can be divided into a number of stages:

- Stage 1: Treatment of active disease
- Stage 2: Prevention of further dental disease

- Stage 3: Re-evaluation of the dental condition
- Stage 4: Treatment related to hypodontia
- Stage 5: Maintenance

STAGE 1: Treatment of active disease

When managing the older patient with hypodontia, there is an increased likelihood of other dental disease such as periodontitis, caries or tooth wear being present. Although the patient's prime objective may be to treat spacing caused by the absence of teeth, it is important that a healthy oral environment is achieved prior to commencing the definitive phase of hypodontia care. Treatment of active disease may involve:

- Caries removal and restoration
- Periodontal therapy
- Repair or replacement of existing restorations or prostheses
- Initial treatment of tooth wear
- Occlusal analysis and adjustment if there is occlusal trauma
- Endodontic treatment
- Extraction of teeth with a poor prognosis

The older patient with hypodontia is more likely to have received restorative treatment to teeth in a manner more destructive of tooth structure than is currently recommended. For example, crowns or veneers may have been placed instead of composite restorations, and conventional bridges used instead of resin-bonded bridgework. This may have been due to the prevailing treatment philosophy at the time or because the materials were inferior to those available now. This more extensive restorative work may require replacement or repair, which can further reduce the amount of tooth structure remaining. A decision may therefore need to be made on the tooth's long-term prognosis and the advisability of its extraction.

STAGE 2: Prevention of further dental disease

Once active disease has been controlled it is important the dentition remains in a healthy condition (Hobkirk *et al.*, 1995). It is often difficult to change a patient's habits unless the patient appreciates the reason for the change and is sufficiently motivated to introduce these changes into their lifestyle. Therefore, a dental professional may need to constantly remotivate a patient and emphasise the importance of maintaining a healthy oral environment so that definitive management of the hypodontia can take place. Prevention of further disease may involve:

- Instruction in appropriate oral hygiene procedures
- Dietary analysis and advice
- Fluoride therapy
- Smoking cessation advice
- Provision of an occlusal splint

STAGE 3: Re-evaluation of the dental condition

Once initial stabilising treatment has been provided, a period of re-evaluation is required to ensure that the dental condition does not deteriorate. This is an important phase in the overall management of a patient with hypodontia as it gives the clinician an opportunity to assess their commitment to treatment. At this stage a decision can be made on whether it is appropriate to continue with an initial treatment plan that may have involved complex care. If a patient fails to demonstrate a sufficiently high level of dental care, a simplified treatment strategy may be more appropriate (Shafi *et al.*, 2008).

Where teeth with a questionable prognosis have received treatment, this period of re-evaluation is crucial in determining whether the treatment has been successful. The re-evaluation period may vary depending on the individual circumstances, but three months is generally considered a suitable *minimum* time interval in most cases.

STAGE 4: Treatment related to hypodontia

Once a stable oral environment has been attained, consideration can be given to the management of the hypodontia-related issues of the treatment plan. Patients may have already received significant amounts of treatment in the early and mixed dentition phases of therapy as outlined in Chapters 7 and 8. On the other hand, some patients present relatively late with an established dentition where simple monitoring has occurred previously, but a change in the dental condition, such as the loss of retained primary teeth, has stimulated a desire to seek treatment (Laing *et al.*, 2008). In the established dentition stage, treatment decisions are often made with a view to the treatment lasting for a considerable number of years, without constantly requiring replacement. However, the longevity of various treatment modalities needs to be balanced with the desire to conserve as much healthy tooth structure as possible. Therefore, while a full-coverage metal-ceramic anterior crown may last longer and have a reduced burden of maintenance compared to composite restorations, the latter are often a more appropriate form of treatment due to their lower biological cost to a tooth (Bishop *et al.*, 2006; Nohl *et al.*, 2008).

The management of hypodontia in the established dentition may involve orthodontic treatment and surgical interventions as well as a wide range of restorative procedures (Dhanrajani, 2002; Carter *et al.*, 2003; Hobson *et al.*, 2003; Jepson *et al.*, 2003; Meechan *et al.*, 2003; Forgie *et al.*, 2005; Thind *et al.*, 2005; Bishop *et al.*, 2006, 2007a, b; Noble *et al.*, 2007; Nohl *et al.*, 2008).

Orthodontic treatment

It is generally more socially convenient to undergo orthodontic treatment in the adolescent and teen-aged years than in later life. Patients in the older age group may have a tendency to opt for a treatment pathway that does not involve orthodontic care but it is still important they are made aware of the benefits of orthodontic treatment and whether this would significantly improve the outcome. Many adult patients do decide to commit to orthodontic therapy if they perceive the benefit to be sufficiently great.

Challenges facing the orthodontist may vary according to the severity of the hypodontia. For patients with mild to moderate hypodontia, these may differ little from those for routine orthodontic procedures especially where space closure is considered appropriate. In these circumstances, correction of tooth alignment, overjet and overbite

with the establishment of good buccal interdigitation is required in order to produce a functional occlusion (Timm *et al.*, 1976; Goodman *et al.*, 1994; Clark and Evans, 2001; Carter *et al.*, 2003; Kokich and Kinzer, 2005; Thind *et al.*, 2005).

Where hypodontia is more severe, orthodontic treatment can sometimes be more complex. In discussion with the restorative dentist, decisions will have been made in relation to the ultimate location and size of edentulous spaces. The orthodontist will then be called on to ensure that there is accurate positioning of the teeth, particularly those that are to act as bridge abutments or will be adjacent to implant sites. The sizes of spaces intended for prostheses must be accurately determined both at crown level and gingival level, especially where implant treatment is planned. Adjacent roots will need to be paralleled or made divergent to avoid encroachment into implant sites (Bishop *et al.*, 2006, 2007a, b). The vertical relationships between the arches will need to be idealised, to reduce deep overbites and to prevent opposing teeth encroaching into edentulous spaces. Overbite reduction in particular may be difficult in the absence of buccal segment teeth, since the extrusion of these contributes greatly to the orthodontic levelling of the curve of Spee. Where premolars are absent, the orthodontist may need to rely on segmental mechanics with utility arches to produce true intrusion of labial segment teeth for overbite reduction.

Anchorage may be a problem for the orthodontist in patients with severe hypodontia. Where there is an absence of posterior teeth, it may be difficult to idealise the position of anterior teeth, especially canines with their large root surface area without supplementing anchorage. In such cases, temporary anchorage devices can be very useful to provide absolute anchorage for both anteroposterior tooth protraction and retraction, or tooth intrusion (Nohl *et al.*, 2008). In contrast, some severe hypodontia patients have so few permanent teeth that the orthodontist may be merely called on to produce relatively simple tooth movements such as closure of a large midline diastema prior to extensive restorative replacements (Figure 9.14).

It is important to ensure that the edentulous spaces are of an acceptable size, and the adjacent roots are positioned satisfactorily prior to removal of the orthodontic appliances. For these reasons,

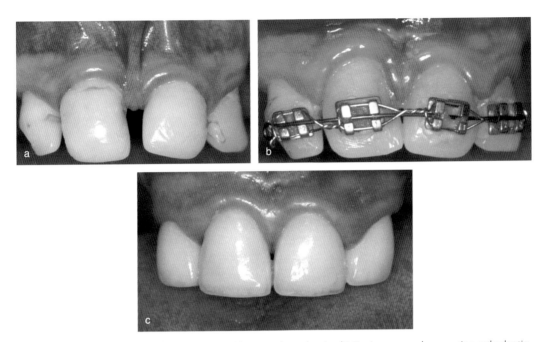

Figure 9.14   (a) Spacing between teeth in a patient with severe hypodontia. (b) During space closure using orthodontic therapy following a maxillary labial fraenectomy. (c) Teeth restored with labial porcelain veneers.

the restorative dentist and orthodontist should review the patient together before fixed appliances are removed (Nohl *et al.*, 2008). Once this has been done the patient will require orthodontic retainers to maintain corrected tooth positions until the restorative phase of care is completed. These are often removable retainers, which can carry pontics in edentulous spaces to provide an improved appearance. In cases where large spaces have been closed, it is often prudent to supplement these with fixed retainers (Zachrisson, 2007), although care should be taken not to encroach on intended abutments for resin-retained bridges. In view of the potential for the unwanted relapse of tooth positions that still exists after the placement of bridges or implants, it is often advised that patients continue the long-term use of retainers that have been made to fit over their fully restored dental arches (Littlewood *et al.*, 2006a, b).

Surgical intervention

In patients with an established dentition who have hypodontia, surgical interventions are most com-

monly associated with the exposure of unerupted and ectopic teeth or the provision of implant treatment. Other surgical procedures that may be necessary in the management of hypodontia include those associated with orthognathic surgery. Patients with severe hypodontia, and particularly those in whom hypodontia is associated with clefts of the lip or palate or with syndromes such as the ectodermal dysplasias, have an increased tendency to a Class III skeletal relationship (Roald *et al.*, 1982; Woodworth *et al.*, 1985; Nodal *et al.*, 1994; Chung *et al.*, 2000; Bondarets *et al.*, 2002; Endo *et al.*, 2004, 2006). Sometimes this is severe enough to warrant orthognathic surgery to reposition either or both jaws into a Class I relationship (Meechan *et al.*, 2003). The timing of surgery needs to be carefully coordinated because often pre-surgical orthodontic therapy is necessary followed by post-surgical orthodontics to refine the tooth positions and the occlusion. Surgical treatment is usually postponed until growth of the jaws is complete, which is normally in the late teenage years. There may be difficulties in ascertaining the appropriate amount of surgical jaw movement where severe hypodontia exists as there may be insufficient teeth to provide stable occlusal contacts. In these circumstances it may be necessary to construct removable dentures that provide the optimum post-surgical occlusion and which the maxillofacial surgeon can use to reposition the jaws at the time of surgery.

Restorative care

Restoring tooth form

Patients with hypodontia frequently also have a discrepancy in the size and/or shape of some of the remaining teeth (Goodman *et al.*, 1994; Jepson *et al.*, 2003; Bishop *et al.*, 2006; Nohl *et al.*, 2008). Restoring their correct form, either to enhance the appearance of the teeth or to improve occlusal contacts, can be achieved in several ways:

● Resin-based composite restorations
● Veneers
● Occlusal onlays
● Crowns

Resin-based composite restorations

The developments in composite materials in recent years have enabled them to be used in situations that previously would have necessitated indirect porcelain restorations. The greatest advantage of composite resins over other materials is that sound tooth structure can be conserved because minimal or no tooth preparation is required (Goodman *et al.*, 1994; Bishop *et al.*, 2006; Nohl *et al.*, 2008). The use of resin-based composite materials to build teeth up has already been detailed in Chapters 7 and 8. In some situations it may be preferable to improve the size of microdont teeth with composite resin additions prior to orthodontic treatment to align the arch. This enables the orthodontist to ensure that the correct degree of space closure is achieved. However, it is important the restorative dentist does not mask any malposition of the tooth with the build-up in this situation as this would make it much more difficult for the orthodontist to correctly position the tooth. Thus, features of a tooth such as rotations, uneven incisal edges or tilting of the crown should not be corrected restoratively at this stage unless deemed appropriate by the orthodontist. In addition to this, composite resin can be usefully employed to increase the

OVD by placing it on several teeth and allowing the discluded teeth to overerupt and thus re-establish occlusal contacts at the new vertical dimension. Although directly placed composite restorations are the most common method of utilising this material, indirect techniques can also be employed in situations such as restoring the occlusal aspects of infra-occluded primary molar teeth that are to be retained (Noble *et al.*, 2007).

Veneers

Veneers are restorations that are bonded to the whole of the buccal or lingual/palatal surface of a tooth. Directly placed veneers include the direct use of composite resin but in many cases indirect laboratory-made veneers are used, often made from porcelain, composite resin or metal alloys (Bishop *et al.*, 2006). Labial porcelain veneers were commonly used to improve the appearance of the anterior teeth, but with developments in composite restorative materials they are no longer the method of choice for initially building up a tooth. However, where extensive composite resin restorations have previously been placed and have shown signs of deterioration or repeated failure, labial porcelain veneers are used in the older patient. Modern advances in composite resin technology also allow the use of indirect composite veneers with comparable aesthetics to their porcelain counterparts, but with the added advantage of being easier to repair intraorally if the need arises. Currently, however, the medium- to long-term aesthetics of porcelain are superior to those of composite resin. Veneer restorations can also be used palatally in the management of hypodontia, particularly where there is a deep overbite and there is insufficient inter-occlusal space for restoration of the spaces resulting from hypodontia. As mentioned above, composite resin can be utilised to increase the vertical dimension of occlusion, but in situations of moderate to severe hypodontia with multiple missing posterior teeth, greater control of anterior tooth contacts may be necessary to establish the appropriate anterior guidance to protect the posterior restorations. Furthermore the wear characteristics of indirect veneers are superior to those of directly placed composite restorations which is especially important if there is evidence of tooth wear caused by bruxism. Veneers constructed from metallic alloys are ideal in this situation as

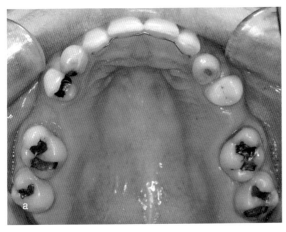
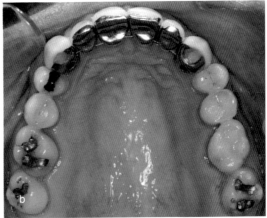

Figure 9.15   (a) A patient with retained URC and ULC and missing UR3, UR5, UL3 and UL5 following orthodontic treatment with a bonded spiral wire ('Twistflex') retainer to prevent relapse of the maxillary incisor teeth. Post-operative result (b) with implant replacement of the missing permanent teeth and palatal gold veneers on the maxillary incisors to provide anterior guidance in the new re-organised occlusion at an increased OVD. The design of the implant crowns UR3, UL3 and the castings on the maxillary incisor teeth allow the continued use of a Twistflex-type orthodontic retainer.

they have adequate strength, are not abrasive to the opposing teeth and can easily be cast to provide the correct morphology using techniques that are readily available in most dental laboratories (Figure 9.15).

Occlusal onlays

Onlay restorations cover the occlusal surfaces of posterior teeth and can be cemented fixed restorations or part of a removable partial denture. Cemented onlay restorations are normally made from metal alloys, composite resin or porcelain and are often used to restore a retained infra-occluded primary molar or to establish occlusal contacts where the OVD has been increased. When cemented onlay restorations are to be used the wear and abrasion characteristics of the material need to be taken into consideration. Composite resin and nickel chromium alloys usually wear in preference to tooth structure, gold alloys wear at a similar rate to enamel, but 'unpolished' porcelain can have a highly abrasive action on the opposing tooth. Patients with more severe hypodontia may require a relatively large increase in the OVD in relation to the often small size of the natural teeth. This can significantly increase the crown to root ratio and the demands on the supporting structures. Removable onlay dentures are particularly useful

where a number of teeth are being replaced at a raised OVD and the patient wishes to avoid more extensive treatment.

Crowns

The provision of crowns usually involves the loss of significant quantities of tooth structure during preparation and therefore the appropriateness of these restorations should be carefully evaluated. In the older patient with hypodontia, the decision to place a crown on a tooth is made easier if the tooth has already been extensively restored. In this situation a crown may be beneficial in splinting the remaining walls of the tooth. The placement of crowns is also generally considered advisable in posterior endodontically treated teeth where one or more marginal ridges have been lost. Tooth preparation for the placement of crowns on microdont teeth may not be as destructive of tooth structure as normally would be the case because the shape of a microdont tooth may be very similar to that of a crown preparation (Figure 9.16). Often only a finishing line is required together with some reduction of the incisal or occlusal surface. In this situation, a crown is likely to be more durable than other restorations and may therefore be the preferred option. However where a microdont tooth is severely tapered, a crown may not be the most

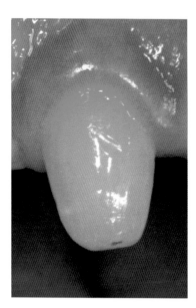

Figure 9.16   Tapered tooth requiring little modification to receive a crown.

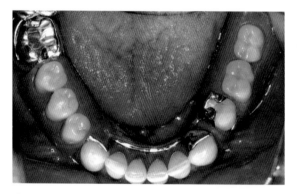

Figure 9.17   Crowns with guide planes and rest-seats to aid the retention and stability of a removable prosthesis.

appropriate choice as the lack of resistance form of the preparation may compromise the success of a crown restoration. Metal-ceramic or all-metal crowns are particularly useful where a removable partial denture is to provide the definitive prosthetic replacement of the missing teeth, because features such as guide-planes, rest-seats and appropriate undercuts can be incorporated into the crowns to aid the retention and stability of the denture (Figure 9.17). Furthermore, precision attachment components can be included in crown

restorations to provide additional retention for a removable prosthesis.

Replacing missing teeth

In the established dentition, there are four main methods of replacing missing teeth (Bishop *et al.*, 2006, 2007a, b):

- Resin-bonded bridges
- Implants
- Removable dentures
- Conventional bridges

Resin-bonded bridges
Detailed considerations relating to treatment with resin-bonded bridgework have been described in Chapter 8. Success requires careful case selection, coverage of a large tooth surface area by the bridge's retaining components, framework rigidity and careful management of the occlusion. Of equal significance are appropriate preparation of the bonding surface of the bridge retainer, adequate moisture control during cementation and the use of an appropriate adhesive cement.

Implants
Dental implants are often the optimal method of tooth replacement (Bishop *et al.*, 2007b). Their greatest advantage is that adjacent teeth do not need to be prepared nor are they required to offer support for the replacement tooth. Often, however, the provision of implant treatment in hypodontia is complicated by the lack of bone and/or soft tissue, and careful planning is essential. This typically involves a diagnostic wax-up or trial tooth set-up from which a radiographic template is generated. The radiographic template is inserted when cross-sectional images such as those from a CT scan are being recorded so that the ideal position of the replacement teeth can be identified on the scan. Anatomical landmarks such as neurovascular structures, the maxillary sinus and the lingual contour of the mandible become increasingly important as the bone volume reduces. If implants of adequate size are to be used, a careful assessment of their proximity to these anatomical structures needs to be made. Often, replacement of the upper second premolar teeth is complicated by a

low maxillary sinus at this site, and implant treatment in the posterior mandible may be restricted by the position of the inferior alveolar and mental nerves. Furthermore, loss of buccal bone volume in the mandible may tempt the clinician to insert an implant in a more lingual position to avoid the need for bone grafting. Care needs to be taken if this is performed to ensure that the lingual cortex is not perforated as this can lead to post-operative haematoma formation in the floor of the mouth, and subsequent airway obstruction. Therefore, the lingual contour and presence of a lingual concavity in the mandible should be assessed in detail on the CT scan. The data from a CT scan can be formatted for analysis by one of the several software programs that are available for planning implant selection and placement (Arai *et al.*, 1999; Fortin *et al.*, 2002; Nohl *et al.*, 2008). The cross-sectional images also allow the quantity of bone to be assessed so that bone augmentation procedures can be planned if necessary.

It is generally accepted that implant treatment should be postponed until growth has been completed, to avoid infra-occlusion of the implant restorations relative to the adjacent teeth and tissues as their positions alter with further growth. For the purposes of implant treatment, growth is considered to be complete by approximately age 17–18 years for females and 18–19 years for males. However where there is anodontia of one or both dental arches, earlier provision of implant treatment in that arch may be considered, as there is unlikely to be further development of the affected jaw (Bergendal *et al.*, 1996). More controversially, implants have been placed in children with Ectodermal Dysplasia, with periodic changes of the implant abutments for longer ones as growth of the adjacent teeth progresses. In some of these cases implants have required removal and replacement. While it is not thought that implants in children inhibit growth, it is not recommended that implants placed on either side of the mid-line be splinted together as this may prevent transverse jaw development (Cronin and Oesterle, 1998; Nohl *et al.*, 2008). The impact and benefits of early implant placement have been suggested as a key area for future clinical research (Hobkirk *et al.*, 2006).

A common feature in patients with hypodontia is a lack of alveolar ridge width at the sites where teeth are missing. This may be sufficiently severe

that it is decided other restorative treatment options would be preferable to implant provision. However, if implant treatment is still deemed to be appropriate, a variety of options exist. It may be possible to utilise narrow diameter implants or to use procedures that surgically expand the ridge prior to implant placement. This normally involves splitting the buccal and lingual plates longitudinally to allow instruments of increasing size to be inserted to enlarge the separation of the plates. Alternatively, the technique of distraction osteogenesis can be employed if there is sufficient patient cooperation to adjust the distraction device. However, if the ridge is markedly osteopenic that expansion is unlikely to be successful and should distraction osteogenesis be unacceptable to the patient then bone augmentation is commonly necessary.

Where bone augmentation procedures are required, a number of materials are available. Autogenous bone is still generally accepted as the gold standard for grafting procedures (Tolman, 1995). Bone can be harvested from local sites such as the maxilla, mandible (Figure 9.18) or cranium, or from more remote sites such as the iliac crest of the hip. The greatest disadvantage of the use of autogenous bone is the increased morbidity associated with the donor site. Where a small bony deficiency is present, bone harvested when preparing the implant site(s) can be used at the time of implant placement to repair the deficit. If a large volume of bone grafting is necessary, the deficient area is usually augmented as an initial phase and then the graft is allowed to integrate before the implant is inserted (Figure 9.19).

In an attempt to overcome the surgical complications that may arise through the use of autogenous bone, a number of materials have been developed which claim to offer comparable bone gain. Bone allografts allow the use of human tissue without the associated morbidity of autogenous bone. A variety of alloplastic materials are also available, such as those based on calcium phosphate or hydroxyapatite crystals (Misch and Dietsh, 1993). These do not carry the risk of transmission of agents that may cause disease, as is the case with the non-synthetic materials. However, at the present time the risk of disease transmission through the use of commercially available grafting materials is felt to be almost non-existent.

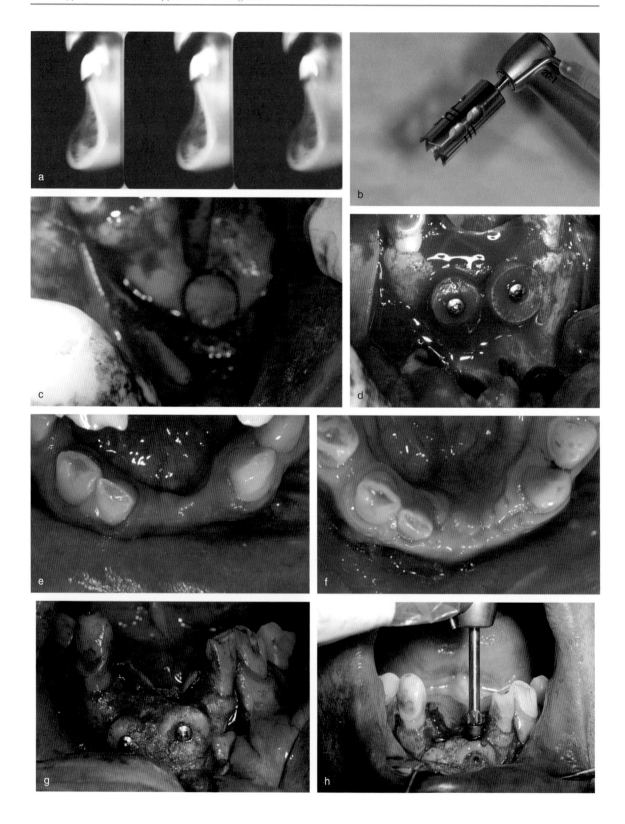

Figure 9.18   Labial augmentation of an anterior mandibular concavity (a) using block grafts to permit implant insertion. (b) Trephine used to harvest block grafts from the chin (c). Blocks in situ (d). The mandibular ridge before (e) and 3 months after grafting (f). Implant placement in grafted site (g)–(h).

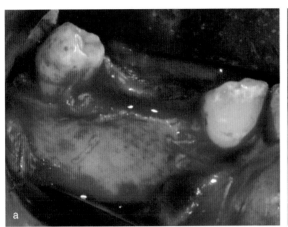
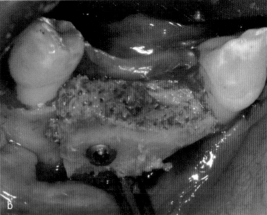

Figure 9.19   (a)–(b) Bony defect in the lower right premolar region reconstructed with a corticocancellous block graft harvested from the iliac crest. The graft will be allowed to integrate prior to implant placement, which will be performed as a separate procedure.

Therefore, xenograft bone augmentation substances have gained increasing popularity (Figure 9.20). They are more readily available than bone allografts and are claimed to support bone formation through osseoconductive mechanisms (Zitzmann *et al.*, 1997).

When implants have been placed in grafted bone it is conventional to submerge the implant fixture by suturing the gingiva over the implant head. After a period of osseointegration that may range from 3 to 12 months, the implant is uncovered to allow its restoration. If bone augmentation has not been necessary and there is sufficient stability of the implant within its osteotomy site, it may be possible to place a transgingival component onto the implant fixture head or even a provisional restoration at the same appointment as implant placement (Cannizzaro *et al.*, 2008).

The buccolingual angle at which an implant fixture is inserted depends on factors such as the contour of the bone and the method to be used to retain the superstructure to the fixture. The contour of the bone at potential implant sites in patients with hypodontia is often deficient but the degree of deficiency can vary considerably. In some instances there may be a minor lack of bone, particularly if the root of the retained primary tooth is of reasonable length. In these circumstances it may be possible to place the implant fixture within the bony envelope, thus avoiding grafting procedures. However, the angle of the fixture may result in its long axis being outside the prosthetic envelope of the potential restoration (Figure 9.21). Therefore, during functional loading of the restoration, the occlusal force will be transmitted in a non-axial direction along the implant-bone interface, which may exacerbate bone loss around the implant fixture. In addition, the implant long axis will pass through the buccal or labial aspect of the prosthetic tooth and therefore where crowns or bridges are being supported by the implant fixture, the restoration may need to be cemented onto an angled abutment rather than screw-retained directly onto the fixture. Cemented restorations do offer an aesthetic advantage over their screw-retained counterparts, and the cement is said to have stress breaking or 'damping' properties to reduce the loading at the implant-bone interface. However, the retrievability

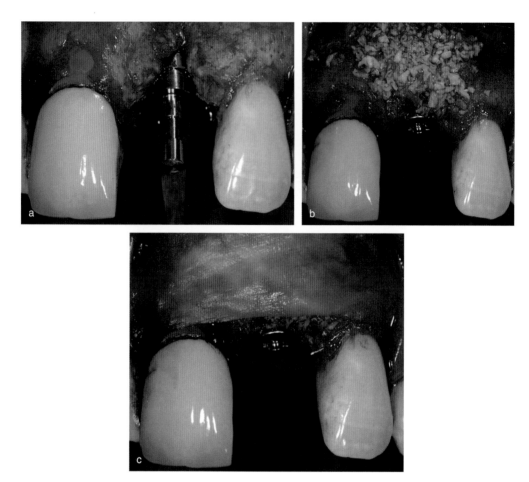

Figure 9.20   (a) Small buccal bone deficiency following preparation of the implant osteotomy. Implant direction indicator in situ. (b) A combination of autogenous bone chips and xenograft bone (Bio-Oss™) material covering the bony defect. (c) A layer of xenograft protective membrane (BioGide™) in place. A second layer was then used to cover the implant in an apicocoronal direction.

of screw-retained restorations is far simpler than that of cemented ones (Michalakis *et al.*, 2003). If the restoration requires repair or replacement, one which has been screwed to the fixture can readily be removed by unscrewing it whereas a cemented restoration may need sectioning before it can be removed, necessitating a new replacement.

Where most or all of the teeth are absent, fixed implant restorations can be very effective in restoring oral function and the appearance. Metal substructures veneered with acrylic resin teeth and flanges have conventionally been used to provide successful implant-based restorations (Figure 9.22).

However, deterioration of the acrylic resin may necessitate repair of what are often long-span bridges. This usually involves removal of the whole bridge and fitting of a temporary removable prosthesis until the implant restoration has been refurbished. Therefore if sufficient implant sites are available, multiple small implant bridges, based on conventional fixed prosthodontic materials such as precious metal alloys and ceramic, can be used. Thus, if one of the bridges requires replacement or repair the remaining restorations may be left in situ thereby reducing the need to construct a temporary appliance.

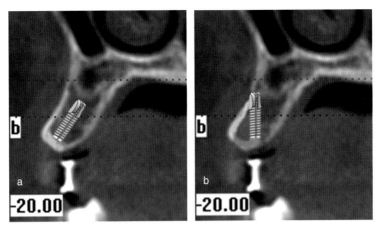

Figure 9.21 (a) CT scan with a simulated implant positioned within the bony envelope. This would result in non-axial loading of the fixture and may require a screw access hole in the buccal aspect of the restoration. (b) Position of simulated implant adjusted to the central long axis of the proposed restoration. This would result in buccal fenestration.

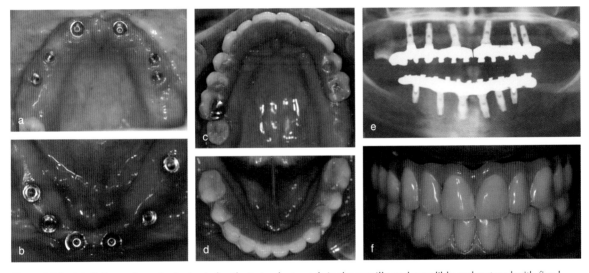

Figure 9.22 (a)–(f) Severe hypodontia treated with six implants each in the maxilla and mandible and restored with fixed metal–acrylic bridges.

Implants can also be used to stabilize removable prosthetic restorations which are particularly useful where there is significant loss of hard and soft-tissue volume. The flanges of the removable denture will restore large tissue deficits in a straightforward manner and obviate the need for extensive grafting procedures (Figure 9.23). Removable implant prostheses are also very useful where there are fewer potential implant sites than would be needed for fixed restorations. Full arch

removable implant-stabilised restorations can be planned with only four implants in the maxilla and two in the mandible. A variety of methods exist to attach the denture to the implants, such as a bar-clip system, a ball and socket arrangement, and numerous semi-precision or precision attachments. The space requirements of these methods vary but generally speaking the bar-clip and ball-socket types are bulkier than many of the precision or semi-precision attachments, especially in a vertical

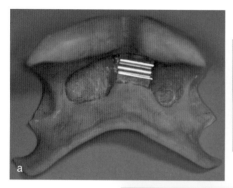
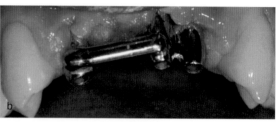
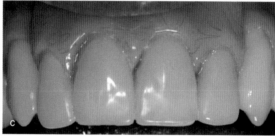

Figure 9.23   (a) Flanges of a removable prosthesis can restore lip support and deficits of hard and soft tissues. A clip is used to retain the prosthesis on an implant bar (b). Removable prosthesis in situ (c).

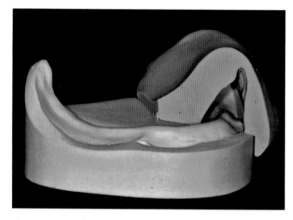

Figure 9.24   Silicone index of a lower denture to allow evaluation of the prosthetic envelope.

direction. Therefore, a careful evaluation of the prosthetic envelope needs to be made to ascertain which method of attachment can be employed (Figure 9.24). Bars however can be robust and do offer the advantage of splinting the implant fixtures together, thus distributing occlusal forces between the splinted fixtures and reducing the risk of bone or fixture overload (Guichet *et al.*, 2002).

Removable dentures

Removable prostheses, or dentures, offer a number of advantages in the management of hypodontia in the established dentition as well as for younger age groups (see chapters 7 and 8). Spaces can be relatively quickly restored and treatment is less invasive than implant therapy. Healthy tooth structure does not need to be removed as is the case with conventional bridgework and a removable denture can readily replace deficiencies of the hard and soft tissues, which may otherwise require complex grafting. Removable dentures can be used as interim or definitive prostheses in the management of hypodontia in the established dentition.

Interim prostheses are often used during the course of implant treatment, particularly where there are multiple missing teeth. They are usually made of acrylic resin to allow multiple adjustments and relining of the base-plate as required. This is often the case following implant surgery if the anatomy of the ridge has altered with implant treatment. Although it may be preferable to avoid micro-movement of the implant fixture during osseointegration, this is not always possible in severe hypodontia where the edentulous span is large or where saddles that are not bounded by teeth exist due to the absence of posterior abutment teeth. In these circumstances interim removable dentures can be invaluable in restoring aesthetics and function for a patient. It is usually helpful to design the denture with flanges around the denture teeth, rather than employing a flangeless 'gum-fitted' design, because this allows more scope to adjust the prosthesis. For example, following implant surgery, it may be possible to significantly adjust the fitting surface of a flanged denture in the region of the surgery so that a reduced load is exerted on the surgical site. As healing proceeds during the post-operative phase there may be a degree of gingival re-contouring over the ridge of the implant area such that the retention and stability of the prosthesis is compromised. This can be resolved by localised relining, which is more straightforward where flanges are present. The OVD may need to be increased during treatment due to a lack of interocclusal space for restorations, correction of an uneven occlusal plane or to improve orofacial appearance. This can be relatively easily achieved with an interim prosthesis, particularly if a significant increase is required (Figure 9.25). This increase may be achieved by the denture teeth occluding at a raised OVD or by extending acrylic resin onto the occluding surfaces of a number of natural teeth, thereby forming onlays. However, careful monitoring is necessary as acrylic onlays are prone to wear or fracture, which may compromise the increase in vertical dimension gained (Figure 9.26). When utilising interim removable prostheses where a definitive fixed restoration is to be made, care needs to be taken to ensure the aesthetics gained with the denture can actually be achieved with the subsequent fixed reconstruction. It is very easy to improve the lip support by thickening the flange of a denture, but a fixed restoration will not achieve the same facial support and a patient may be disappointed with the final result if they have not been fully informed beforehand.

Removable prostheses are also valuable as definitive restorations in the management of hypodon-

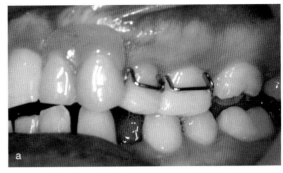
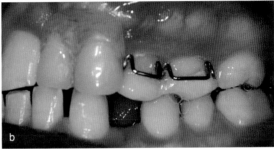

Figure 9.25   (a) Removable onlay prosthesis for increasing the OVD. (b) Note further eruption of the permanent teeth after 6 months.

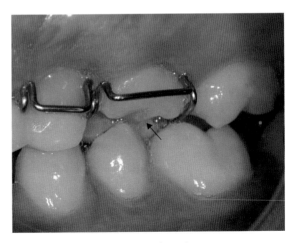

Figure 9.26   Fracture of an acrylic onlay (arrow).

tia. Metal-based dentures are usually used due to their superior physical properties. The provision of stable and retentive dentures is more challenging where microdont or conical teeth exist in combination with hypodontia because the tooth undercuts

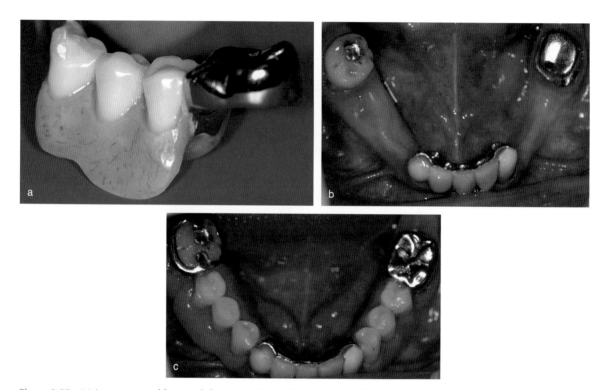

Figure 9.27   (a) Lower removable partial denture with a coping incorporated into the prosthesis. (b) Telescopic crown providing support for the prosthesis, together with rest-seats incorporated into the anterior resin-bonded bridge casting. (c) Removable partial denture in situ.

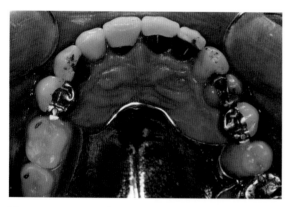

Figure 9.28   Try-in of removable partial denture retained with precision attachments in UR4, UL5 and UL7.

may be inadequate for the effective use of clasps. In these situations it may be possible to modify the tooth contour with bonded restorative materials, such as composite resin, or with cast restorations. The latter allow the ideal tooth contours to be

created for removable prosthesis stabilisation (Figure 9.27), such as guide planes, rest seats and correctly sized undercuts. Alternatively precision attachments may be incorporated into the denture, which fit onto the corresponding component in the mouth (Figure 9.28). These attachment components may be sited on teeth or be implant-based. Enhancing the retention and stability through the use of idealised cast restorations or with precision attachments may also be necessary if the denture-bearing area is poorly formed due to a lack of alveolar development.

In cases of severe hypodontia, or where there is significant microdontia, overdentures may be used to restore one or both dental arches at an appropriate OVD. These are removable dentures whose base covers one or more teeth, roots of teeth or implants. Use of overdentures with implants has been discussed above under the section 'Dental Implants', but teeth can also be used to help stabilise the prosthesis by virtue of the support and

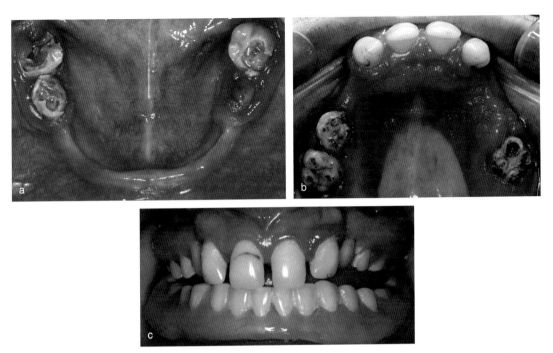

Figure 9.29   (a)–(c) Denture-related stomatitis, caries and periodontal disease associated with the wearing of overdentures in the absence of adequate oral care.

retention which they provide via their occlusal/ incisal surfaces and friction with their vertical surfaces. Much of the retention in the maxillary denture will be obtained by ensuring that there is an adequate peripheral seal, but this can be difficult if significant soft tissue undercuts exist, as it may not be possible to extend the flange into the full depth and width of the functional sulcus. Where overdentures are to be utilised in the management of a patient, scrupulous oral hygiene measures are of paramount importance to prevent dental or soft tissue disease. Teeth covered by overdentures will be prone to caries and periodontal disease (Ettinger and Qian, 2004), whereas candidal infections may affect the mucosa (Figure 9.29). Patients must therefore be educated about these risks and informed of strategies to prevent disease (Keltjens *et al.*, 1994). These may include the use of topical fluoride on tooth abutments and chlorhexidine gel on the fitting surface of the prosthesis, in addition to normal cleaning methods such as tooth brushing and flossing/interproximal cleaning.

Conventional dental bridges

While implant bridges and resin-bonded bridges are commonly used in the management of hypodontia, conventional bridge restorations are infrequently utilised due to their destruction of tooth structure (Bishop *et al.*, 2007a). However, where the potential abutment tooth has already been restored with a reasonably large restoration, conventional bridgework can be an appropriate method of replacing missing teeth. A further advantage of conventional bridges is that it is possible to replace teeth and alter the size, shape and colour of the adjacent teeth at the same time as providing the bridge. Conventional bridges have also been used to provide a fixed option in severe cases of hypodontia where adhesive bridges are impractical and implant treatment would involve grafting which the patient wishes to avoid. Thus, extensive bridges may have to be constructed on relatively few abutments. Careful planning and management of the occlusion is required and in some cases gold copings are bonded to the prepared teeth with the bridge superstructure then being cemented onto the copings with temporary cement. This provides a degree of retrievability and simplifies maintenance, as it is often possible to remove the bridge superstructure to enable repairs or replacement to occur as necessary.

STAGE 5: Maintenance

An important consideration when planning the management of a patient is the maintenance requirements of the proposed treatment. Often patients with hypodontia will seek treatment at a relatively early stage and therefore any work that is performed may require maintenance for many years. It is imperative a patient understands this from the outset and appreciates their own role in optimising the oral environment to achieve a successful long term outcome. Recall intervals will vary between patients depending on the complexity of treatment and their susceptibility to dental disease. Often the frequency of recall is high for a period of time after treatment has been completed and then reduces if the oral condition is stable. Although maintenance issues will be artificially separated in this chapter, it is important to stress that a holistic approach is necessary to identify potential complications at an early stage. Important aspects relating to maintenance include the following:

Periodontal maintenance

A stable periodontal condition is key to the successful outcome of most treatment plans (Drisko, 2001). Before active treatment commences any periodontal disease should be treated and the patient be able to demonstrate an ability to achieve an adequate level of oral cleanliness. At the completion of treatment, additional oral hygiene advice may need to be given to enable a patient to maintain this level of oral cleaning. For example, where a spaced dentition has been corrected by orthodontic and/or restorative treatment, a patient may need to be instructed on the use of dental floss, which may not have been required prior to treatment. Similarly, additional oral hygiene measures such as the use of interdental brushes, 'Superfloss™'

or intraoral water irrigation devices may need to be employed where bridgework, either tooth or implant-supported, has been used.

Periodontal indices should be recorded at least annually so that the condition of the periodontium can be monitored. BPE scores in each sextant where teeth are present would be the minimum requirement but additional information such as a full pocket chart and bleeding, plaque and mobility scores may also be advisable in periodontally-susceptible patients.

Maintenance of remaining teeth

In addition to maintaining periodontal health, the remaining teeth themselves should be kept in a healthy condition. Therefore regular clinical examination, with adjunctive radiographs where appropriate, should identify conditions such as dental caries, pulpal pathology and toothwear at an early stage. Teeth or roots that are serving as overdenture abutments are at a particular risk of developing caries and periodontal disease and therefore appropriate preventative advice should be provided when delivering the prosthesis to the patient. This may include the application of fluoride pastes and antimicrobial gels (such as chlorhexidine) in addition to regular toothbrushing.

Orthodontic maintenance

Relapse due to the propensity of teeth to move back to their original positions is invariably a risk factor of orthodontic treatment. There tends to be a greater likelihood of orthodontic relapse immediately after active treatment has been completed but tooth alignment can still fall back several years later. Therefore retention is an important component when considering orthodontic treatment, which should be emphasised to the patient at the outset. Orthodontic retention can be achieved using fixed or removable devices. A fixed method that is commonly used involves bonding a length of spiral wire to the palatal or lingual surfaces of a number of teeth with composite resin (Zachrisson, 2007). This needs to be carefully monitored to ensure bond failure of the retainer does not occur, as this may result in the development of caries beneath the wire if failure is undetected or relapse of tooth position. The presence of a spiral wire retainer means that oral hygiene procedures will need to be modified by using interdental brushes, 'Superfloss™' or a floss threader rather than conventional dental floss. Removable orthodontic retainers come in a variety of designs but all require adequate patient motivation and cooperation to ensure they are worn as prescribed. A common timetable involves 3–6 months of full-time wear followed by a 6–9 months period of nighttime-only wear. After this, the patient is usually advised that the removable retainer should be worn several nights per week indefinitely to ensure relapse does not occur (Littlewood et al., 2006a, b). If the retainer breaks or is lost, the patient should be instructed to seek its replacement as soon as possible.

Restorative maintenance

Composite restorations

Composite resin is an excellent material to conservatively improve the shape and appearance of teeth. However, a certain degree of deterioration can be expected in the medium term that necessitates refurbishment of the restoration. This may involve re-polishing a stained area, re-surfacing superficial regions of deterioration or repairing chips. Wear of the occluding surfaces of these restorations should also be carefully monitored to ensure a stable occlusal relationship remains. If frequent repair becomes necessary, it may be decided that alternative restorations will be more appropriate, even though they may be more destructive of tooth tissue (Manhart et al., 2004).

Veneers and cast restorations

These restorations invariably involve a certain degree of tooth preparation and a definite margin is usually required. The restoration needs to fit sufficiently well to inhibit micro-leakage of bacteria or their products that may cause caries or pulpal pathology (Bergenholtz et al., 1982; Triadan, 1987). Margins that have been placed sub-gingivally require particularly careful monitoring because direct visual inspection is not possible. Tactile methods utilising a dental probe combined with radiographs where appropriate have to be relied on to detect deterioration or disease at the margin. Various studies have shown a 10–20% incidence of apical pathology associated with full coverage cast restorations and therefore periodic radiographs may need to be taken to assess the apical status of these teeth (Valderhaug et al., 1997, Saunders and Saunders, 1998).

Bridgework

Resin-bonded bridges generally tend to have fewer maintenance issues compared with conventional bridges, unless there is a problem with debonding of the restoration. The margins of the bridge retainer can be placed supra-gingivally with resin-bonded bridgework and therefore the effect on the periodontium is negligible (Rashid et al., 1999, Pjetursson et al., 2008). The margins of conventional bridges may need to be placed sub-gingivally for aesthetic reasons, or because the desire to obtain a ferrule beyond the limits of the core restoration requires the extension of the retainer margin into the gingival crevice. These sub-gingival margins are more difficult for a patient to keep clean and combined with any discrepancy of fit, can lead to gingival inflammation or periodontal disease.

The early detection of caries is important for the continued survival of a bridge restoration. Fixed-fixed designs of resin-bonded bridge carry the risks of debonding of one retainer potentially leading to leakage and the development of caries (Gilmour, 1989), since the bridge often remains in place so that the patient is unaware of the bridge failure and does not seek professional treatment (Figure 9.30). Hence, whenever fixed-fixed resin-bonded bridges are constructed the patient should be advised of the importance of regular recall and at each appointment the dental professional should actively look for any signs of the bridge debonding. Conventional bridges of cantilever, fixed-fixed or other designs have the risk of caries forming at the retainer margins (Walton, 2003) and therefore these areas require particular examination during recall visits. Conventional bridges also have a higher risk for the development of pulpal disease than single unit full coverage cast restorations and this needs to be carefully assessed at review

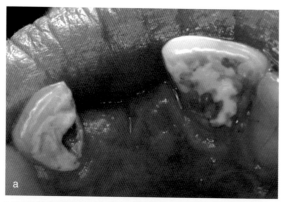

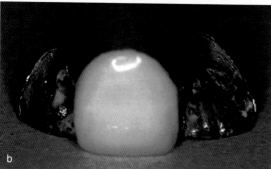

Figure 9.30 (a)–(b) Repeated failure of a fixed-fixed resin-bonded bridge with subsequent dental caries of the abutment teeth.

appointments. In contrast, the risk of pulpal disease from resin-bonded bridges is insignificant.

Most definitive bridges involve the use of porcelain veneered over a metal or toughened ceramic substructure. This veneering porcelain is highly aesthetic but inherently brittle if unsupported. Therefore a portion may fracture and this can be difficult to repair in situ. Various porcelain repair kits are available that allow the use of hydrofluoric acid intraorally to etch the surrounding porcelain surface so that bonded composite resin can be used to effect the repair. Alternatively, the remainder of the porcelain in that unit of the restoration can be removed, an impression taken and a laboratory-made porcelain veneer cemented to the existing substructure. If these methods are unsuccessful, the whole restoration may need to be replaced.

Where patients with hypodontia have microdont teeth which have been used as bridge abutments,

the potential long-term survival of the restoration may be adversely affected. The decreased surface area for bonding can lead to increased failure rates in resin-bonded bridges and the smaller abutments will compromise the resistance and retention form of the tooth preparation for conventional bridges (Bishop *et al.*, 2007a).

Removable dentures

Acrylic dentures are prone to wear or fracture if there is a reduced bulk of acrylic resin or an increased occlusal load from an intact opposing dentition or one that has been reconstructed with a fixed restoration. As a result, prostheses such as acrylic onlay dentures require their occlusal surfaces to be carefully monitored to ensure occlusal stability is maintained. Fortunately acrylic dentures are relatively easy to repair, refurbish or replace. Metal-based prostheses are inherently stronger and metal occluding surfaces on dentures less likely to wear, however, metal-based dentures are more difficult to modify after they have been fitted. If precision attachments have been utilised it is likely that the male and/or female components will wear over time. Where these are made from metal, the wear will occur at a much slower rate than systems where one of the components is constructed from a softer polymeric material, although the non-metallic component of such systems is often easily replaced without the need to fabricate a new denture (Ku *et al.*, 2000). Where all-metal attachments have been used a completely new prosthesis is usually required when metal attachment components have worn significantly, although this may not be necessary for a considerable time.

Implants

Dental implants consist of two main components – the implant *fixture* and the *superstructure*. The *fixture* is that portion which is inserted into the bone of the maxilla or mandible and onto which the *superstructure* is attached. The maintenance requirements of the implant fixture relate to the interface between the fixture surface and the surrounding bone. Currently the gold standard for this is osseointegration, the loss of which may occur around an implant body but is more commonly observed as a gradual apical progression of the level of the bone around the fixture. A number of factors have been associated with this, however its precise aetiology is not well understood. Current good practice emphasises the maintenance of good oral hygiene, control of occlusal loads and regular monitoring of mucosal health and bone levels around the implant.

Clinical examination involves assessing the bleeding tendency of the gingivae around the implant, measuring probing depths, evaluating the width of keratinized gingiva, determining the effectiveness of plaque control and analysing the peri-implant sulcus fluid (Salvi and Lang, 2004). However, some of these parameters are difficult to measure accurately because of the discomfort generated even by gentle probing forces. Therefore, radiographs are frequently used to assess bone levels around implants and to monitor these over time. There is no consensus on the intervals at which radiographs should be taken but a common protocol involves baseline radiographs at the time of restoration placement, further films 3–6 months later and again at the 1-year time period from baseline. Subsequent radiographs are usually taken every 12–24 months, but the frequency may need to be individualised depending on clinical circumstances. Radiographs however only provide limited information on the surface area of bone contact and buccal or lingual bony defects are not always apparent on radiographs. Therefore, more sophisticated methods such as resonance frequency analysis are increasingly being used (Kessler-Liechti et al., 2008) although their clinical significance has been questioned (Hobkirk and Wiskott, 2006).

Implant superstructures include a wide variety of restorations from single unit crowns to full-arch fixed or removable restorations. Much of the maintenance centres on effective oral hygiene procedures and the mechanical integrity of the materials used (Palmer and Pleasance, 2006). In the latter case there is some similarity with non-implant restorations, for example repair of fractured porcelain or replacement of worn precision attachments. Where screw-retained restorations have been used, loosening of the screw may necessitate re-tightening and torquing to the correct value, and screw fracture will require removal of the broken portions together with replacement of the screw. Restorations that have been cemented may become de-bonded,

and if this occurs frequently it may be necessary to use increasingly strong cements and accept the reduced likelihood of being able to remove the restoration intact if ever needed.

Concluding remarks

The effective management of hypodontia relies upon a well-integrated multidisciplinary team to develop an appropriate long-term treatment plan. This will need to take into account the patient's expectations and objectives of treatment, their commitment to maintain a healthy oral environment and the ability to attend for treatment. A thorough assessment of the mouth will highlight any issues that may complicate the provision of the desired treatment so that this can be discussed with the patient and an alternative plan sought if necessary. An important aspect of the management of patients with hypodontia is the maintenance requirements of the treatment that is performed. This often requires lifelong care.

The psychosocial impact of missing teeth should not be under-estimated and many patients with hypodontia will undergo extensive treatment over a prolonged period of time (Figure 9.31). However, the end result can be immensely gratifying for them and for all the clinicians involved in their management.

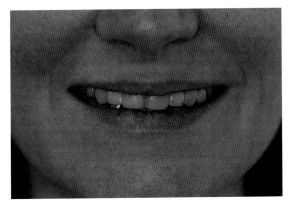

Figure 9.31   Same patient as in **Figure 9.8** after comprehensive multidisciplinary care involving orthodontics, bone grafting, implant surgery and prosthodontics over a 4-year period.

Key Points

Managing missing maxillary lateral incisor(s)
- Consider space closure if possible to reduce the restorative maintenance in the long term
- A detailed assessment of the canine tooth in relation to its size, contour, colour, shape and gingival margin level will aid the decision on whether the canine can be successfully disguised as a lateral incisor tooth
- The long-term prognosis of the lateral incisor(s) should be taken into consideration
- A symmetrical dentition is often aesthetically pleasing
- Where spacing exists in the labial segment, this can be localised into the missing lateral incisor site whereas space closure is usually preferable in a crowded dentition
- Consider space closure in a Class II malocclusion and space opening in a Class III incisor relationship
- Good interdigitation of the posterior teeth with a Class I canine relationship often requires opening of the lateral incisor space
- Assess the position of the root apex of the canine tooth
- Evaluate any bony deficiencies and whether movement of the canine can aid development of the alveolar ridge

Preparing a treatment plan
- Identify the patient's motivations and expectations and relate these to what is achievable with treatment
- A multidisciplinary team approach should be used when developing a treatment plan
- Identify the patient's ability to attend for appointments and their commitment to the treatment plan
- An improvement in the orofacial appearance is often a strong motivating factor
- Assess space in all dimensions:
  - Mesiodistal – Measure at crown *and* root level if implants are being considered. Approximately 7 mm of space is adequate for a regular-sized implant but 6–6.5 mm can be sufficient for a narrow-platform implant
  - Buccolingual – Assess the buccolingual volume beyond the crest of the ridge to evaluate any deficiencies in the bone
  - Vertical – Assess the current OVD and whether this should be altered for the final restorations

Management of narrow ridges
- Restore using an alternative option to implant treatment
- Use narrow diameter implants
- Utilise techniques that expand the alveolar ridge
- Localised bone augmentation with xenograft/allograft materials and/or bone harvested from the surgical area
- Block onlay grafting with autogenous bone or allografts
- Distraction osteogenesis
- Use a combination of the above

Providing treatment
- The effective management of hypodontia in the established dentition relies on a well-integrated multidisciplinary team to develop an appropriate long-term treatment plan
- This will need to take into account the patient's expectations and objectives of treatment, their commitment to maintain a healthy oral environment and the ability to attend for treatment
- A thorough assessment of the mouth will highlight any issues that may complicate the provision of the desired treatment so that this can be discussed with the patient and an alternative plan sought if necessary
- A variety of treatment options exist but when developing a treatment plan it is important any active disease is initially treated and the patient provided with appropriate advice on the prevention of further disease. After a period of re-evaluation definitive treatment may be performed. Once this has been completed, a patient should enter into a recall programme so that the optimum environment is provided for long-term success
- The orthodontic anchorage requirements need to be particularly carefully assessed in patients with severe hypodontia to ensure the roots as well as the crowns of teeth are correctly positioned
- The orthodontist and restorative dentist should liaise regularly during the course of treatment to ensure the teeth are in the correct positions to allow the provision of long-term restorative care
- When restoring tooth form a balance often needs to be achieved between minimising the biological cost to a tooth and providing a restoration that does not require significant maintenance in the long-term
- In the established dentition missing teeth may be replaced by:
  - Resin-bonded bridges
  - Implant crowns
  - Implant bridges
  - Implant-stabilised removable dentures
  - Conventional removable dentures
  - Conventional bridges
- Patients often require maintenance care over many years as considerable treatment may be necessary at a relatively young age

References

Açikgöz A, Kademoglu O, Elekdag-Tűrk S, Karagöz F. Hypohidrotic ectodermal dysplasia with true anodontia of the primary dentition. *Quintessence Int* 2007;38: 853–858.

Addy L, Bishop K, Knox J. Modern restorative management of patients with congenitally missing teeth: 2. Orthodontic and restorative considerations. *Dent Update* 2006;33:592–595.

Arai Y, Tammisalo E, Ikwai K, Hashimoto K, Shinoda K. Development of a compact computed tomographic apparatus for dental use. *Dentomaxillofac Radiol* 1999; 28:245–248.

Arvystas M. *Orthodontic Management of Agenesis and Other Complexities: An Interdisciplinary Approach to Functional Esthetics.* Martin Dunitz, London and New York, 2003.

Bergendal B, Bergendal T, Hallonsten AL, *et al.* A multidisciplinary approach to oral rehabilitation with osseointegrated implants in children and adolescents with multiple aplasia. *Eur J Orthod* 1996;18:119–129.

Bergenholtz G, Cox CF, Loesche WJ, *et al.* Bacterial leakage around dental restorations: Its effect on the dental pulp. *J Oral Pathol* 1982;11:439–450.

Bishop K, Addy L, Knox J. Modern restorative management of patients with congenitally missing teeth: 1. Introduction, terminology and epidemiology. *Dent Update* 2006;33:531–537.

Bishop K, Addy L, Knox J. Modern restorative management of patients with congenitally missing teeth: 3. Conventional restorative options and considerations. *Dent Update* 2007a;34:30–38.

Bishop K, Addy L, Knox J. Modern restorative management of patients with congenitally missing teeth: 4. The role of implants. *Dent Update* 2007b;34:79–84.

Bondarets N, Jones RM, McDonald F. Analysis of facial growth in subjects with syndromic ectodermal dysplasia: a longitudinal analysis. *Orthod Craniofac Res* 2002;5: 71–84.

Cannizzaro G, Leone M, Consolo U, Ferri V, Esposito M. Immediate functional loading of implants placed with flapless surgery versus conventional implants in partially edentulous patients: A 3-year randomised controlled clinical trial. *Int J Oral Maxillofac Implants* 2008;23:867–875.

Carter NE, Gillgrass TJ, Hobson RS, *et al.* The interdisciplinary management of hypodontia: orthodontics. *Br Dent J* 2003;194:361–366.

Chung LK, Hobson RS, Nunn JH, *et al.* An analysis of the skeletal relationships in a group of young people with hypodontia. *J Orthod* 2000;27:315–318.

Clark JR, Evans RD. Functional occlusion: I. A review. *J Orthod* 2001;28:76–81.

Costa A, Raffaini M, Melsen B. Miniscrews as orthodontic anchorage: A preliminary report. *Int J Adult Orthodon Orthognath Surg* 1998;13:201–209.

Cronin RJ, Oesterle LJ. Implant use in growing patients, treatment planning concerns. *Dent Clin North Am* 1998; 42:1–34.

Dhanrajani PJ. Hypodontia: Etiology, clinical features, and management. *Quintessence Int* 2002;33:294–302.

Drisko CH. Nonsurgical periodontal therapy. *Periodontol 2000* 2001;25:77–88.

Endo T, Yoshino S, Ozoe R, *et al.* Association of advanced hypodontia and craniofacial morphology in Japanese orthodontic patients. *Odontology* 2004;92:48–53.

Endo T, Ozoe R, Yoshino S, *et al.* Hypodontia patterns and variations in craniofacial morphology in Japanese orthodontic patients. *Angle Orthod* 2006;76: 996–1003.

Esposito SJ, Cowper TR. Overdentures in partial anodontia: Simple solutions for complex problems. *Compendium* 1991;12:172–177.

Ettinger RL, Qian F. Abutment tooth loss in patients with overdentures. *J Am Dent Assoc* 2004;135:739–746.

Forgie AH, Thind BS, Larmour CJ, *et al.* Management of hypodontia: restorative considerations. Part III. *Quintessence Int* 2005;36:437–445.

Fortin T, Champleboux G, Bianchi S, *et al.* Precision of transfer of preoperative planning for oral implants based on cone-beam CT-scan images through a robotic drilling machine. *Clin Oral Implants Res* 2002;13:651–656.

Francischone CE, Oltramari PV, Visconcelos LW, *et al.* Treatment for predictable multidisciplinary implantology, orthodontics, and restorative dentistry. *Pract Proced Aesthet Dent* 2003;15:321–326.

Gaggl A, Schultes G, Kärcher H. Distraction implants: A new operative technique for alveolar ridge augmentation. *J Craniomaxillofac Surg* 1999a;27:214–221.

Gaggl A, Schultes G, Kärcher H. Distraction implants: A new possibility for augmentative treatment of the edentulous atrophic mandible: A case report. *Br J Oral Maxillofac Surg* 1999b;37:481–485.

Gill DS, Naini FB, Tredwin CJ. Smile aesthetics. *Dent Update* 2007;34:152–158.

Gilmour AS. Resin-bonded bridges: A note of caution. *Br Dent J* 1989;167:140–141.

Goodman JR, Jones SP, Hobkirk JA, *et al.* Hypodontia: 1. Clinical features and the management of mild to moderate hypodontia. *Dent Update* 1994;21:381–384.

Guichet DL, Yoshinobu D, Caputo AA. Effect of splinting and interproximal contact tightness on load transfer by implant restorations. *J Prosthet Dent* 2002;87: 528–535.

Hobkirk JA, Brook AH. The management of patients with severe hypodontia. *J Oral Rehabil* 1980;7:289–298.

Hobkirk JA, Goodman JR, Jones SP. Presenting complaints and findings in a group of patients attending a hypodontia clinic. *Br Dent J* 1994;177:337–339.

Hobkirk JA, King PA, Goodman JR, *et al.* Hypodontia: 2. The management of severe hypodontia. *Dent Update* 1995;22:8–11.

Hobkirk JA, Nohl F, Bergendal B, *et al.* The management of ectodermal dysplasia and severe hypodontia. International conference statements. *J Oral Rehabil* 2006;33: 634–637.

Hobkirk JA, Wiskott HW. Working Group 1. Biomechanical aspects of oral implants. Consensus report of Working Group 1. *Clin Oral Implants Res* 2006; 17(Suppl.2):52–54.

Hobson RS, Carter NE, Gillgrass TJ, *et al.* The interdisciplinary management of hypodontia: the relationship between an interdisciplinary team and the general dental practitioner. *Br Dent J* 2003;194:479–482.

Jepson NJ, Nohl FS, Carter NE, *et al.* The interdisciplinary management of hypodontia: restorative dentistry. *Br Dent J* 2003;194:299–304.

Keltjens HM, Creugers TJ, Mulder J, *et al.* Survival and retreatment need of abutment teeth in patients with overdentures: a retrospective study. *Community Dent Oral Epidemiol* 1994;22:453–455.

Kesling HD. The diagnostic set-up with considerations of the third dimension. *Am J Orthod* 1956;42:740–748.

Kessler-Liechti G, Zix J, Mericske-Stern R. Stability measurements of 1-stage implants in the edentulous mandible by means of resonance frequency analysis. *Int J Oral Maxillofac Implants* 2008;23:353–835.

Kinzer GA, Kokich VO Jr. Managing congenitally missing lateral incisors. Part III: Single tooth implants. *J Esthet Restor Dent* 2005;17:202–210.

Kokich VO Jr, Kinzer GA. Managing congenitally missing lateral incisors. Part I: Canine substitution. *J Esthet Restor Dent* 2005;17:5–10.

Ku YC, Shen YF, Chan CP. Extracoronal resilient attachments in distal-extension removable partial dentures. *Quintessence Int* 2000;31:311–317.

Laing ER, Cunningham SJ, Jones SP, *et al.* The psychosocial impact of hypodontia in children. *J Orthod* 2008;35:225.

Lee JS, Kim JK, Park YC, *et al. Applications of Orthodontic Mini Implants.* Quintessence Publishing, Chicago, 2007.

Littlewood SJ, Millett DT, Doubleday B, *et al.* Retention procedures for stabilising tooth position after treatment with orthodontic braces. *Cochrane Database Syst Rev* 2006a, 25, CD002283.

Littlewood SJ, Millett DT, Doubleday B, *et al.* Orthodontic retention: a systematic review. *J Orthod* 2006b;33: 205–212.

Manhart J, Chen H, Hamm G, *et al.* Buonocore Memorial Lecture. Review of the clinical survival of direct and indirect restorations in posterior teeth of the permanent dentition. *Oper Dent* 2004;29:481–508.

McKeown HF, Robinson DL, Elcock C, *et al.* Tooth dimensions in hypodontia patients, their unaffected relatives and a control group measured by a new image analysis system. *Eur J Orthod* 2002;24:131–141.

Meechan JG, Carter NE, Gillgrass TJ, *et al.* Interdisciplinary management of hypodontia: Oral surgery. *Br Dent J* 2003;194:423–427.

Michalakis KX, Hirayama H, Garefis PD. Cement-retained versus screw-retained implant restorations: A critical review. *Int J Oral Maxillofac Implants* 2003; 18:719–728.

Millar BJ, Taylor NG. Lateral thinking: the management of missing upper lateral incisors. *Br Dent J* 1995;179: 99–106.

Misch CE, Dietsh F. Bone grafting materials in implant dentistry. *Implant Dent* 1993;2:158–167.

Morgan C, Howe L. The restorative management of hypodontia with implants: 1. Overview of alternative treatment options. *Dent Update* 2003;30:562–568.

Naini FB, Gill DS. Facial aesthetics: 1. Concepts and canons. *Dent Update* 2008a;35:102–107.

Naini FB, Gill DS. Facial aesthetics: 2. Clinical assessment. *Dent Update* 2008b;35:159–170.

Noble J, Karaiskos N, Wiltshire WA. Diagnosis and management of the infraerupted primary molar. *Br Dent J* 2007;203:632–634.

Nodal M, Kjaer I, Solow B. Craniofacial morphology in patients with multiple congenitally missing permanent teeth. *Eur J Orthod* 1994;16:104–109.

Nohl F, Cole B, Hobson R, *et al.* The management of hypodontia: Present and future. *Dent Update* 2008;35: 79–90.

Ostler MS, Kokich VG. Alveolar ridge changes in patients with congenitally missing mandibular second premolars. *J Prosthet Dent* 1994;71:144–149.

Palmer RM, Pleasance C. Maintenance of osseointegrated implant prostheses. *Dent Update* 2006;33:84–86, 89–92.

Peck S, Peck L, Kataja M. Prevalence of tooth agenesis and peg-shaped maxillary lateral incisor associated with palatally displaced canine (PDC) anomaly. *Am J Orthod Dentofacial Orthop* 1996;110:441–443.

Peck S, Peck L, Kataja M. Concomitant occurrence of canine malposition and tooth agenesis: evidence of orofacial genetic fields. *Am J Orthod Dentofacial Orthop* 2002;122:657–660.

Pjetursson BE, Tan WC, Tan K, *et al.* A systematic review of the survival and complication rates of resin-bonded bridges after an observation period of at least 5 years. *Clin Oral Implants Res* 2008;19:131–141.

Rashid SA, Al-Wahadni AM, Hussey DL. The periodontal response to cantilevered resin-bonded bridgework. *J Oral Rehabil* 1999;26:912–917.

Richardson G, Russell KA. Congenitally missing maxillary lateral incisors and orthodontic treatment considerations for the single tooth implant. *J Can Dent Assoc* 2001;67:25–28.

Ricketts RM. The biologic significance of the divine proportion and Fibonacci series. *Am J Orthod Dentofacial Orthop* 1982;81:351–370.

Roald KL, Wisth PJ, Böe OE. Changes in cranio-facial morphology of individuals with hypodontia between the ages of 9 and 16. *Acta Odontol Scand* 1982;40:65–74.

Salvi GE, Lang NP. Diagnostic parameters for monitoring peri-implant conditions. *Int J Oral Maxillofac Implants* 2004;19 (Suppl.):116–127.

Santos LL. Treatment planning in the presence of congenitally absent second premolars: A review of the literature. *J Clin Pediatr Dent* 2002;27:13–17.

Saunders WP, Saunders EM. Prevalence of periradicular periodontitis associated with crowned teeth in an adult Scottish subpopulation. *Br Dent J* 1998;185:137–140.

Shafi I, Phillips JM, Dawson MP, *et al.* A study of patients attending a multidisciplinary hypodontia clinic over a five year period. *Br Dent J* 2008;205:649–652.

Shroff B, Siegel SM, Feldman S, *et al.* Combined orthodontic and prosthetic therapy. Special considerations. *Dent Clin North Am* 1996;40:911–943.

Simeone P, De Paoli C, De Paoli S, Leofreddi G, Sgrò S. Interdisciplinary treatment planning for single tooth restorations in the esthetic zone. *J Esthet Restor Dent* 2007;19:79–88.

Stephen A, Cengiz SB. The use of overdentures in the management of severe hypodontia associated with microdontia: A case report. *J Clin Pediatr Dent* 2003;27:219–222.

Swartz B, Svenson B, Palmqvist S. Long-term changes in marginal and periapical periodontal conditions in patients with fixed prostheses: A radiographic study. *J Oral Rehabil* 1996;23:101–107.

Thind BS, Stirrups DR, Forgie AH, *et al.* Management of hypodontia: Orthodontic considerations(II). *Quintessence Int* 2005;36:345–353.

Timm TA, Herremans EL, Ash MM Jr. Occlusion and orthodontics. *Am J Orthod* 1976;70:138–145.

Tolman DE. Reconstructive procedures with endosseous implants in grafted bone: A review of the literature. *Int J Oral Maxillofac Implants* 1995;10:275–294.

Triadan H. When is microleakage a real clinical problem? *Oper Dent* 1987;12:153–157.

Valderhaug J, Jokstad A, Ambjørnsen E, Norheim PW. Assessment of the periapical and clinical status of crowned teeth over 25 years. *J Dent* 1997;25:97–105.

Walton TR. An up to 15-year longitudinal study of 515 metal-ceramic FPDs: Part 2. Modes of failure and influence of various clinical characteristics. *Int J Prosthodont* 2003;16:177–182.

Woodworth DA, Sinclair PM, Alexander RG. Bilateral congenital absence of maxillary lateral incisors: A craniofacial and dental cast analysis. *Am J Orthod Dentofacial Orthop* 1985;87:280–293.

Yao CC, Lee JJ, Chen HU, *et al.* Maxillary molar intrusion with fixed appliances and mini-implant anchorage studied in three dimensions. *Angle Orthod* 2005;75:754–760.

Zachrisson BU. Long-term experience with direct-bonded retainers: update and clinical advice. *J Clin Orthod* 2007;41:728–737.

Zitzmann NU, Naef R, Scharer P. Resorbable versus non-resorbable membranes in combination with Bio-Oss for guided bone regeneration. *Int J Oral Maxillofac Implants* 1997;12:844–852.

Glossary of Terms

This glossary contains descriptions of some of the terms used in this book and is intended to aid readers who may be less familiar with terminology outside their own speciality. It is not intended as a definitive list or to serve as a medical dictionary, for which readers should consult standard reference works.

Allograft: A graft between genetically dissimilar members of the same species.

ANB: An angular measurement constructed from a lateral cephalometric radiograph by subtracting angle *SNB* from angle *SNA*, reflecting the relative relationships of the maxilla and mandible to each other. It is a means of assessing skeletal pattern. In Caucasians the norm is 3° (SD 2°).

Anchorage: Resistance to unwanted three-dimensional forces generated in reaction to the active components of an orthodontic appliance.

Angle's Class I malocclusion: A malocclusion in which the buccal groove of the mandibular first permanent molar occludes with the mesiobuccal cusp of the maxillary first molar.

Angle's Class II malocclusion: A malocclusion in which the buccal groove of the mandibular first permanent molar occludes *posterior* to the mesiobuccal cusp of the maxillary first molar. A Class II division 1 malocclusion describes this relationship when the maxillary central incisors are proclined or normally inclined and the overjet is increased. A Class II division 2 malocclusion describes this relationship when the maxillary central incisors are retroclined.

Angle's Class III malocclusion: A malocclusion in which the buccal groove of the mandibular first permanent molar occludes *anterior* to the mesiobuccal cusp of the maxillary first molar.

Angle's classification: A classification of malocclusion introduced by Edward Angle defined by the anteroposterior relationship of the first permanent molars rather than by the incisor relationship.

Angulation: The mesiodistal angulation of the long axis of a tooth in relationship to a line drawn perpendicular to the occlusal plane. (Compare with *Inclination*.)

Hypodontia: A Team Approach to Management, First Edition
© J.A. Hobkirk, D.S. Gill, S.P. Jones, K.W. Hemmings, G.S. Bassi, A.L. O'Donnell and J.R. Goodman
Published 2011 by Blackwell Publishing Ltd

Ankylosis: An abnormal fusion between two bones or between a tooth and bone.

Anodontia: The developmental absence of all teeth.

Anterior guidance: The influence of the contacting surfaces of the anterior teeth on limiting mandibular movements.

Archwire: A wire engaged into orthodontic brackets to provide the active forces for tooth movement and/or a stable platform for bodily tooth movement.

Autograft: Tissue transplanted from one site on an individual's body to another site.

Balanced occlusion: The bilateral, simultaneous, anterior and posterior occlusal contact of teeth in centric and eccentric positions.

Bolton (tooth size) discrepancy: A mismatch between the sum of mesiodistal widths of the maxillary and mandibular dentition that makes it difficult to achieve an ideal occlusal fit.

Border movement: Mandibular movement at the limit dictated by anatomical structures, as viewed in a given plane.

Buccal segment: The canine, premolar and molar teeth.

Camouflage (orthodontic): Occlusal compensation of mild or moderate skeletal discrepancies by orthodontic tooth movement.

Canine-guided occlusion: A form of mutually protected articulation in which the vertical and horizontal overlap of the canine teeth disengage the posterior teeth in the excursive movements of the mandible.

Centric occlusion (intercuspal position): The position of maximum intercuspation.

Centric relation (retruded contact position): The relationship between the mandible and maxilla with the condyles in an unstrained retruded position within the glenoid fossae.

Class I incisor relationship: The lower incisor edges occlude on or directly beneath the cingulum plateau of the upper incisors (British Standards Classification).

Class II division 1 incisor relationship: The lower incisor edges lie posterior to the cingulum plateau of the upper incisors, the overjet is increased, and the upper central incisors are normally inclined or proclined (British Standards Classification).

Class II division 2 incisor relationship: The lower incisal edges occlude posterior to the cingulum plateau of the upper incisors and the upper central incisors are retroclined (British Standards Classification).

Class II intermaxillary traction: Intermaxillary anchorage provided by placing elastics between the maxillary incisors and mandibular molars.

Class III incisor relationship: Two or more of the lower incisal edges occlude anterior to the cingulum plateau of the upper incisors (British Standards Classification).

Class III intermaxillary traction: Intermaxillary anchorage provided by placing elastics between the maxillary molars and mandibular incisors.

Composite resin: A highly cross-linked polymeric material reinforced by a dispersion of amorphous silica, glass, crystalline, or organic resin-filler particles and/or short fibres bonded to the matrix by a coupling agent. Sometimes referred to colloquially as 'composite'.

Curve of Spee: A convex curve, when viewed in the sagittal plane, produced by the curvature of the cusps and incisal edges of the mandibular teeth. The depth of the curve positively correlates with the depth of an overbite.

Decompensation: The removal of adaptive occlusal changes within the dentition that mask the severity of a skeletal discrepancy. It is undertaken prior to orthognathic surgery.

Dental implant abutment: A dental implant component used to join a dental implant (body) to a fixed or removable dental prosthesis (See also dental implant connecting component). Frequently dental implant abutments, especially those used with endosteal dental implants, are changed to alter abutment design or use before a definitive dental prosthesis is fabricated. Such a preliminary abutment is termed an interim (dental implant) abutment. The abutment chosen to support the definitive prosthesis is termed a definitive (dental implant) abutment. Dental implant abutments are often described by their form, the material of construction or any special design features.

Dental implant body: See *Dental implant*.

Dental implant connecting component: That part of a dental implant system designed to be placed on a dental implant body to enable its connection to a prosthetic superstructure.

Dental implant system: A set of premanufactured components designed to be employed together when providing treatment with dental implants. A system typically includes a range of components and the clinical and laboratory devices necessary for their use.

Dental implant: A prosthetic device made of one or more alloplastic materials that is implanted into the oral tissues beneath the mucosal or periosteal layer, and on or within the bone to provide retention and support for a fixed or removable dental prosthesis. They may be classified by their relationship with the bone as lying on its surface (eposteal or subperiosteal), lying within the bone (endosseous or endosteal) or penetrating the bone (transosseous or transosteal). The term is often understood to mean an endosseous device and may also be used to describe only the intra-bony component (implant body) or the fully assembled implant body and connecting component or abutment that is mounted on it, as well as sometimes the prosthetic superstructure.

Diagnostic (Kesling) set-up: A diagnostic laboratory procedure in which the teeth are sectioned from a duplicate model and realigned into their desired positions in order to assess the occlusal outcome of a proposed treatment plan.

Diastema: A naturally occurring space between teeth.

Dilaceration: The presence of an abnormal bend or curve in the root or crown of a tooth commonly as a result of dental trauma.

Displacement (mandibular): A sagittal and/or lateral movement of the mandible on closing from centric relation into centric occlusion as a result of an occlusal interference.

Distraction osteogenesis: A surgical technique for lengthening bones, and their associated soft tissue envelope, involving corticotomy followed by gradual separation (distraction) of the bone segments (typically 1 mm per day) and osseous infill.

Dysfunction: The presence of functional disharmony between a morphologic form (teeth, occlusion, bones, joints) and function (muscles, nerves) that may result in pathological changes in the tissues or produce a functional disturbance.

Facemask: An extra-oral appliance, commonly used in Class III malocclusion, that uses anchorage from the chin and forehead to exert anterior forces on the maxillary dentition and/or max-

illa. It can be used to provide increased anterior anchorage for molar protraction in patients with hypodontia.

Fixed appliance: An orthodontic appliance cemented or bonded onto the teeth that cannot be removed by the patient.

Fixture: A colloquial synonym for a dental implant body.

Fraser guidelines: See *Gillick competency*.

Functional appliance: A removable or fixed orthodontic appliance, commonly used in patients with a Class II malocclusion, that alters the posture of the mandible, stretching the facial soft tissues to produce a combination of dental and skeletal changes.

Functional mandibular movements: All the normal, proper, or characteristic movements of the mandible made during speech, mastication, yawning, swallowing and other associated movements.

Functional occlusion: The occlusal contacts of the maxillary and mandibular teeth during mastication and deglutition.

Gillick competency: Together with the Fraser guidelines, this relates to a UK legal case that looked specifically at whether doctors should give contraceptive advice or treatment to under 16-year-olds without parental consent. Since then, the guidelines have been more widely used to help assess whether a child is mature enough to make his or her own decisions and to understand their implications. The Fraser guidelines were set out by Lord Fraser in his judgement of the Gillick case in the House of Lords in 1985, and apply specifically to contraceptive advice (Wheeler, 2006).

Group function: Multiple contact relations between maxillary and mandibular teeth in lateral movements on the working side, whereby simultaneous contact of several teeth acting as a group distribute occlusal forces.

Growth rotation: A rotation of the core of the mandible and maxilla in relation to the cranial base that occurs with normal growth. Growth rotations are described as being clockwise (backward) or counterclockwise (forward).

Headgear: An extraoral orthodontic appliance utilising cervical or cranial anchorage to apply forces to the teeth or jaws for tooth movement or growth modification.

Hypodontia: The developmental absence of one or more teeth excluding the third molars.

Impaction: Failure of a tooth to erupt due to insufficient space or an obstruction.

Inclination: The labiolingual or buccolingual angulation of the long axis of a tooth in relationship to a line drawn perpendicular to the occlusal plane (Compare with *Angulation*.)

Informed consent: The process of providing the patient (or carer in the case of children) with relevant information regarding the treatment options, their relative advantages and disadvantages and the consequences of no treatment.

Infra-occlusion: The positioning of a tooth below the occlusal plane.

Intercuspal position (ICP): The complete intercuspation of opposing teeth independent of condylar position.

Interference: Any tooth contact that interferes with or hinders harmonious mandibular movement.

Interproximal enamel reduction: The removal of interproximal enamel for space creation.

Labial segment: The incisor teeth.

Le Fort I osteotomy: A surgical maxillary procedure in which the maxilla is osteotomised just above the tooth apices and used to advance or vertically reposition the maxilla.

Levelling: A stage of orthodontic treatment aimed at flattening the curve of Spee for overbite reduction.

Lower anterior facial height: The soft-tissue lower anterior face height is the linear distance between the columella and inferior border of the chin. The hard-tissue lower anterior facial height is the linear distance between the maxillary plane and Menton.

Malocclusion: Any deviation from normal occlusion.

Masticatory cycle: A three-dimensional representation of mandibular movement produced during the chewing of food.

Mutually protected occlusion: An occlusal scheme whereby the posterior teeth prevent excessive contact of the anterior teeth in maximum intercuspation and the anterior teeth disengage the posterior teeth in all mandibular excursive movements.

Nasolabial angle: The angle between a line drawn at a tangent to the columella of the nose and a line connecting the subnasale to the mucocutaneous border of the upper lip.

Non-working side: The side of the mandible that moves towards the median line in a lateral excursion.

Occlusal interference: An occlusal contact occurring during mandibular closure from centric relation into centric occlusion that results in a mandibular displacement.

Onlay denture: A denture that covers the occlusal or incisal surface of a tooth for the primary purpose of modifying its contours.

Orthodontic site development: The development of alveolar bone by orthodontic tooth movement.

Orthognathic surgery: Surgical repositioning of the mandible and/or maxilla for the correction of a dentofacial deformity.

Osteotomy: A surgical bone cut.

Overbite: The degree of vertical overlap of the mandibular incisors by their maxillary counterparts measured perpendicular to the occlusal plane and with the teeth in occlusion (normally 2–4 mm).

Overdenture: A complete or partial denture that completely covers an underlying tooth or teeth or one or more dental implants which enhance its stability, often by means of precision attachments.

Overjet: The horizontal distance between the labial surfaces of the mandibular incisors and the maxillary incisal edges measured parallel to the occlusal plane to the most prominent point on the maxillary central incisal edges (normally 2–4 mm).

Overlay denture: See *Onlay denture*.

Precision attachment: *1*. A pre-manufactured retainer consisting of a metal receptacle (matrix) and a close-fitting part (patrix). The matrix is usually contained within the normal or expanded contours of a crown on an abutment tooth/dental implant and the patrix is attached to a pontic or removable dental prosthesis framework. 2. An interlocking device with one component fixed to an abutment or abutments, and the other integrated into a removable dental prosthesis in order to stabilise and/or retain it.

Presurgical orthodontics: Orthodontic treatment carried out in preparation for orthognathic surgery.

Prosthetic envelope: Space within the oral cavity that is potentially available for the placement of a fixed or removable prosthetic device. The term is commonly used in relation to treatment with dental implants.

Prosthodontics: The dental specialty pertaining to the diagnosis, treatment planning, rehabilitation and maintenance of the oral function, comfort, appearance and health of patients with clinical conditions associated with missing or deficient teeth and/or maxillofacial tissues using biocompatible substitutes.

Protrusion: A position of the mandible anterior to centric relation.

Pubertal (adolescent) growth spurt: The acceleration in growth associated with puberty.

Relapse: The return of the original features of a malocclusion following treatment.

Removable appliance: An orthodontic or prosthodontic appliance that can be removed by the patient for the maintenance of oral hygiene.

Restorative dentistry: A dental specialty recognised in the UK that comprises the study, examination and treatment of diseases of the oral cavity and the teeth and their supporting structures. It includes the dental monospecialties of endodontics, periodontics and prosthodontics (including implantology) and is based on how these interact in the management of patients requiring multifaceted care.

Retention: *1.* The final phase of orthodontic treatment aimed at stabilisation of corrected tooth positions. *2.* The resistance of a removable prosthesis to movement away from its supporting tissues.

Retrognathia: Retrusion of the maxilla and/or mandible in relationship to the cranial base.

Retruded contact: Contact of a tooth, or teeth, along the retruded path of closure. A retruded contact position (RCP) is a guided occlusal relationship occurring at the most retruded position of the condyles in the joint cavities.

Retrusion: Movement towards the posterior.

Scissor-bite (lingual crossbite): This occurs when the buccal cusps of the lower premolars/molars occlude palatal to their opposing counterparts.

Skeletal pattern: The three-dimensional relationship between the maxilla and mandible.

SNA: An angular measurement constructed from a lateral cephalometric radiograph by joining the centre of the sella turcica (sella, S), the frontonasal suture (nasion, N) and the greatest concavity of the maxillary alveolus adjacent to the roots of the maxillary incisors (A-point). Angle SNA is a representation of maxillary skeletal protrusion or retrusion. In Caucasians the norm is 81° (SD 3°).

SNB: An angular measurement constructed from a lateral cephalometric radiograph by joining the centre of the sella turcica (sella – S), the frontonasal suture (nasion – N) and the greatest concavity of the mandibular alveolus adjacent to the roots of the mandibular incisors (B-point). Angle SNB is a representation of mandibular skeletal protrusion or retrusion. In Caucasians the norm is 78° (SD 3°).

Supernumerary tooth: Any tooth in excess of the normal series.

Surgical envelope: The space potentially available within a bone for the placement of an endosseous dental implant body.

Temporary anchorage device: A biocompatible device inserted into bone for the purpose of moving teeth orthodontically and subsequently removed after treatment.

Transeptal fibres: Periodontal fibres interconnecting adjacent teeth.

Traumatic overbite: Contact between the lower incisors and palatal mucosa and/or the mandibular labial gingivae that results in discomfort, inflammation, recession and/or ulceration.

Working side (WS): A side towards which the mandible moves in a lateral excursion.

Xenograft: Tissue or organs from an individual of one species transplanted into or grafted onto an organism of another species, genus or family.

Reference

Wheeler R. Gillick or Fraser? A plea for consistency over competence in children. Gillick and Fraser are not interchangeable. *BMJ* 2006;332:807.

Index

Page numbers in *italics* represent figures, those in **bold** represent tables.

abrasion 86–7, **86**
abutment alignment 67–8
aesthetics 14, 153
age
 occlusal changes with 65, *65*
 and treatment planning 55
agenesis 3
 prevalence by gender **5**
allografts 96, 188
alveolar atrophy 132
alveolar development, reduced 20–1, *20*, 94
ameloblasts 8
amelogenesis imperfecta 8, 23
ANB 22, 188
anchorage 188
anchorage control 130, **131**
Angle's classification 61, 188
 class I malocclusion 61, 188
 class II malocclusion 61, 188
 class III malocclusion 61, 188
angulation 89–90, *89*, *90*, 133, 188

ankylosis 51, *51*, 189
anodontia 3, **4**, 189
 partial 4
 permanent dentition *16*
anterior guidance 60, 66, 72, 74, 75, 141, 168, 188
anteroposterior incisor relationship 157
appearance 23, *23*
appliance breakage 135
arch coordination 133–4
arch relationship 157
archwires 129, 132, *132*, 133, 135, **136**, 188
Association Français des Dysplasies Ectodermiques 33
attrition **86**, 87
Australian Ectodermal Dysplasia Support Group 32
autogenous grafts 96
autografts 96, 189
autotransplantation 145–6, **146**
Axin2 gene 8

Hypodontia: A Team Approach to Management, First Edition
© J.A. Hobkirk, D.S. Gill, S.P. Jones, K.W. Hemmings, G.S. Bassi, A.L. O'Donnell and J.R. Goodman
Published 2011 by Blackwell Publishing Ltd

balanced occlusion 63–5, *64*, *65*, 189
    bilateral 63–4
bilateral absence of teeth **6**
Bio-Oss 98
bioactive glasses 96
block grafts 98
Block–Sulzberger syndrome **10**
Bmp gene 8
Bolk's Theory of Terminal Reduction 7
Bolton (tooth size) discrepancy 49, *49*, 189
bond failure 131
bone 93–5, 163
    buccal contour 157
    children 108
    reduced alveolar development 20–1, *20*, 94
    retained primary teeth 94
    ridge narrowing 94–5, *94*, *95*
bone grafting 95–9
    allografts 96, 188
    autogenous grafts 96
    autografts 189
    block grafts 98
    distraction osteogenesis 99, *99*, 190
    efficacy of 98
    graft materials 95–7
    guided bone regeneration 97, 98–9
    particular grafts 98
    techniques 97
    xenografts 96, 192
bone morphogenetic proteins 97
Book syndrome **10**
border movement 63, 72, 189
bridges
    conventional 74, 144–5, 180
    maintenance 181–2, *182*
    resin-bonded 73–4, 142–4, *142–4*, 170
buccal segment 166, 189
buccolingual space 161, *162*
Butler's Field Theory 7

calcium carbonate-based materials 97
calcium phosphate-based alloplasts 96–7
camouflage (orthodontic) **56**, 189
Canadian Dermatology Association 32
canine-guided occlusion 64, 67, 189
canine-protected occlusion 64, *64*
canines
    colour 155–6
    contour 154–5
    eruption 53

gingival margins 154, *155*
    movement of *46*
    repositioning of 66–7, *67*
    shape 156
    simulation of lateral incisors 137, *138*
    size 154, *155*
care pathway 36–9, *38*, *39*
care provision 28–41
cast restorations 181
cementoblasts 8
centric occlusion (intercuspal position) 63, 189, 191
cetric relation (retruded contact position) 63, 189, 192
cheeks 83–5, *84*, *85*
children
    establishing relationship 106–7, *107*
    implants 118–20
    initial examination 107
        hard tissues 108
        soft tissues 107–8
    investigations 108–11
    oral health 112–13
    surgery 117–18, *117*
    treatment 111–18
    treatment planning 111–12
    see also primary dentition; late mixed/early permanent dentition
Children Act 1989 112
class I incisor relationship 157, 189
class II incisor relationship 157, 189
    division 1 157, 189
    division 2 157, 189
class III incisor relationship 157, 189
cleft lip/palate-ectodermal dysplasia syndrome **10**
clinical geneticists 35
clinical psychologists 35
composite resin 73, 189
    maintenance of restorations 181
    re-contouring 136
computerised clinical databases 37
conical teeth 17–18, *17*, *23*, *89*
consent to treatment 112, 191
    Gillick competence 112, 190
conventional bridges 74, 144–5, 179
counselling 30–1
cranial base–mandibular plane angle 22
craniofacial morphology 22
cross bite 67–8
crown angulation (tooth tip) 62
crown inclination (tooth torque) 62

crowns 73, *73*, 169–70, *170*
    in children 114–15
curve of Spee 62, 129, 166, 189

Dahl appliance 57, 69, *69*, *70*
data collection 32
decompensation **56**, 189
dens invaginatus 154, *154*
dental caries 50, 92
    treatment 165
dental implants 74–5, *75*, 93, 145, 170–6, *172–6*,
        189–90
    abutment 67–8, 189
    in children 118–20
    maintenance 183, *183*
    systems 189
dental nurses 33–4
dental practitioners 33
dentinogenesis imperfecta 8, 23
dentition 15–16
dentures 140, *141*, 176–79, *176–9*
    complete, in children 116
    maintenance 182–3
    occlusion on 73, *74*
    partial, in children 115
dermatologists 35–6
developmental stage, and treatment choice **125**
diagnosis 30
diagnostic (Kesling) set-up 54, 135, *136*,
        164, 190
diastema 190
    median 137–8, *138*
dilaceration 161, 190
disclusion 64
displacement (mandibular) 190
distraction osteogenesis 99, *99*, 190
Down syndrome (trisomy 21) **10**
drifting 53
dysfunction 190

ectodermal dysplasia 32, *106*
ectodysplasin-A 9
ectopic eruption 18, *18*
ectrodactyly, ectodermal dysplasia and cleft lip/
        palate syndrome **10**
edentulousness, long-term 132
environmental factors 7
erosion **86**, 87
eruption 87, *87*, *88*
    abnormal 53

Essix retainers *134*, 135

facemask 190
facial growth *52*
facial profile **56**
family, counselling 30–1
Fgf gene 8
fissure sealants 113
fixed retainers 135, *135*, 190
fixtures *see* dental implants; implant body
fluoride 113
fraena 108
    surgery 118
Frankfort–mandibular plane angle 22
Fraser guidelines *see* Gillick competence
freeway space 20, 53
    increased 21, 23, *84*
    primary dentition 110
functional appliance 68–9, 124, 129–30, 190
functional mandibular movements 190
functional occlusion 190

gender **5**, 16
genetic factors 7
Gillick competence 112, 190
glass-ionomer cements 96
graft materials 95–7
    bone morphogenetic proteins 97
    calcium carbonate-based 97
    calcium phosphate-based 96–7
    silicate-based 96
group function occlusion 64, *64*, 190
growth rotation 22, 53, *54*, 129, 190
guidance theory 53
guided bone regeneration 97, 98–9

Hawley retainers *134*
headgear 141–2, **143**, 170, 190
health-related issues 151
Hertwig's root sheath 8
Hg gene 8
holoprosencephaly **10**
homeobox genes 8
hydroxyapatite 97
hypodontia 3, **4**, 190
    aetiology 7–11
    environmental and genetic factors 7
    inheritance patterns 7–8
    permanent dentition 5–6, **5**, **6**
    prevalence 4–6

primary dentition 4–5
  severe **4**
  severity of 47, *47*
  sites and frequency of missing teeth 6, **6**
  syndromic associations 9, **10**
hypodontia team
  collaboration with patient support groups
    32–3
  composition of 33–6
  diagnosis and interdisciplinary treatment
    planning 30
  outreach care provision 31
  patient and family counselling 30–1
  referral to 28–9, *29*
  roles of 29–33
  teaching, research and data collection 32
  treatment within unit 31–2
  see also individual team members
hypohidrotic ectodermal dysplasia 9, **10**, 30

ideal occlusion 61
  balanced 63–5, *64, 65*
  normal 61–3, *62*
impaction 29, **61**, 104, 190
implant body 31, 96, 190, 195, 203
implant site development 128, *128*
implant-connecting component 191
implants *see* dental implants
incisors, maxillary lateral, missing 66–7, *67*
inclination 71, 72, 145, 149, 173, 191
incontinentia pigmenti **10**
Index of Orthodontic Treatment Need 4
informed consent *see* consent to treatment
infra-occlusion 50–3, *51, 52*, 191
  consequences of **51**
  orthodontic treatment 139–40
  primary dentition 110–11, *110, 111*
inheritance patterns 7–8
  genetics of odontogenesis 8
  tooth development 8
inter-arch relationships 61–2
inter-arch space 57
intercuspal position *see* centric occlusion
interdisciplinary treatment planning 30
interference 72, 75, 82, 101, 128, 146, 191
intermaxillary traction
  class II 189
  class III 189
interproximal enamel reduction 133, 191
intraoral forces 85–6

intraoral space 86–93
  horizontal dimension 86
  vertical dimension 86–7, **86**
isolated hypodontia/oligodontia 3

Kesling set-up 54, 135, *136*, 164, 190

labial segment 168, 169, 178, 191
laboratory technicians 35
late mixed/early permanent dentition 124–49
  developmental stage 124–6, **125**
  orthodontic treatment 126–46
late tooth development 134
Le Fort I osteotomy 191
levelling 68, 166, 191
lips 83–5, *84, 85*
lower anterior facial height 63, 191

maintenance post-treatment 180–4
  bridgework 181–2, *182*
  dental implants 182–3, *183*
  dentures 182
  orthodontic 180–1, *182*
  periodontal 180
  remaining teeth 180
malocclusion 191
  Angle's Class I 61, 188
  Angle's Class II 61, 188
  Angle's Class III 61, 188
mastication difficulties 24–5
masticatory cycle 191
masticatory problems 88
median diastema 137–8, *138*
mesiodistal dimension 160–1, *160*
metal occlusal surfaces 73, *73*
microdont teeth 16–17, *17*, 47–8, *48*
  children *114*
  occlusal variations 67, *67*
  orthodontic problems 133–4
  orthodontic treatment 138–9, *139*
  prognosis 154, *154*
  tooth positioning 127, *128*
missing teeth 15–16, 157–8, *158, 159*
  dentition 15–16
  gender 16
  number 15, *15, 16*
  patterns within jaws 16
  racial group 16
  replacement 170–80, *172–9*
  tooth form 16

molars
    relationship of **56**
    tilted 127
Msx1 gene 8
mucosa 85
    children 107
multidisciplinary approach 37, 54–5
multiple dental agenesis 3
mutually protected occlusion 62, 64, 191

nasolabial angle 191
National Foundation for Ectodermal Dysplasia 33
necking 45
Nemo gene 9
non-working side 63, 65, 191
normal occlusion 61–3, *62*
    crown angulation (tooth tip) 62
    crown inclination (tooth torque) 62
    curve of Spee 62
    inter-arch relationships 61–2
    rotations 62
    tight contacts 62

occlusal interference 89, 116, 134, 191
occlusal onlays 169
occlusal pathology 76
occlusal philosophies 61–6
occlusal vertical dimension 18, 65, 86
    reduction of 69–70, *71*
occlusion 60–81
    age changes 65, *65*
    balanced 63–5, *64*, *65*, 189
    canine-guided 64, 67, 189
    centric 63, 189
    functional 190
    group function 64, *64*, 190
    hypodontia 66–72, *66*
    microdontia 67, *67*
    mutually protected 191
    normal 61–3, *62*
    restoration of 72–6
odontoblasts 8
odontogenesis 8
oligodontia 3, **4**
onlay dentures 191
    in children 114–15
oral care, commitment to 151–2, *152*, **152**
oral cavity 82–5
    cheeks, lips and tongue 83–5, *84*, *85*
    mucosa 85

oral function 153
oral health **56**, 112–13
oral and maxillofacial surgeons 35
oral–facial–digital syndrome **10**
orthodontic appliances 128–9
    see also individual appliances
orthodontic assessment 109–10
orthodontic maintenance 180–1, *182*
    composite restorations 181–2
    veneers and cast restorations 181
orthodontic site development 53, 191
orthodontic space redistribution 55, **56**
orthodontic treatment 126–46
    benefits of 126–8, *126*, *127*
    children 116–17
    long-term maintenance 157
    permanent dentition 166–7, *167*
    problems of 129–35, *130–2*, **131**, *134*
    restorative management of patients 135–40,
        136, **136**
    tooth movement 157
    tooth replacement 140–6
orthodontists 34
orthognathic surgery 21, 22, 35, 55, **56**, **125**, 166, 191
osteotomy 191
outreach care provision 31
overbite 53–4, *54*, 191
    correction of 127
    deep 129–30, *130*
    reduction 68–9, *69*, *70*
    traumatic 192
overdentures 140–2, *141*, *142*, 191
    in children 115, *116*
overerupted teeth 127
overjet 191
overlay denture *see* onlay denture

paediatric dentists 34
pain 25
patient support groups 32–3
patients
    age of 55
    children *see* children; primary dentition
    commitment to oral care 151–2, **152**
    counselling 30–1
    expectations of treatment 151
    treatment concerns 55, **56**
patients' complaints 22–5, *22*
    appearance 23, *23*
    excessive freeway space 23

mastication difficulties 24–5
pain 25
spacing 23, *23*
speech problems 24
Pax9 gene 8
pericision 132
periodontal examination **152**
periodontal maintenance 180
periodontal tissues 107–8
permanent dentition 150–87
    abnormal eruption 53
    age of eruption **90**
    anodontia *16*
    delayed eruption 21–2
    extraction of 117–18, *117*, *118*
    health-related issues 151
    hypodontia 5–6, **5**, **6**
    maintenance 180–4
    orthodontic treatment 166–7, *167*
    patient expectations 151
    restorative care 168–80
    sizes **91**
    social issues 151
    surgical treatment 167–8
    treatment objectives 150–1, 164
    treatment planning 150–66
Pitx2 9
plastic restorations 73
pontics 132, *132*
porcelain 73
presurgical orthodontics 191
primary dentition 105–23
    age of eruption **90**
    extraction of 117
    freeway space 110
    hypodontia 4–5
    infra-occlusion 110–11, *110*, *111*
    initial examination 108
    orthodontic assessment 109–10
    periodontal tissues 107–8
    radiography 108–9
    retained 18–20, *19*, *20*, 48–50, *49*, *50*, 71–2, 94,
        132–3
    root resorption 90–3, **90**, **91**, **93**
    sizes **91**
    vitality testing 109
prosthetic envelope *19*, 45, 83, *88*, *90*, 173, 176,
        176, 192
prosthodontics 34, 192
protrusion 192
pubertal (adolescent) growth spurt 192

racial group 16
radiography, primary dentition 108–9
re-contouring 136–7, **136**
referral 28–9, *29*
relapse 75–6, 192
removable appliance 192
research 32
resin-based composite restorations 168
resin-bonded bridges 73–4, 142–4, *142–4*, 170
rest vertical dimension 86
restorative dentistry 192
    permanent dentition 168–80
    primary dentition 113–16
    see also individual treatment options
retained primary dentition 18–20, *19*, *20*
retainers 75–6
retention 134–5, *134*, 192
retrognathia 192
retruded contact *see* centric relation
retrusion 22, 192
ridge narrowing 94–5, *94*, *95*
Rieger syndrome 9, **10**
root paralleling 126–7, 133
root resorption *19*, 50–3, *50*, 90–3, **90**, **91**, **93**
    local factors 92–3
    systemic factors 92
root separation 126–7
rotated teeth 62, 67–8, *68*, 131–2

scissor-bite (lingual crossbite) 192
shimstock foil 75, *75*
shortened dental arch 70, *72*
silicate-based alloplasts 96
skeletal pattern **56**, 192
SNA 22, 192
SNB 22, 192
social issues 151
soft tissues 163–4
    examination in children 107–8
    surgery 118
space closure 55, *56*, *57*, 127
space distribution 126, *127*
space requirements 156–7, *156*, 158–63
spacing 23, *23*, 45–59, **56**
    acceptance of space distribution 57
    between dental arches 53–4, *54*
    inter-arch space 57
    mesiodistal 45
    transverse 45
    treatment planning 54–7
    uneven distribution 45–7, *46*

vertical 45
within dental arches 45–7, *46*
speech 88–9
speech and language therapists 36
speech problems 24
splinting 75–6
Superfloss 180
supernumerary tooth 8, 48, 192
supporting tissues 82–101
  bone 93–5
  bone grafting 95–9
  intraoral forces 85–6
  intraoral space 86–7
  oral cavity 82–5
  teeth 87–93
surgery
  children 117–18, *117*, *118*
  orthognathic 21, 22, 35, 55, **56**, **125**, 166, 191
  permanent dentition 167–8
  soft tissue 118
  see also orthodontic treatment
surgical envelope 34, 45, 58, 82, 88, 90, *90*, 95, *95*,
    128, 192
symmetry 156
syndromic associations 9, **10**
syndromic hypodontia/oligodontia 3

taurodontism 89, *89*
teaching 32
teeth 87–93
  angulation 89–90, *89*, *90*
  appearance 88
  eruption 87, *87*, *88*
  form and size 89, *89*
  masticatory problems 88
  missing *see* missing teeth
  root resorption *19*, 50–3, *50*, 90–3, **90**,
    91, **93**
  speech 88–9
temporary anchorage devices 130, *131*, 192
  deep overbite *130*
temporomandibular joints 63
terminology **4**
thalidomide 7
tight contacts 62
tilting 67–8
tissue response to treatment 152–3, *153*
tongue 83–5, *84*, *85*
tooth development 8

tooth form 16, 153–7, *154*, *155*
tooth movement 157
tooth and nail syndrome **10**
tooth replacement 140–6
  autotransplantation 145–6, **146**
  conventional bridges 74, 144–5
  dental implants *see* dental implants
  dentures *see* dentures
  overdentures *see* overdentures
  resin-bonded bridges 73–4, 142–4, *142–4*
tooth size 153–7, *154*, *155*
tooth surface loss 20, *20*, 86, **86**
transeptal fibres 132, 192
traumatic overbite 192
treatment 15
  children 111–18
  consent to 112, 190, 191
  multidisciplinary approach 37
  orthodontic 116–17
  relapse 75–6
  restorative dentistry 113–16, 168–80, 192
  within unit 31–2
treatment planning 31
  active disease 165
  children 111–12
  developmental stage **125**
  multidisciplinary 37, 54–5
  permanent dentition 150–66
  prevention of further disease 165
  re-evaluation 165
  spacing 54–7, **56**
tricalcium phosphate 97

UK Ectodermal Dysplasia Society 32

van der Woude syndrome (lip-pit syndrome) **10**
veneers 73, 168–9, *169*
  maintenance 181
vertical space 161–3, *163*
vitality testing 109

wagon-wheel effect 133
waisting 20–1, 45
Witkop syndrome **10**
Wnt gene 8
working side 192

X-linked hypodontia 9
xenografts 96, 192